P9-APX-513

Acquired Apraxia of Speech in
Aphasic Adults

Brain Damage, Behaviour and Cognition

Developments in Clinical Neuropsychology

Series Editors:
Chris Code, Leicester Polytechnic, and Dave Muller, Suffolk College of Further and Higher Education

Brain Damage, Behaviour and Cognition
Developments in Clinical Neuropsychology

Acquired Apraxia of Speech in Aphasic Adults:

Theoretical and Clinical
Issues

Edited by
Paula Square-Storer

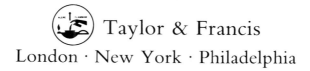 Taylor & Francis
London · New York · Philadelphia

UK   Taylor & Francis Ltd, 4 John St., London WC1N 2ET

USA   Taylor & Francis Inc., 242 Cherry St., Philadelphia,
         PA 19106-1906

Copyright © Taylor & Francis 1989

*All rights reserved. No part of this publication may be reproduced,
stored in a retrieval system, or transmitted, in any form or by any
means, electronic, electrostatic, magnetic tape, mechanical, photocopying,
recording or otherwise, without the prior permission of the copyright
owner.*

First published 1989

British Library Cataloguing in Publication Data

Acquired apraxia of speech in aphasic adults.
  1. Man. Speech disorders
  I. Square-Storer, Paula II. Series
  616.85′5

  ISBN 0-85066-449-7
  ISBN 0-85066-468-3 Pbk

Typeset in 11 on 13 point Bembo by
Mathematical Composition Setters Ltd, 7 Ivy Street,
Salisbury, UK

*Printed and bound in Great Britain by
Redwood Burn Ltd Trowbridge Wiltshire*

to Frederic L. Darley, mentor and friend

Contents

Contents

Contributing Authors

Amy R. Clark
355 Fairview Street
Danville, California
USA

Michael J. Collins
Director, Speech and Language
Pathology
Dean Clinic
Madison, Wisconsin
USA

Lee Ann C. Golper
Audiology and Speech Pathology
Service
Veterans' Administration Medical
Center
Portland, Oregon
USA

Deborah (Chumpelik) Hayden
Bell Children's Centre
Speech Foundation of Ontario
Toronto, Ontario
Canada

Yvan Lebrun
Neurolinguistics Department
Vrije University
Brussels
Belgium

Kevin G. Munhall
Department of Communicative
  Disorders
Elborn College
University of Western Ontario
London, Ontario
Canada

Richard K. Peach
Department of Communication
  Sciences and Disorders
University of Georgia
Athens, Georgia
USA

Marie T. Rau
Audiology and Speech
  Pathology Service
Veterans' Administration Medical
  Center
Portland, Oregon
USA

Eric A. Roy
Department of Kinesiology
University of Waterloo
Waterloo, Ontario
Canada

Contributing Authors

Marianne M. Simpson
Speech Pathology Service
Veterans' Administration Medical
  Center
Long Beach, California
USA

Elaine R. Stevens
PO Box 362
Waterville, Maine
USA

Paula Square-Storer
Graduate Department of Speech
  Pathology and
Department of Rehabilitation
  Medicine
University of Toronto
Canada

John D. Tonkovich
Detroit Rehabilitation Institute
Detroit, Michigan
USA

Patricia F. Waugh
Department of Rehabilitation
  Medicine
University of Washington
Seattle, Washington
USA

Kathryn M. Yorkston
Department of Rehabilitation
  Medicine
University of Washington
Seattle, Washington
USA

Foreword

Two decades have passed since Darley and his colleagues rekindled our interest in a specific type of speech disorder due to brain damage, a time-honored subject of controversy for over a century since the days of Broca. They called our attention to its specific patterns of articulatory and prosodic features which are distinct from aphasia and dysarthria and designated it as apraxia of speech.

The past twenty years have witnessed a resurgence of inquiries into the nature of this syndrome, explanatory concepts of its underlying mechanisms, and better ways to treat patients afflicted with the disorder. A wide spectrum of research strategies have been developed and used to answer these inquiries, out of which not only a substantial gain in our knowledge but also a series of further questions have emerged.

This fervor in the investigation of apraxia of speech was high-lighted by the publication of two books in 1984, *Apraxia of Speech: Physiology, Acoustics, Linguistics, Management* edited by Rosenbek, McNeil, and Aronson, and *Apraxia of Speech in Adults: The Disorder and Its Management* edited by Wertz, LaPointe, and Rosenbek. The former was prepared as a Festschrift for Dr. Darley to honor his timeless contributions to the subject, with the major emphasis of many papers focused upon verification of the abnormalities by presenting hard data derived from measurements of physiologic, acoustic, or anatomic alterations in apraxia of speech. The latter, on the other hand, is primarily an introductory textbook on the subject for clinicians, with a comprehensive overview of the characteristics of the problem followed by state-of-the-art treatment methodologies for the patients with different severity levels of apraxic disorders.

Now, four years later, another volume entitled *Acquired Apraxia of Speech in Aphasic Adults: Theoretical and Clinical Issues* by Dr. Square-Storer and her colleagues joins its two predecessors. This book has been conceived of as a 'forum' for a number of leading clinicians/researchers representing various disciplines and with expertise on the subject of apraxia of speech, to present their own perspectives, standpoints, and working hypotheses regarding the nature of the disorder and its treatment. Specific step-by-step procedures for new and innovative treatment strategies, each with its theoretical basis, are also presented with empirical evidence of their effectiveness. In other words, unlike its predecessors, the uniqueness of the volume lies in the divergencies, rather than convergencies, of viewpoints and approaches, while maintaining a consistent emphasis on better and improved clinical management of the patients themselves. The overall combination, therefore, provides not only a rational structure for current understanding of apraxia of speech but also the unsolved issues and uncertainties. There is no doubt that this book will be broadly useful to clinicians and researchers, and will serve as the basis for many future inquiries into the disorder, which in turn will bring about further improvement in treatment procedures for the patients.

I am particularly happy that this important volume is going to be dedicated to our mentor, Frederic L. Darley, and that I can join in this dedication in a small but very special way by contributing this foreword.

Sumiko Sasanuma
1988

Series Editors' Preface

From being an area primarily on the periphery of mainstream behavioural and cognitive science, neuropsychology has developed in recent years into an area of central concern for a range of disciplines. We are witnessing not only a revolution in the way in which brain–behaviour–cognition relationships are viewed, but a widening of interest concerning developments in neuropsychology on the part of a range of workers in a variety of fields. Major advances in brain imaging techniques and the cognitive modelling of the impairments following brain damage promise a wider understanding of the nature of the representation of cognition and behaviour in the damaged and undamaged brain.

Neuropsychology is now centrally important for those working with brain damaged people, but the very rate of expansion in the area makes it difficult to keep up with findings from current research. The aim of the *Brain Damage, Behaviour and Cognition* series is to publish a wide range of books which present comprehensive and up-to-date overviews of current developments in specific areas of interest.

These books will be of particular interest to those working with the brain-damaged. It is the Editors' intention that undergraduates, postgraduates, clinicians and researchers in psychology, speech pathology and medicine will find this series a useful source of information on important current developments. The authors and editors of the books in this series are experts in their respective fields working at the forefront of contemporary research. They have produced texts which are accessible and scholarly. We thank them for their contribution and their hard work in fulfilling the aims of the series.

Chris Code and Dave Müller
Leicester and Ipswich

Preface

It is the purpose of this book to provide a forum for a number of 'authorities' from various clinical and research disciplines such as speech/language pathology, neuropsychology, and speech science, to present their philosophies, perspectives, tenets, and working constructs regarding the disorder, apraxia of speech. Revealed in a salient way are the divergencies of opinions and various vantage points from which the disorder may be viewed. The information presented hopefully will provide a catalyst for further basic and clinical research and the advancement of hypotheses which will aid our understanding of brain behavior and damage, generally, and apraxia of speech, specifically.

That there is little consensus of opinion regarding underlying disrupted mechanisms and symptomatology, and no definitive guidelines for the selection of the most efficacious treatment procedures for individual verbally apractic patients, will be apparent to the reader from the outset. Yet, this lack of consensus is viewed as both healthy and good for the advancement of science and clinical practice. Various opinions are expressed, for example, to questions such as the following. May we think of some forms of perseveration as apractic in nature and thus amenable to apraxia of speech (AOS) treatment procedures for aphasic patients with recurrent stereotypies? May some forms of mutism be apractic in nature and how, when, and why would we treat this disability as a disorder of praxis? When may we consider 'conduite d'approche' behaviors as motorically rather than linguistically based? What underlying disrupted psychological processes may result in similar 'surface' articulatory errors? What aspects of the interactions of language and motor speech programming must be considered when treating aphasic/apractic patients? Although no definitive answers are provided for these questions and numerous others which arise, these issues are discussed differently by different contributors.

With the mandates of this text being to encite original thinking and advanced clinical practice and research, it is obvious that it would not fulfil the purpose of an introductory text. We, instead, most strongly recommend Wertz, Lapointe, and Rosenbek (1984) as a foundation. But for the graduate student, postgraduate, academician, advanced clinician, and researcher, it is felt this volume will provide most meaningful discussions of apraxia of speech and a bank of knowledge not found within one volume elsewhere.

In no way has this volume been designed to be comprehensive. Instead, selected areas of interdisciplinary interest are presented. The book consists of eleven chapters organized in four parts. Part I is directed toward general perspectives. Chapter 1 by Lebrun provides a review of the history of the 'concept' of apraxia of speech. Square-Storer and Roy, in Chapter 2, review the commonalities and differences among verbal, nonverbal oral, and limb apraxia. Symptomatology, as traditionally defined in the literature, provides the major perspective from which the apraxias are compared. In Chapter 3, Munhall directs his discussion to research issues, particularly valid methods of measuring articulatory variability, a symptom of apraxia traditionally thought to be paramount.

Discussions in Part II are directed towards common clinical concerns and issues, specifically, the differential diagnosis of apraxia of speech from aphasic syndromes by Collins in Chapter 4, what the focus of treatment should be, motor speech or language, in aphasic/apractic individuals by Tonkovich and Peach in Chapter 5, and selection criteria for appropriate traditional methods of AOS treatment by Square-Storer in Chapter 6. In Part III of this volume, three novel approaches to intervention not discussed at length elsewhere, are presented. Empirical data are pro-offered for two. Rau and Golper discuss in Chapter 7 the criteria for selection of and efficacious use of cueing to facilitate verbal expression in aphasic/apractic individuals. In Chapter 8, Square-Storer and Hayden explain a dynamic motokinesthetic approach for remediation of apraxia of speech, developed by Hayden originally for treating apractic children. Data are presented which indicate that for some apractic/agrammatic patients, this approach may be extremely effective for 'programming in' functional phrases. In Chapter 9, Stevens explains and provides some persuasive data which indicate that some verbal perseverations may be motically based and that a method of treatment which 'breaks' the pathological motor loop may be efficacious even for global aphasic individuals with severe AOS.

Two chapters are included in Part IV. Both discuss treatment programs. The focus of Chapter 10 by Simpson and Clark is a discussion of apractic mutism and the clinical management of it. To our knowledge, no in-depth discussion of this area has appeared heretofore in the literature. Finally, in Chapter 11, Yorkston and Waugh discuss principles of the burgeoning area of augmentative communication as applied to verbally apractic patients. For the speech/language pathologist, aphasiologist, speech scientist, and neuropsychologist, areas of relevance and interest to the understanding, study, and treatment of apraxia of speech are presented.

I wish to thank Dr Robert Marshall for his original suggestion that I edit such a volume and for his continued confidence and support in bringing this project to fruition. For their helpful suggestions and various contributions towards fostering the growth of this project, the following are recognized: Dr Harris Winitz, Dr Norman Lass, and Dr Margaret Stoicheff. For their suggestions regarding content and organization: Dr Chris Code, Professor Dave Muller, Dr Reg Warren, Dr Richard Peach, and Ms Frances Ezerzer are acknowledged. For their contributions along the way, Dr Tony Mlcoch and Mr Ronald Thacker are thanked.

For their support and resources provided, the Graduate Department of Speech Pathology and Department of Rehabilitation Medicine, Faculty of Medicine, University of Toronto are most gratefully acknowledged. To my husband, Jack, for his wise counsel, patience, vision, and support, I am eternally grateful.

Paula Square-Storer

WERTZ, R.T., LAPOINTE, L.L. and ROSENBEK, J.C. (1984) *Apraxia of Speech in Adults: The Disorder and Its Management*, New York, Grune and Stratton.

Abbreviations

Amer-Ind	American Indian gestural code
AOS	Apraxia of speech, verbal apraxia, speech apraxia
BDAE	Boston Diagnostic Aphasia Examination
cv	Coefficient of variation
HELPSS	Helm Elicited Language Program for Sentence Stimulation
LA	Limb apraxia
LHD	Left-hemisphere damage
MIT	Melodic Intonation Therapy
OA	Oral apraxia, buccofacial apraxia, buccolingual facial apraxia
PICA	Porch Index of Communicative Abilities
PROMPTS	Prompts for Restructuring Oral Muscular Phonetic Targets
WAB	Western Aphasia Battery

PART ONE
General Perspectives

Chapter 1

Apraxia of Speech:
The History of a Concept

Yvan Lebrun

From Aphemia to Apraxia of Speech

In 1825 in a paper read at the French Academy of Medicine and subsequently published in the *Archives Générales de Médecine*, the French physician, Jean-Baptiste Bouillaud, mentioned the case of a patient, Catherine Thirion, who suddenly lost the ability to speak. Her speech organs were not paralyzed, however. Moreover, she could easily understand spoken and written language and express herself in writing. Bouillaud contrasted her impairment of speech production with an impairment of verbal memory and suggested that the former resulted from damage to the white matter and the latter from damage to the gray matter of the frontal lobes. He further pointed out that speech movements are learned movements which may be impaired while other more automatic movements, such as those of suction and deglutition, remain totally preserved.

Early in 1861, a patient called Leborgne was transferred to Paul Broca's surgical department in the Parisian hospital, Bicêtre. This man had been in Bicêtre for 21 years. During all this time, he had been unable to speak. All he could say was 'tan', a syllable which he usually uttered two times in succession. It was only when he was very angry that the expletive, 'Sacré nom de Dieu', would pass his lips instead of his syllabic stereotypy. In addition to his severe reduction of speech production, the patient had right-sided hemiplegia. Leborgne came under Broca's care because a large phlegmon had developed in his paralyzed leg. He died of gangrene after a few days, and Broca autopsied him.

A few months later in the *Bulletin de la Société d'Anatomie* Broca reported on this case, which he construed as an instance of 'aphemia'. According to Broca, aphemia was a selective disturbance of articulate speech due to an acquired brain lesion. The patient with aphemia had no comprehension difficulty and, if literate, could express himself in writing, but he had lost the ability to perform the complex movements which bring about the words of spoken language. Although the speech musculature was not paralyzed, it could no longer be made to produce speech sounds, with the possible exception of a stereotypy, which was then invariably and incoercibly uttered whenever the patient attempted to speak. Non-verbal movements performed by the oral muscles were unimpaired.

A few years later, Armand Trousseau, in his *Clinique Médicale de l'Hôtel-Dieu de Paris* (1861–1864), described what he considered a rare form of 'aphasia' characterized by an inability to speak but with preservation of comprehension and of writing skills. In addition, intelligence was totally spared which, in Trousseau's view, was never the case in other types of aphasia.

In 1877 Adolf Kussmaul described a special form of what he called 'ataxic aphasia'. Patients with this particular syndrome could no longer speak, even when shown the articulatory movements to be performed. They were unable to utter speech sounds. The oral musculature was not paralyzed, however. The intellect was fully preserved, as was inner speech. Writing skills were unabated. In 1885 Ludwig Lichtheim expressed the view that this type of aphasia was by no means rare and that many instances of it had already been reported. He specified that patients with this disorder could no longer speak spontaneously, repeat words, or read aloud. They had preserved full comprehension of both spoken and written language, could express themselves in writing, and could copy and write to dictation.

Shortly after the publication of Lichtheim's paper, Carl Wernicke (1885) proposed to call this speech disorder 'subcortical motor aphasia' and contrasted it with 'cortical motor aphasia', in which inner speech was disturbed. The dichotomy proposed by Wernicke was generally admitted. Subcortical motor aphasia came to be known also as 'pure motor aphasia', and cortical motor aphasia as 'Broca's aphasia', despite the fact that the condition originally described by Broca under the name 'aphemia', in reality, corresponded to pure motor aphasia.

In 1901, Jules Dejerine pointed out that in pure motor aphasia singing was as impaired as spontaneous speech or repetition, while in Broca's aphasia it could be remarkably preserved. On the other hand, Dejerine believed that articulatory disorders were identical in the two types of aphasia. Indeed, he thought that with the passing of time Broca's aphasia could turn into pure motor aphasia. Dejerine contrasted the two motor aphasias with dysarthria, which in his view resulted from the paralysis of the speech musculature. He insisted that motor aphasic patients could freely use their oropharyngeal musculature for all movements which were not verbal. He further denied that these patients could be apractic for speech movements. [1]

In the first decade of the twentieth century, Pierre Marie contended that 'pure motor aphasia' was a misnomer, since the condition it denoted was neither aphasic nor motor in nature. He therefore recommended to substitute 'anarthria' for pure motor aphasia. While he stressed that anarthria was neither an aphasic nor a motor disorder, Marie did not clearly say what it actually was. In a paper published in May 1906, he suggested that anarthria might be akin to pseudobulbar palsy. However, in October of the same year, he contended that anarthria was a disorder of the coordination of speech movements and was completely different from pseudobulbar or paralytic deficits. Less than a year later (1907), he disclaimed any knowledge of the pathophysiology of anarthria. However, in May 1908, he agreed with Gilbert Ballet (1908) that anarthria was a form of apraxia.

On the other hand, Marie (1906, a and b) was emphatic that articulatory disorders were identical in anarthria and in Broca's aphasia. Indeed, he maintained that Broca's aphasia was a combination of anarthria and genuine aphasia. Nonetheless, he doubted that Broca's aphasia could ever evolve into anarthria. [2] Marie (1906b) also insisted that anarthria resulted from a subcortical lesion in or near the lenticular nucleus, the caudate nucleus, the internal, or the external capsule. The lesion could be on the left or on the right, whereas aphasia could only be caused by a left-sided injury. Finally, Marie thought that the prognosis of anarthria was better than that of aphasia, except when anarthria resulted from a bilateral lesion.

At a meeting of the 'Société de Neurologie' in May 1908, and again in June of the same year, Gilbert Ballet proposed to abandon the word 'anarthria' and to revert to the term 'aphemia' introduced by Broca, because, he said, 'anarthria' tended to call a motor disorder to mind, whereas what patients actually had was an apractic impairment. [3]

Dupré thought that the term 'pure motor aphasia' was the most appropriate because in the condition it denoted inner speech was not intact. The patient had what Dupré called 'a psychomotor disorder', i.e., a disturbance that occurred at the border between internal and external language: the mental image of the word could no longer be properly exteriorized. [4]

In the 1920s Kurt Goldstein substituted the terms 'central' and 'peripheral motor aphasia' for 'Broca's aphasia' and 'pure motor aphasia' or 'anarthria', but he failed to clearly define the nosological entities to which these labels referred. Indeed, he expressed the view that the symptomatology of motor aphasia was extremely complex (1933) and to some extent varied from patient to patient. For instance, in 1948 (p. 79), he remarked that in some motor aphasic patients all voluntary movements of the oropharyngeal structures were impaired, while in others only verbal movements were, and in still others only nonverbal movements. Furthermore, he claimed that in a few patients the speech disorder was apractic in nature while in the majority of the cases it was due 'to a defect of the learned specialized motor speech performances'. Although he insisted that it was very important to distinguish between the two etiologies in order to use the appropriate therapy, he did not explain how one could tell them apart, nor what the difference was between apraxia and a disturbance of 'learned specialized motor speech performances' (1948, p. 80).

In the 1950s Eberhart Bay (1957) revived Marie's basic opinion about anarthria and Broca's aphasia. However, he proposed to speak of 'cortical dysarthria' when oral comprehension, reading, writing skills, and inner speech were found to be preserved. Moreover, on the basis of glossographic recordings, he claimed that in cortical dysarthria all fine movements of the oropharyngeal musculature were impaired. He called this impairment apraxic but considered it to be spastic in nature, 'analogous to spastic pareses of the limbs'. He further believed that cortical dysarthria could only result from damage to the dominant hemisphere (Bay, 1964).

In the late 1960s and early 1970s, Fred Darley and his team at the Mayo Clinic kindled interest in the problem in the United States. In a series of publications they endeavoured to characterize a syndrome which they called 'apraxia of speech' and which corresponded to 'aphemia', also named 'cortical dysarthria' (Johns and Darley, 1970). As a result, in recent years, a sizeable number of papers and several books, including a monograph by Wertz, LaPointe and Rosenbek (1984) and a volume edited by Rosenbek, McNeil and Aronson (1984), have been devoted to apraxia of speech (also called 'verbal apraxia'), testifying to the interest speech pathologists are taking in the condition.

Does Apraxia of Speech Really Exist?

Although the notion of a selective impairment of articulate speech was introduced more than 160 years ago and, under various names, has been passed down to the present time, the reality of an isolated disturbance of articulation has been repeatedly questioned. For instance, Head (1926, p. 200) doubted that articulate speech could be selectively impaired. He considered that all patients with so-called pure motor aphasia or anarthria on close examination proved to have additional deficits of an aphasic nature, particularly as regards written language. Head's doubts were shared by Weisenburg and McBride (1935, p. 56) who found that reports of pure motor aphasia were all incomplete in one respect or another. As a consequence, the existence of the condition could not be regarded as established.

A few years later, Alajouanine, Ombredane and Durand (1939) submitted that cases of pure anarthria did exist but were rare. Moreover, the adjective 'pure' was but relative: it indicated that the patient had a conspicuous articulatory disorder (which Alajouanine and co-workers called a 'syndrome of phonetic disintegration') and minor aphasic deficits which generally could only be discovered on close examination.

In 1974, Martin raised questions as to the appropriateness of the term 'apraxia of speech' either as a descriptive or explanatory label. He found that it reflected an outdated dichotomous model of language functioning. He argued that aphasia could be defined as 'an inefficient processing of linguistic units' and that the disorder referred to as apraxia of speech could be construed as an impairment of the selection and combination of linguistic units at the phonological level. Martin further claimed that experiments with so-called speech apraxics had failed to demonstrate that in these patients phonological perception was unimpaired and that perceptual disturbances did not play any role in the occurrence of the speech errors. In other words, Martin upheld the view that there did not exist a separate nosological entity featuring a selective motor speech impairment, but simply a variety of aphasia in which the processing of linguistic units was particularly impaired at the phonological level.

This view had been anticipated by Hécaen (1972, pp. 12–20) who posited the existence of a 'phonematic aphasia', which he described as a disturbance of phonological programming, and which he equated with the classical notion of motor aphasia and with Marie's conception of anarthria. According to Hécaen, in phonematic aphasia, there is nearly always some degree of agraphia, but the errors in writing do not parallel the errors in speaking. Hécaen's notion of a phonematic aphasia can, in fact, be traced back to Froment who considered motor aphasia to be essentially a phonological disorder characterized by defective recall and discrimination of speech sounds (Froment and Feyeux, 1934).

Has the Syndrome of Speech Apraxia any Specificity?

In view of the above divergence of opinions, it may well be wondered whether anarthria or, alternatively, apraxia of speech has any specificity. Is anarthria a distinct syndrome or is it an attenuated form of Broca's aphasia in which oral comprehension, reading and writing happen to be but slightly impaired? One way to answer this question might be to compare classical descriptions of Broca's aphasia with detailed reports of pure anarthria (apraxia of speech) in which:

1 The patient has reached the 'phase d'état', i.e., the stage following the acute period and characterized by a relative stability of the symptoms
2 The patient is not mute
3 Aphasic disorders such as agraphia, alexia, or telegraphic style are absent or minimal.

In fact, such a comparison strongly suggests that there are differences between pure anarthria and the output difficulties of Broca's aphasic patients. To begin with, at the 'phase d'état', pure anarthric patients can utter any word. To be sure, they may have to try several times before they can say the whole word, especially if it is a long one, and despite their repeated efforts they may fail to say the word correctly. But they will get it out. For instance, when asked to reproduce the French adverb *philosophiquement*, Joseph, the French-speaking anarthric patient described by Lebrun (1976), said: 'philo-philos-philosoph-ph-s-philosophiquement'. Broca's aphasic patients, on the contrary, may find it impossible to utter a particular word. They get stuck even before the first sound of the word is emitted. As an example, an excerpt reproduced by Martin (1974) may be quoted. In an attempt to say the word 'wife', his patient blurted: 'You know what I mean ... The other one ... not him, her ... Goddammit, this is awful ... The one with him ... Her ... her ... the Mrs ... That's it ... The other one ... The Mrs, the Mrs ... Jesus Christ, the wife... his wife.' This patient seemed to be having a lexical access problem. He knew that there was a word to denote a married woman but could not immediately get at it in his mental dictionary. Pure anarthrics do not seem to have such lexical access problems. What they apparently find difficult is to have the chosen lexical entry properly activate the verbo-motor pattern that implements the audible production of the word.

Both anarthric and Broca's aphasic patients make phonemic paraphasias. However, there seems to be at least one quantitative difference between these errors. It has been repeatedly observed (for example, see

Alajouanine, Pichot and Durand, 1949; Lebrun, Buyssens and Hen-eaux, 1973; Lapointe and Johns, 1975; Itoh and Sasanuma, 1984) that in the verbal output of anarthric patients anticipations by far outnumber perseverations. In the speech of Broca's aphasic patients, on the contrary, perseverations are more numerous, it would seem, than anticipations. For instance, in the patients with Broca's aphasia whom they tested, Nespoulous *et al.* (1983) found more perseverations than anticipations. Moreover, in Broca's aphasia, anticipations seem to occur rarely across word boundaries, whereas in anarthria they often do.

A study by Nespoulous, Lecours and Joanette (1982) suggests that there may exist a second quantitative difference between the phonemic paraphasias of patients with speech apraxia and those of patients with Broca's aphasia. Comparing the phonemic substitutions made by four patients with Broca's aphasia with the phonemic substitutions made by one anarthric patient, they found that the former replaced voiced plosives by homorganic voiceless plosives far more frequently than the latter. If this finding could be confirmed, there would be yet another criterion for distinguishing between apraxia of speech and the output difficulties of patients with Broca's aphasia.

It has repeatedly been noted (for example, see Johns and Darley, 1970; Lebrun, 1976) that anarthric patients make proportionally more errors in longer than in shorter words. This does not seem to be necessarily the case in Broca's aphasia. For instance, Nespoulous, Lecours and Joanette (1983) found that Broca's aphasic patients made proportionally more errors in mono- than in polysyllabic items when reading aloud lists of words.

A further difference lies in the omnipresence of the anarthric disorder. The speech apraxic is impaired irrespective of the kind of expressive activity he engages in. The severity of his condition remains constant, whether he holds a conversation, recites series he knows by rote, or repeats words pronounced by the examiner (Alajouanine, Pichot and Durand, 1949; Pilch and Hemmer, 1970; Nebes, 1975; Lebrun, 1976; Puel *et al.*, 1980; Washino *et al.*, 1981). Indeed, even singing is impaired (Nebes, 1975). In Broca's aphasia, on the other hand, output difficulties more often than not, vary with the type of expressive activity. Not infrequently repetition is markedly better than spontaneous speech. The recitation of automatized series may be fluent and singing remarkably preserved. Within spontaneous speech, islands of fair fluency may alternate with stretches of laboriously enunciated words. An instance of Broca's aphasia in which this variability could be clearly observed was reported by Lebrun in 1976. Such variability is not observed in cases of pure anarthria. Interestingly, as early as the beginning of this century, Dejerine (1901) pointed out that in pure motor aphasia, the disorder of articulation is present in every mode of speech. He further noted that singing is disturbed in pure motor aphasia, while it may be largely preserved in Broca's aphasia (Wernicke's cortical motor aphasia). A corollary of this is that Melodic Intonation Therapy often proves useful in deblocking the output of motor aphasic patients but does not seem to benefit pure speech apraxics (Wertz, Lapointe and Rosenbek, 1984, p. 227).[5]

Again, immediately after onset the anarthric patient may be totally unable to speak, but this mutism does not last. After some time the possibility to say words returns. However, articulation is defective and may remain so for many years (see, for instance, the patient of Itoh and Sasanuma, 1984). In Broca's aphasia, on the contrary, oral output may be extremely limited, and sometimes even inexistent, for many months. As early as 1933 Froment and Feyeux underscored this difference. Reporting on a female who a year after onset was still completely unable to speak, they rejected the diagnosis of anarthria which other physicians had proposed, and classified the patient as a motor aphasic. In their view, the patient had a language rather than a speech disorder. This was confirmed by the fact that she had writing and reading difficulties. Patient No. 2 in the chapter Simpson and Clark have contributed to this volume is a further case in point. A year and a half post-stroke this man was still mute. Then, under the influence of therapy he slowly started to recover the ability to whisper and at times to speak with voice. He also showed gains in auditory comprehension, sentence and paragraph reading, and writing. After he was discharged from therapy, written expression continued to improve. However, five years later, it had not completely normalized. This case then proves to be one of motor aphasia, as could have been predicted on the basis of the long-lasting mutism.

All this seems to legitimize the conclusion that anarthria is a separate nosological entity that does not coincide with the oral expression difficulties in Broca's aphasia. Consequently, patients who at the *phase d'état* can utter only a few words should probably not be diagnosed as having anarthria or speech apraxia, even if they can express themselves relatively better in writing than in speaking (for example, see De Morsier's second case, 1949). These patients are most likely to have a special form of Broca's aphasia in which writing is less impaired than speaking. By the same token, aphasia with recurrent utterance (Lebrun, 1986) should be radically separated from anarthria. The two conditions have widely different symptomatologies and should be considered two totally distinct nosological entities.

This leaves us with a double paradox. The description which Broca gave of 'aphemia' did not fit the impairment of Leborgne, although it was the Leborgne case which prompted the description. The syndrome of 'aphemia' does not fit in the picture of Broca's aphasia either. Broca then depicted a condition which was not that of the patient who inspired the description. Nor is the condition a component of the aphasia that bears Broca's name.

A recent study by Square-Storer, Darley and Sommers (1988) gives indirect support to the view upheld here that apraxia of speech is not an integral symptom of Broca's aphasia. The authors studied the performances of four patients with pure apraxia of speech, ten patients who were considered to have aphasia without apraxia of speech, ten patients who were considered to have aphasia in addition to speech apraxia, and eleven normals on a variety of nonspeech and speech auditory processing tasks and internal language processing tasks. They found that in all cases, the patients with speech apraxia performed as normal subjects, while only few differences were observed among the aphasic patients with and the aphasic patients without speech apraxia. From these findings the authors derived the conclusion that 'apraxia of speech and aphasia are mutually exclusive disorders' (p. 80). Such a conclusion could hardly have been reached if apraxia of speech were a regular component of an aphasic syndrome. As a matter of fact, if speech apraxia were such a component, the four patients with pure apraxia of speech in the study by Square-Storer, Darley and Sommers (1988) would have had a mild form of aphasia rather than a disorder distinct from aphasia. Their test scores might accordingly have been expected to lie between those of the normal subjects and those of the patients with clear aphasia rather than being indistinguishable from those of normals.

The Nature of Apraxia of Speech

Since anarthria (apraxia of speech) appears to be a syndrome in its own right, one may wonder what the exact nature of it is. One might argue, as Martin (1974) did, that the core of the disorder is a disturbance of the selection and combination of phonological units and that the condition accordingly has to be considered aphasic in nature. However, since anathric patients are generally able to recognize their errors, i.e., to discriminate between correct and faulty production of words, it may be assumed that they still know the phonological composition of words. This knowledge enables them to perform metalinguistic tasks implying the mental comparison of spoken words. For instance, Joseph, even in the acute phase, when he could not say a single word, could in an array of five objects point to the two whose names began with the same sound (Lebrun, 1976). And Nebes' patient (1975) could, in a list of five written words, find the two which rhyme in spoken language despite their diverging spellings, e.g. 'through' and 'new'.

These abilities suggest that what is disturbed in anarthria is the implementation of phonological knowledge. The patient knows what the word should sound like but he is no longer able to properly organize the sequence of articulatory gestures which produces the desired sound complex. This seems to be a typically apraxic problem. In fact, patients with apraxia, provided they are not demented at the same time, know what the goal is which they want to reach, but no longer know how to reach it. They do not remain inactive, though. They act, but do so inadequately, with many trials and errors, with anticipations, perseverations, and transpositions of part-movements. Though frequent, their gestural mistakes are erratic, unsystematic, and unpredictable. A comparable behaviour can be observed in speech apraxics at the 'phase d'état'. They speak but with many articulatory errors, including anticipations, perseverations, and metatheses. These errors are numerous, irregular, and unforeseeable (Alajouanine, Pichot and Durand, 1949; Johns and Darley, 1970; Lebrun, Buyssens and Henneaux, 1973).

Because they know that their articulation tends to go astray, anarthric patients endeavour to control it at every step. This may be one reason why in anarthria the rate of delivery is abnormally slow and phonemes are often protracted (Alajouanine, Ombredane and Durand, 1939, patient Elodie; Alajouanine, Pichot and Durand, 1949; Shankweiler *et al.*, 1966; Lebrun, Buyssens and Henneaux, 1973; Washino *et al.*, 1981). When patients are tired, this control can no longer be properly exerted and articulation disintegrates (Lebrun, 1982). Lecours and Lhermitte's patient (1976) explained how strenuous speech had become as a result of anarthria: 'In the normal state, thought is expressed through speech, automatically. One gives very little attention, if any, to articulation; by the strength of habit, articulation has become mechanical... My articulation ... is no longer automatic but has to be commanded, directed. I have to think of the word I am going to utter, and of the way in which to utter it. If I want to say "bonjour", I can no longer do so out of habit; it is no longer automatic. If I am not very attentive, I might say "beuseu". If I wish to say "le", "la", without being attentive, I might say "de", "da". For this reason, I must articulate each vowel, each consonant, in short each syllable' (p. 93).

It seems reasonable to assume that when he learns to speak his mother-tongue a child forms articulatory habits, i.e., verbomotor patterns. These patterns, or neuronal circuits, in adolescence and in adulthood ensure a smooth, fluent pronunciation, which the speaker, as Lecours and Lhermitte's patient aptly pointed out, has not constantly to be concerned and to care about. In apraxia of speech these patterns are disturbed. As a result, pronunciation is chaotic and disheveled, and requires constant conscious control and checking on the part of the speaker.

It may further be assumed that in fluent bilinguals there exist two separate sets of verbo-motor patterns, one for each language. Following brain damage, one set may be more impaired than the other. As a consequence, pronunciation is more disturbed in one language than in the other, as was observed in the bilingual patient described by Alajouanine, Pichot and Durand (1949).

However, it would seem that in apraxia of speech there is more than a disturbance of the individual verbomotor patterns. In addition to being internally impaired, the patterns tend to interfere with one another when they are being prepared for use. In particular, patterns which are going to be used a little later in the sentence and are therefore, in all likelihood, pre-excited even before the sentence begins (Lebrun, Brihaye and Lebrun, 1971), tend to influence the unreeling of the patterns used earlier in the sentence and thus to cause anticipations across word boundaries. The interference of verbomotor patterns to be used later in the sentence is a praxic deficit. As a matter of fact, a comparable sequencing disorder has been noted in the behaviour of patients with limb apraxia (Poeck and Lehmkuhl, 1980).

It appears then that apraxia of speech really is what its name implies, a praxic disorder of articulation: the complex, multifaceted gestures which externalize words, phrases, and clauses can no longer be properly organized because the verbomotor patterns which were formed during language acquisition are individually disturbed. Moreover, when being prepared for use, they tend to interfere with one another.

The Dejerine-Marie-Controversy in Retrospect

At the turn of the century, Marie (e.g. 1906a, b) published a series of provocative papers in which he advocated a complete revision of traditional views of aphasia. These papers caused such a commotion in French neurological circles that in 1908 the French Neurological Society decided to devote three special meetings to a debate on aphasia.

These meetings took place on June 11, July 9, and July 23 1908, and the proceedings were published in the *Revue Neurologique* for the same year. The two main protagonists were Jules Dejerine and Pierre Marie. Dejerine reproached Marie for confusing dysarthria with motor aphasia. Marie retorted that what he called 'anarthria' was different both from dysarthria and from aphasia. The two disputants failed to come to an agreement. Dejerine kept claiming that Marie's anarthria was, in fact, a motor disorder and Marie kept repeating that anarthric patients had no paralysis of the speech musculature and therefore were totally different from patients with bulbar or pseudobulbar dysarthria.

Maybe the whole issue was obscured by the fact that there exist patients who evidence a total inability to speak together with some reduction of the oropharyngeal motility. Such a case was reported by Jude and Trabaud in 1928. The patient was a right-handed male who, following a cerebrovascular accident in the right hemisphere, lost the ability to speak while retaining the ability to understand both spoken and written language and to express himself in writing. He had severe left hemiplegia and facial paralysis on the same side. According to Jude and Trabaud, this case was a typical instance of pure anarthria. However, the patient was unable to blow out a burning match or to whistle. He could move his tongue but only slowly, and he had difficulty in chewing and in swallowing. How can these additional deficits be accounted for? It has repeatedly been observed that oral apraxia may accompany anarthria (for example, see Tissot, Rodriguez and Tissot, 1970, and LaPointe and Wertz, 1974). Perhaps the patient of Jude and Trabaud had oral apraxia in addition to his speech disorder, and this may account for his inability to blow out a match and to whistle. But what about his reduced tongue agility and his dysphagia? These impairments seem to have been really motor in nature, and this is difficult to reconcile with the view that patients with anarthria or apraxia of speech show no 'significant weakness (or) slowness of the speech musculature' (Johns and Darley, 1970).

The case reported by Alajouanine *et al.* in 1959 raises similar problems. The patient was a 27-year-old male who suddenly presented with right-sided hemiplegia and total inability to utter speech sounds. In addition, he could hardly move his lips or tongue voluntarily and could not firmly close his eyes on request. No movement of the velum could be observed and the palatal reflex was abolished. The patient had difficulty in drinking through a straw. On the other hand, he had no dysphagia and the gag reflex could be elicited. Spontaneous laughing was normal, but, for the rest, facial expression tended to be void. Oral comprehension, reading, and writing with the left hand were unimpaired. Arteriography pointed to a left-sided vascular lesion involving the lenticular nucleus, the caudate nucleus and the internal capsule, which is precisely the region where Marie thought the lesion causing anarthria typically was. Alajouanine *et al.* construed their case as an instance of aphemia but were careful to point out that the speech disorder was associated with disturbances of the voluntary and reflex activity of the orofacial musculature.

It appears, then, that in the acute stage, speech apraxia may be accompanied by oropharyngeal motor problems which may confuse the picture and render diagnosis difficult. Indeed, if the patient is totally speechless, it may be at first impossible to safely distinguish between anarthria (or aphemia or apraxia of speech) and pseudobulbar dysarthria, since the latter condition not infrequently features a total inability to speak accompanied by reduced tongue motility and dysphagia, the palatal and pharyngeal reflexes being sometimes abolished and sometimes preserved (compare De Morsier's first case, 1949, and Lebrun's patient Mathilde V., 1976). Accordingly, it may be necessary to wait for the patient to recover some ability to speak before anarthria or apraxia of speech can be safely diagnosed. Then, on the basis of the types of articulatory errors, it becomes possible to distinguish between apractic and purely motor disorders of pronunciation (see also Chapter 8).

The difficulty in classifying mute patients at the acute stage may account in part for the persistent disagreement between Dejerine and Marie. Both neurologists undoubtedly had seen mute patients. But Dejerine may have been more sensitive to the accompanying disorders of oropharyngeal motricity and may have been inclined to classify patients with such disorders as having bulbar or pseudobulbar, i.e., paralytic, dysarthria. Indeed, the presence of motor disorders of the speech musculature may have been for Dejerine a sure indication that the patient had dysarthria, and not aphasia, as he believed that in motor aphasia all oropharyngeal movements which were not verbal could be easily performed.[6]

Conclusion

At the meeting of the American Speech and Hearing Association in Denver, Colorado in 1968, Darley presented a paper entitled 'Apraxia of Speech: 107 years of terminological confusion'. The present review shows that the history of the concept of speech apraxia is not only one of terminological but also of semiological confusion. If patients had been examined more carefully and their symptoms — verbal and nonverbal — analyzed more accurately, much arguing could probably have been avoided. In 1904, Joseph Babinski began a series of lectures with the following remark: 'Diagnostic errors result far more frequently from imperfect observation of the symptoms than from faulty interpretation of them. Diagnostic mistakes proceed from semiological mistakes. The study of neurological symptomatology therefore is of cardinal importance'. If Babinski's recommendation had been constantly minded in investigations of apraxia of speech, perhaps less confusion would have arisen.

Notes

1 See *Revue Neurologique* (1908) **16**, pp. 626 and 1030.
2 See *Revue Neurologique* (1908) **16**, p. 634.
3 See *Revue Neurologique* (1908) **16**, p. 628.
4 See *Revue Neurologique* (1908) **16**, p. 632.
5 In the case reported by Keith and Aronson (1975) singing therapy proved helpful not because the case was 'exceptional' (Wertz, Lapointe and Rosenbek, 1984, p. 227) but because the patient, in fact, had Broca's aphasia.
6 See *Revue Neurologique* (1908) **16**, p. 626.

References

ALAJOUANINE, T., OMBREDANE, A. and DURAND M. (1939) *Le Syndrome de Désintégration Phonétique dans l'Aphasie*, Paris, Masson.
ALAJOUANINE, T., PICHOT, P. and DURAND, M. (1949) 'Dissociation des altérations phonétiques avec conservation relative de la langue la plus ancienne dans un cas d'anarthrie pure chez un sujet français bilingue', *L'Encéphale*, **28**, pp. 245–65.
ALAJOUANINE, T., LHERMITTE, F., CAMBIER, J., RONDOT, P. and LEFEVRE, J. (1959) 'Perturbations dissociées de la motricité facio-bucco-pharyngée avec aphémie dans un ramollissement sylvien profound partiel', *Revue Neurologique*, **101**, pp. 493–8.
BABINSKI, J. (1904) Introduction à la sémiologie des affections du système nerveux, *Gazette des Hôpitaux* (11 October, 1904).
BALLET, G. (1908) 'Apraxie faciale (impossibilité de souffler) associée à de l'aphasie complexe (aphasie motrice et aphasie sensorielle). Apraxie et aphémie', *Revue Neurologique*, **16**, pp. 445–7.
BAY, E. (1957) 'Die corticale Dysarthrie und ihre Beziehungen zur sogenannten motorischen Aphasie', *Deutsche Zeitschrift für Nervenheilkunde*, **176**, pp. 553–91.

BAY, E. (1964) 'Principles of classification and their influence on our concepts of aphasia', in DE REUK, A. and O'CONNOR, M. (Eds) *Disorders of Language*, London, Churchill, pp. 112–39.

BOUILLAUD, J. (1825) 'Rescherches cliniques propres à démontrer que la perte de la parole correspond à la lésion des lobules antérieurs du cerveau, et à confirmer l'opinion de M. Gall sur le siège de l'organe du langage articulé', *Archives Générales de Médecine*, **8**, pp. 25–45.

BROCA, P. (1861) 'Remarques sur le siège de la faculté de langage suivies d'une observation d'aphémie', *Bulletin de la Société d'Anatomie*, **6** (2e série), pp. 330–57.

DE MORSIER, G. (1949) 'Les troubles de la déglutition et des mouvements de la langue dans l'anarthrie (aphasie motrice)', *Practica Oto-Rhino-Laryngologica*, **11**, pp. 125–33.

DEJERINE, J. (1901) 'Sémiologie du système nerveux', in Bouchard (Ed.) *Traité de Pathologie Générale*, Paris, Masson, **5**, pp. 391–471.

FROMENT, J. and FEYEUX, A. (1934) 'Aphasie motrice pure: simili-anarthrie rééduquée sans redressement aucun des coordinations articulaires par simple sommation de la mémoire des sons', *Revue Neurologique*, **42**, pp. 1058–66.

GOLDSTEIN, K. (1933) 'L'analyse de l'aphasie et l'étude de l'essence du langage', *Journal de Psychologie Normale et Pathologique*, **30**, pp. 430–96.

GOLDSTEIN, K. (1948) *Language and Language Disturbances*, New York, Grune and Stratton.

HEAD, H. (1926) *Aphasie and Kindred Disorders of Speech*, Cambridge, Cambridge University Press.

HECAEN, H. (1972) *Introduction à la Neuropsychologie*, Paris, Larousse.

ITOH, M. and SASANUMA, S. (1984) 'Articulatory movements in apraxia of speech', in ROSENBEK, J., MCNEIL, M. and ARONSON, A. (Eds.) *Apraxia of Speech*, San Diego, College-Hill Press; London, Taylor and Francis, pp. 135–65.

JOHNS, D. and DARLEY, F. (1970) 'Phonemic variability in apraxia of speech', *Journal of Speech and Hearing Research*, **13**, pp. 556–83.

JUDE and TRABAUD (1928) 'Hémiplégie gauche avec anarthrie. Accès de fourire contrastant avec la correction de la mimique douloureuse', *Revue Neurologique*, **36**, pp. 726–8.

KEITH, R. and ARONSON, A. (1975) 'Singing as therapy for apraxia of speech and aphasia: Report of a case', *Brain and Language*, **2**, pp. 483–8.

KUSSMAUL, A. (1877) 'Die Störungen der Sprache', in *Ziemssen's Handbuch der speziellen Pathologie und Therapie*, **11**, pp. 1–300, Reprinted separately as *Die Störungen der Sprache. Versuch einer Pathologie der Sprache*, Leipzig, Vogel (1881).

LAPOINTE, L. and JOHNS, D. (1975) 'Some phonemic characteristics in apraxia of speech', *Journal of Communication Disorders*, **8**, pp. 259–69.

LAPOINTE, L. and WERTZ, R. (1974) 'Oral-movement abilities and articulatory characteristics of brain-injured adults', *Perceptual and Motor Skills*, **39**, pp. 39–46.

LEBRUN, Y. (1976) 'Neurolinguistic models of language and speech', in Whitaker, H. (Ed.) *Studies in Neurolinguistics*, **1**, New York, Academic Press, pp. 1–30.

LEBRUN, Y. (1982) 'Aphasie de Broca et anarthrie', *Acta Neurologica Belgica* **82**, pp. 80–90.

LEBRUN, Y. (1986) 'Aphasia with recurrent utterance: A review', *British Journal of Disorders of Communication*, **21**, pp. 3–10.

LEBRUN, Y., BRIHAYE, J. and LEBRUN, N. (1971) 'On expressive agrammatism', *Journal of Communication Disorders*, **4**, pp. 126–33.

LEBRUN, Y., BUYSSENS, E. and HENNEAUX, J. (1973) 'Phonetic aspects of anarthria', *Cortex*, **9**, pp. 126–35.

LECOURS, R. and LHERMITTE, F. (1976) 'The pure form of the phonetic disintegration syndrome (pure anarthria): Anatomo-clinical report of a historical case', *Brain and Language*, **3**, pp. 88–113.

LICHTHEIM, L. (1885) 'On aphasia', *Brain*, **7**, pp. 433–84.

MARIE, P. (1906a) 'La troisième circonvolution frontale gauche ne joue aucun rôle spécial dans la fonction du langage', *Semaine Médicale*, **26**, pp. 241–7.

MARIE, P. (1906b) 'Que faut-il penser des aphasies sous-corticales?', *La Semaine Médicale*, **26**, pp. 493–500.

MARIE, P. (1907) 'Présentation de malades atteints d'anarthrie par lésion de l'hémisphère gauche du cerveau', *Bulletins et Mémoires de la Société Médicale des Hôpitaux*, pp. 864–5.

MARTIN, D. (1974) 'Some objections to the term "apraxia of speech"', *Journal of Speech and Hearing Disorders*, **39**, pp. 53–64.

NEBES, R. (1975) 'The nature of internal speech in a patient with aphemia', *Brain and Language*, **2**, pp. 489–97.

NESPOULOUS, J., LECOURS, A. and JOANETTE, Y. (1982) 'Stabilité et instabilité des déviations phonétiques et/ou phonémiques des aphasiques. Insuffisance d'un modèle statique d'analyse, *La Linguistique*, **18**, pp. 85–97.

NESPOULOUS, J., LECOURS, A. and JOANETTE, Y. (1983) 'La dichotomie 'phonétique-phonémique' a-t-elle une valeur nosologique?', in Messerli, P., Lavorel, P. and Nespoulous, J. (Eds.) *Neuropsychologie de l'expression orale*, Paris, Editions du Centre National de la Recherche Scientifique, pp. 71–91.

PILCH, H. and HEMMER, R. (1970) 'Phonematische Aphasie', *Phonetica*, **22**, pp. 231–9.

POECK, K. and LEHMKUHL, G. (1980) 'Das Syndrom der ideatorischen Apraxie und seine Lokalisation', *Der Nervenarzt*, **51**, pp. 217–25.

PUEL, M., NESPOULOUS, J., BONAFE, A. and RASCOL, A. (1980) 'Etude neurolinguistique d'un cas d'anarthrie pure', *Grammatica (Université de Toulouse-Le Mirail)* **7**, pp. 239–291.

ROSENBEK, J., MCNEIL, M. and ARONSON, A. (1984) *Apraxia of Speech*, San Diego, College-Hill Press; London, Taylor and Francis.

SHANKWEILER, D., HARRIS, K and TAYLOR, M. (1968) 'Electromyographic studies of articulation in aphasia', *Archives of Physical Medicine and Rehabilitation* 49 : 1–8.

SQUARE-STORER, P., DARLEY, F. and SOMMERS, R. (1988) 'Nonspeech and speech processing skills in patients with aphasia and apraxia of speech', *Brain and Language*, **33**, pp. 65–85.

TISSOT, A., RODRIGUEZ, J. and TISSOT, R. (1970) 'Die Prognose der Anarthrie im Sinne von Pierre Marie', in Leischner, A. (Ed.) *Die Rehabilitation der Aphasie in den romanischen Ländern*, Stuttgart, Thieme, pp. 20–43.

TROUSSEAU, A. (1861–1864) *Clinique médicale de l'Hôtel-Dieu de Paris*, Paris, Masson.

WASHINO, K., KASAI, Y., UCHIDA, Y. and TAKEDA, K. (1981) 'Tongue movement during speech in a patient with apraxia of speech: A case study', in Peng, F. (Ed.) *Current Issues in Neurolinguistics: A Japanese Contribution*, Tokyo, The International Christian University, pp. 125–59.

WEISENBURG, T. and MCBRIDE, K. (1935) *Aphasia*, New York, The Commonwealth Fund.

WERNICKE, C. (1885) 'Die neueren Arbeiten über Aphasie', *Fortschritte der Medizin*, **3**, pp. 824–30.

WERTZ, R., LAPOINTE, L. and ROSENBEK, J. (1984) *Apraxia of Speech in Adults*, Orlando, Grune and Stratton.

Chapter 2

The Apraxias: Commonalities and Distinctions

Paula Square-Storer and Eric A. Roy

Apraxia, a disturbance of movement or action not due to neuro-muscular innervation disruption as observed, for example, in paresis or ataxia, but instead to a hypothesized disruption of motor programming, has been identified for the speech, nonverbal oral, and limb motor systems. These three disorders, most commonly referred to as apraxia of speech (AOS) or verbal apraxia; oral, buccofacial, or buccolingual facial apraxia (OA); and limb apraxia (LA), respectively, have received a growing amount of attention in the neurological literature since the late 1800s. Few attempts, however, have been made to evaluate the similarities and distinctions among the apraxias across the three motor systems. One exception has been our recent hypothetical (Roy and Square, 1985a) and empirical work (Roy and Square, 1985b) which has addressed specifically the commonalities and distinctions among the apraxias. It is the purpose of this chapter to elaborate further on our hypotheses, observations, and experimental work. Specifically, we will address the following areas:

1 Definitions of the apraxias
2 Subtypes and their specific behaviors and assumed correlative lesion sites
3 Coexistence of the apraxias
4 Similarities with regard to symptoms as 'traditionally' defined in the literature.

The Apraxias Defined

The contemporary definition of apraxia of speech and the one cited most frequently, derives from the work of Darley (1968). He stated that apraxia of speech is 'an articulatory disorder resulting from impairment, as a result of brain damage, of the capacity to program the positioning of speech musculature and the sequencing of muscle movements for volitional production of phonemes. The speech musculature does not show significant weakness, slowness, or incoordination when used for reflex and automatic acts. Prosodic alterations may be associated with the articulatory problem, perhaps in compensation for it'. Highlighted within this definition are the disabilities for spatial targeting, motor sequencing, 'phasing' of muscle movements (Kent and Rosenbek, 1983), and transitionalization between phones and/or syllables (Trost, 1970). A coexisting inference is that volitional/purposive speech behavior, either self-formulated or as a repeated response to an auditory model, will most probably be more affected than automatic speech. (See Chapter 1 for a discussion of an alternative viewpoint.)

A traditional definition of oral apraxia derives from the early descriptions of the disorder by Jackson (1878) and Wilson (1908). Roy and Square (1985a) defined the disorder '... as the inability to efficiently and immediately produce oral movements on verbal command and/or imitation with preserved ability to produce similar actions semi-automatically' (p. 142). This definition, as some for apraxia of speech, stresses the disparity of performance for the production of automatic and volitional oral behaviors. Although the quality of motor inefficiency is not broached in this definition, it has been in the work of Mateer and colleagues (Mateer and Kimura, 1977; Mateer, 1978; Ojemann and Mateer, 1979), Poeck and Kerschensteiner (1975), De-Renzi, Pieczuro, and Vignolo (1966) and Tognolo and Vignolo (1980) among others. These motor deviances will be described in detail in later sections of this chapter.

Limb apraxia presents as an inability to perform gestures, e.g., show me how to stir coffee, to verbal command or to imitate the same gestures pantomimed by the examiner. Although unable to carry out such gestures in a clinical examination, patients are able to make these gestures in the appropriate environmental context, e.g., when making a cup of coffee. As with many disorders in neurology, limb apraxia is defined both by exclusion and inclusion. By exclusion this impairment to gesturing is defined as apraxia only if generalized impairments to behavioral function (dementia), auditory–verbal comprehension disorders (aphasia), visual recognition disorders, and basic motor control impairments can be ruled out. The definition by inclusion stresses more the types of errors which are characteristic of apraxia. These errors are reviewed at length in later sections of this chapter.

Subtypes of the Apraxias

For each of the apraxias — verbal, oral, and limb — various subtypes have been proposed. The bases for these subclassifications have been neuroanatomical, behavioral, derived from hypothesized underlying disrupted neuropsychological mechanisms, and/or specified with respect to accompanying disorders such as aphasia, and neuroinnervatory motor disturbances. The subclassifications for each of the apraxias as derived from the literature will be reviewed in this section.

Apraxia of speech

Few attempts have been made to identify subgroups of patients with apraxia of speech. Those subclassifications which have been proposed have been based predominately upon locus of lesion and, thus, termed by Buckingham (1979) as center-lesion theories. Luria (1966, 1976) identified two subgroups of 'motor aphasia' — afferent and efferent. Both were characterized not only by linguistic dysfunction, i.e., aphasia, but by impaired motor speech production. Afferent motor aphasia was thought to be a sequelae of parietal lobe damage specifically involving the facial region of the sensory strip of the language-dominant hemisphere. Inferred from this center-lesion subclassification is the disordered mechanism underlying defective speech, namely, the inability to use kinesthetic information for the repetition or self-initiated production of speech. Results of research by Rosenbek, Wertz and Darley (1973), in fact, have lent some credence to Luria's hypothesis that orosensory perception may be disrupted among some apractic speakers. (See Chapter 5 for further discussion of orosensory perceptual deficits in AOS.) Efferent motor aphasia was thought to arise from damage to the third frontal convolution (Broca's area) of the dominant hemisphere. The disrupted mechanism inferred from this site of lesion was loss of kinetic melody as evidenced by the patient's difficulty in transition between individual speech segments. The loss of 'kinetic melody', internalized rhythm, and/or impairment of transitionalization among Brocas's aphasic individuals was demonstrated empirically by Trost (1970) and by Trost and Canter (1974). (See Chapter 6 for further discussion of 'rhythm'.)

Recent empirical evidence for cortical anterior and posterior syndromes of verbal apraxia have been proposed by Deutsch (1984). Canter (1969) also proposed a frontal/posterior center-lesion dichotomy for subclassifications of apraxia of speech. However, inferred disrupted mechanisms differed from those proposed by Luria (1966, 1976). Primary verbal apraxia, due to a lesion to Broca's area, was said to be characterized predominately by segmental errors, i.e., speech sound errors, in which either a substituted or distorted segment close to the intended target with respect to place and manner of production was produced. It seems, then, that Canter (1969) was implicating spatial targeting and malphasing of articulatory features as the mechanisms primarily disrupted in primary verbal apraxia. Secondary verbal apraxia was said to be due to posterior lesions which damaged the sensory association areas or transcortical tracts. Inferred underlying disturbed mechanisms in this subclassification of the disorder appeared to be of a higher order than those proposed for primary verbal apraxia. Canter's belief was that the actual selection and sequencing of phonemes were disrupted. Many aphasiologists would term malselection of phonemes as phonemic or literal paraphasia (for example, Lecours and Lhermitte, 1969; Poncet *et al.*, 1972; or, for a discussion, Roy and Square, 1985a). In fact, even Canter seemed to change his position regarding the underlying mechanism of the disorder he originally termed 'secondary verbal apraxia' in that the disorder was re-termed 'phonemic para-phasia' in later works (Canter, Trost and Burns, 1985), thus, implying that the speech errors were due to a disruption of language processes and not motor speech processes. Darley (1982), however, continued to question the 'phonologic' basis of such errors in the verbal output of left-hemisphere-damaged (LHD) patients. (See Chapter 5 for further discussion.) It has been proposed, however, that, 'acting in the world may involve the operation of two systems' (Roy, 1983): 'a conceptual system which provides an abstract representation of action and a production system which incorporates a sensory motor component of knowledge (generalized action programs) as well as encompassing the perceptual motor processes for organizing and executing actions...' (Roy and Square, 1985a, p. 112). Further, it has been proposed by Roy and Square (1985a) that, because the 'phoneme' can be thought to be an abstract representation of action, speech errors, as a result of acquired brain damage that are not due to disruptions of neuromuscular innervation, i.e., the dysarthrias, may be a form of apraxia in which malfunction of the conceptual-linguistic system interferes with the top-down control of speech movements.

Recent empirical studies of patients with symptoms of apraxia of speech with parietal lobe lesions have implicated behaviors different from those reported by Canter (1969) and Canter, Trost and Burns, 1985. Square, Darley and Sommers (1982) reported that their two parietal-lobe lesioned verbally apractic patients who demonstrated no clinical evidence of aphasia produced perceived speech errors which were similar and which consisted predominately of initiation and transitionalization errors and frank consonantal substitutions. The patients were quite dysfluent in that their speech was marked by repetitions of phonemes, syllables, and words; struggle behavior, both audible and inaudible; groping behavior, and self-correction. Consistent with reports by Canter and colleagues (Canter, 1969; Canter, Trost and Burns, 1985), frank consonantal substitutions predominantly characterized segmental production. When consonantal distortions did appear among the patients studied by Square, Darley and Sommers (1982), glides, fricatives, and affricates were predominately affected.

Itoh and colleagues reported extensively on the motor speech characteristics, measured instrumentally, of a patient with symptoms of apraxia of speech, minimal aphasia, and a subcortical lesion extending to Area 44 of the left hemisphere. Findings indicated that this patient had extreme difficulty regulating temporal coordination of velar movements with lingual articulation (Itoh, Sasanuma and Ushijima, 1979), coordinating several articulators simultaneously including the tongue, lips, and velum (Itoh *et al.*, 1980), and coordinating laryngeal behavior, specifically voicing, with supraglottal articulation (Itoh *et al.*, 1982). The disrupted mechanism inferred from these instrumental results was the temporal programming (integration) of individual muscle movements.

Square, Darley, and Sommers (1982), Square and Mlcoch (1983), and Kertesz (1984) also proposed subclassifications of apraxia of speech based upon site of lesion. These studies identified patients with subcortical lesions to the basal ganglia of the dominant hemisphere as forming a subgroup of verbally apractic patients who presented with symptoms somewhat different than patients with only cortical damage. Kertesz (1984) reported that aphasic/verbally apractic patients with lesions extending to the subcortical areas more often had coexisting symptoms of dysarthria while Square, Darley and Sommers (1982) and Square and Mlcoch (1983) highlighted the predominance of phoneme distortions in their apractic patient with a subcortical lesion. Further, Schiff *et al.* (1983), although acknowledging the typical symptoms of apraxia of speech such as initial gropes, reattempts, and labored speech, preferred to describe the speech disorder in their 'aphemic' patients as 'dysarthric'. As reviewed in Chapter 1, subcortical lesions had been implicated as accounting for the symptoms of 'anarthria' and 'pure motor aphasia' by both Marie (1906) and Wernicke (1885), respectively. These reports, as well as more contemporary ones (Goodglass and Kaplan, 1972; Lecours and Lhermitte, 1976; Mazzocchi and Vignolo, 1979; Naeser *et al.*,

1982), terminological confusion withstanding, have all seemed to describe a subgroup of patients who present with many symptoms of apraxia of speech but who appear to be dysarthric as well, i.e., have a coexisting neuromotor execution disorder (see Chapter 8). The disrupted mechanism responsible for the motor speech disorder would seem to be one of motor programming for spatial targeting and phasing, i.e., temporal coordination of speech movements and muscles or muscle subgroups, compounded by a fine motor control problem.

To summarize, several subtypes of apraxia of speech may exist in that several cortical and subcortical sites appear responsible for the programming of spatial and temporal information requisite for normal motor speech production. Different disordered mechanisms and/or coexisting deficits may underlie or coexist with verbal apractic symptomatology.

Oral apraxia

Disorders of oral praxis are associated with left-hemisphere lesions and have been reported by Kertesz (1984) and DeRenzi, Pieczuro and Vignolo (1966) to be associated always with aphasia. Mateer (1978), however, reported that oral apraxia may occur in the absence of aphasia, just as Square, Darley and Sommers (1988) reported that apraxia of speech may occur in the absence of aphasia. Subclassifications of oral apraxia exist and, similar to verbal apraxia, are also based on site of lesion and correlative symptomatology. It consistently has been reported that patients with presumed frontal lesions, i.e., Broca's aphasic subjects, most commonly show oral apraxia. Further, in this group, production of single postural movements and sequences of those movements are affected (Mateer and Kimura, 1977; Mateer, 1978). Both postural meaningful gestures such as 'smile' and meaningless gestures such as 'tongue out' are affected under both command and imitative modalities (DeRenzi, Pieczuro and Vignolo, 1968). In a CT scan study of oral apraxia associated with imitation of oral gestures, Tognolo and Vignolo (1980) concluded that it is the integrity of the central and frontal opercula which is necessary for the production of single postural gestures. With regard to the production of coordinated gestures, i.e., those which require the coordination of several motor subsystems such as lip rounding with expiration for production of the gesture 'blow', again frontal-lesioned patients, i.e., those with Broca's aphasia, are most impaired (Watamori *et al.*, 1981). This later finding led Watamori and colleagues to speculate that the premotor areas are responsible for the temporal coordination of the subcomponents requisite for the production of coordinated oral gestures.

In their discussion of the disturbed mechanisms underlying oral apraxia, Roy and Square (1985a) speculated that the errors produced by frontal-lesioned patients in the production of isolated oral gestures may be related to spatial disorientation within the vocal tract. Mateer and Kimura (1977) and Mateer (1978) demonstrated that this group of patients usually demonstrated random and continuous amorphous movements when attempting isolated gestures. It appears, then, that frontal-lesioned patients may be searching or groping for a spatial target when attempting to produce single gestures.

With regard to posterior-lesioned patients, the literature is contradictory regarding ability to produce isolated gestures. Mateer and Kimura (1977) and Mateer (1978) reported a relatively well-preserved ability among fluent aphasic patients. DeRenzi, Pieczuro and Vignolo (1966) reported that less than 6 per cent of Wernicke's but more than a third of conduction aphasic subjects were impaired. Poeck and Kerschensteiner (1975), however, reported impairment of oral praxis function for isolated oral gestures among all types of aphasic patients. Further, error profiles did not differ for aphasic classifications. Semantically unrelated substitutions followed by fragmentations and, then, talking instead of producing a movement, characterized behaviors in all subgroups. Surprisingly, amorphous movements, those which Mateer (1978; Mateer and Kimura, 1977) found to prevail for nonfluent subjects, ranked second to last for all aphasic subgroups studied by Poeck and Kerschensteiner (1975). Watamori and colleagues (1981), however, like Mateer noted distinct differences between anterior and posterior aphasic patients. While two subgroups of Broca's patients were considered 'dyspraxic' because of groping behaviors, delays, extraneous noises, and additional movements, the posterior patients were considered to be 'parapraxic' in that the majority of their errors were substitutions. Further the production of meaningless coordinated movements, such as clicking one's teeth, compared to production of meaningful coordinated movements, such as coughing, was strikingly aberrant.

The findings by Watamori *et al.* (1981) have relevance for inferring disturbed underlying mechanisms. Indicated from these later data may be support for the hypothesis that malselection of oral actions signifies a top-down control problem or conceptual disruptions among posterior-lesioned patients (see Roy, 1983; Roy and Square, 1985a). Also, the difficulty for production of meaningless coordinated gestures may lend even more credence in that conception of the meaningless movements provides even less of a governing framework for top-down control of production. On the other hand, the amorphous movements produced by the anterior-lesioned patients may have their grounding in a production disorder in which spatial targeting and/or the temporal coordination of muscle movements is/are deviant. Thus, a nondefinitive, unstructured oral movement occurs.

Production of sequences of nonverbal oral movements has also been examined for left-hemisphere-lesioned patients presumed to have either anterior or posterior lesions based upon type of aphasia demonstrated, i.e., nonfluent versus fluent aphasia, respectively (Mateer and Kimura, 1977; Mateer, 1978). Patients with both sites of lesion were found to be impaired for production of oral sequences. The underlying disturbed mechanism for oral sequencing disorders among left-hemisphere-damaged (LHD) subjects has been studied in our laboratory as well as by Mateer and Kimura (1977). The latter researchers hypothesized that the disability for producing oral sequences among left-hemisphere-damaged subjects was related to a disorder of transitionalization. Since fluent aphasic subjects were able to produce discrete isolated gestures but not sequences, disabilities to reach targets within sequences, i.e., transitionalization, was the implicated disrupted mechanism and the left hemisphere was said to be the regulator of this function. It may be inferred, however, from results reported by LaPointe (1969) and LaPointe and Wertz (1974), that brain damage in general results in oral sequencing disabilities. They studied aphasic, verbally apractic, and dysarthric individuals, the latter group inferentially, but not necessarily, having cortical lesions (see Darley, Aronson and Brown, 1975), and found 75 per cent of their patients to have oral sequencing problems. Such results would seem to implicate brain damage in general and not just damage to the left hemisphere as being responsible for oral sequencing disabilities. Preliminary findings from our work (Roy *et al.*, 1987a) have suggested that a memory disorder may underlie the reduced ability to produce sequences of oral gestures among LHD patients. Our findings are similar to those reported by Jason (1983) for manual sequencing among LHD patients. Further research regarding the disturbed mechanisms underlying oral sequencing disabilities among left-hemisphere-lesioned subjects obviously is needed.

Limb apraxia

Limb apraxias, in a very general sense, may be viewed as involving two major types of disorders: those which affect both limbs (bilateral apraxias) and those which affect only one limb (unilateral apraxias). Considering the bilateral variety, two of the most well-known types are termed ideational and ideomotor apraxia (Liepmann, 1920). Both of these disorders arise from damage to the left hemisphere in the supramarginal gyrus region. Ideational apraxia has been characterized in a number of ways. Poeck (1983) suggested that this apraxia is observed principally in tasks requiring a sequence of actions, particularly those involving the use of multiple objects, e.g., making a cup of coffee. The individual actions, e.g., stirring the coffee, are often performed effortlessly and fluently, although the object may be used inappropriately. Ideational apraxia has also been characterized as an impairment in the use of single objects. In this case, both performances to verbal command, e.g., show how to use a hammer, and actually holding the object, are impaired. In contrast, performance imitating the examiner's demonstration is often much less impaired. Patients with this disorder are frequently impaired even in their home environment.

In contrast to ideational apraxia, ideomotor apraxia is much less severe. This disorder is often described as being much more examination-bound in the sense that it is often observed only in the clinical setting (DeRenzi, 1985). Patients with this disorder exhibit less fluency of movement than those with ideational apraxia. These patients are often able to perform sequences of actions involving real objects but with considerable effort. They appear most impaired in the performance of single gestures. In this case, the patient is unable to perform both to verbal command and imitation but shows improved performance when using the actual object.

The other types of bilateral apraxias have been described by Luria (1980) and are termed frontal and premotor apraxia. These apraxias, involving damage to the frontal and premotor areas, respectively, affect the performance of sequential motor acts and, so, present somewhat like ideational apraxia.

The unilateral apraxias (see Roy, 1978, 1982 for details) involve those which present with characteristics of ideational and ideomotor apraxia, i.e., sympathetic and callosal apraxia, and those which present principally as an impairment in the control of movement, i.e., limb kinetic and kinesthetic apraxia, with little evidence of errors characteristic of the bilateral apraxias.

A number of studies have examined the types of errors observed in limb apraxia and many are analogous to those observed in oral and verbal apraxia. Others are peculiar to limb apraxia. Later in this chapter, the error types traditionally defined in the literature which are common to all forms of apraxia are presented. The error types more typical of only limb apraxia are discussed in the remainder of this section.

Generally the errors observed in limb apraxia may be characterized as errors which relate to the performance of single gestures and those which are apparent in the performance of sequences of gestures. With regard to single gestures, a number of errors have been described (see Roy, 1982 and Roy *et al.*, 1985 for a review). One of the most common types of errors observed in limb apraxia is one termed 'body-part-as-object'. In this case, rather than pantomiming the action requested (e.g., show me how to hammer a nail) by using a hand posture and arm action similar to what would be used if the patient were actually holding the object, the patient uses his hand as if it were the object, i.e., pounding the clenched fist on the table as if it were the hammer. Another type of error involves poor control of the movement used in gesturing. This so-called 'clumsiness' was described by Heilman (1975). However, there is considerable controversy as to whether this impairment to motor control is really part of the limb apractic syndrome (Kimura, 1979; Haaland, Porch and Delaney, 1980).

A third type of error sometimes observed in single-object use involves the patient substituting an action which is associated with the gesture requested rather than the appropriate movement. For example, when a patient was asked to demonstrate how to put lipstick on, she reached into her pocket and pulled out a handkerchief and touched her lips with it. In this case, the patient had substituted an action (blotting her lips) which occurs somewhat later in the act of putting on lipstick, for the correct action of showing how to hold the lipstick and apply it to her lips. These errors may also be observed in oral apraxia. Such errors may be conceptual in nature in that semantic confusions occur. As such they may be analogues to 'verbal paraphasias' in the linguistic system, i.e., semantically related lexical items are substituted for intended words and/or true 'literal perseverations', especially those of sequencing. (See Canter, Trost and Burns, 1985, for a discussion of speech sequencing errors in LHD patients.)

A final type of error observed in single-object use is termed a deictic response in which the patient reaches for and grasps the object manipulating it in a way which suggests that he may be attempting to use the feel of the object to inform him as to its use. This error is frequently observed in young children as the developmentally earliest response to a request to demonstrate how to use an object (Cermak, 1985).

With regard to the underlying disrupted mechanism, limb apraxia has been considered as a disruption to one of a number of processes: a conceptual/symbolic disorder, a disconnection between control centers in the brain, an impairment of the body schema, or a motor control disorder. For the sake of brevity we will examine only the last of these. (See Roy, 1982, for details of all the mechanisms). One view of limb apraxia as a motor disorder was proposed by Kimura (1977, 1982). In this view, apraxia is considered as an inability to make transitions between posture and space. There is an overriding tendency for the patient to perseverate or repeat postures or actions he has just completed. Another view proposed by Roy (1981, 1983, 1985; Roy and Square, 1985a) is that limb apraxia may arise from disruptions to a conceptual and/or a production system. The conceptual system is viewed as a knowledge base for movement specifically related to three areas — object functions, actions, and the serial order of actions. Disruptions to each of these aspects may be associated with one of several types of errors. For example, disruption to the knowledge of the serial order of actions may present as an inability to mediate the production of actions through language. The production system is viewed as important in the actual control of movements. Impairments in this system are thought to result from a deficit in selectively directing attention at key points in the sequence, thereby leading to either perseverations or the production of the wrong action at a given point in the sequence.

Kelso and Tuller (1981) provide a somewhat different account of apraxia. They suggest that the motor system is organized heterarchically, i.e., there is no one executor or controller, and involves a coalitional style of control where there is a dynamic interface between the performer and the environment. One of the key aspects in this view of the motor system is the notion of tuning whereby supraspinal influences bias or change brainstem and spinal organization to provide the 'postural context' in which a circumscribed class of movements may occur. Apraxia, then, may arise from brain insults which disrupt the supraspinal influences, preventing the patient from specifying the appropriate postural context for actions he is requested or volitionally attempting to perform.

Coexistence of the Apraxias

Few studies have been undertaken which specifically have examined the coexistence of verbal, oral, and/or limb apraxia within the same patients. DeRenzi, Pieczuro and Vignolo (1966) were the first to comment upon the coexistence of the apraxias. First, with regard to oral apraxia and speech disorders, it was found that the majority of aphasic patients with severe 'phonemic–articulatory' disorders exhibited oral apraxia and, in two-thirds of these patients, the oral apractic disorder was severe. Even among patients with mild 'phonemic–articulatory' disorders almost one-half demonstrated impaired oral praxis. Conversely, among those aphasic patients with no 'phonemic–articulatory' disorder, oral praxis function was usually rated as normal or near-normal. Finally, the two aphasic syndromes with which impaired oral praxis function was most commonly associated were those in which speech disorders were also most commonly associated — Broca's and phonemic jargon.

The relationship between limb apraxia and oral apraxia was also examined by DeRenzi, Pieczuro and Vignolo (1966). Again, co-occurrence was high but not as high as for oral apraxia and 'phonemic–articulatory' disorders. The one limitation in interpreting the results of this study was that DeRenzi and his colleagues did not distinguish between patients with 'typical' symptoms of apraxia of speech versus those with 'typical' symptoms of phonemic paraphasia. Thus, a definitive statement about the co-occurrences of AOS and OA and LA cannot be made; only general statements about the coexistence of speech disorders due to left-hemisphere damage and oral and limb apraxia can be made.

Trost (1970) studied oral praxis skills among her ten Broca's aphasic subjects. On the imitative test of oral praxis, four of the ten subjects performed as well as normal control subjects. However, on the verbal command test, none of the asphasic subjects performed similarly to normal subjects. These results concurred with those of DeRenzi, Pieczuro and Vignolo (1966) and the hypotheses proposed by Geschwind (1965) in that OA was manifested more when asphasic subjects performed to verbal command. With regard to the relationship of speech errors and oral praxis skills, Trost (1970) reported that as oral praxis skills decreased in proficiency, speech errors in mono- and polysyllabic words and phrases increased; nonetheless, none of these correlations was significant. Trost speculated that because some subjects did well on the oral praxis test but poorly with regard to verbal praxis and vice versa, separate motor areas probably subserve the production of speech and nonverbal oral movements; it was thought, however, that those areas probably were close in proximity.

Poeck and Kerschensteiner (1975) also looked at the co-occurrences of articulatory errors and OA. The relationship between these two disorders was so striking that these researchers stated that '... particularly precise verbal and non-verbal movements are subserved by similar brain mechanisms' (p. 104). Further evidence for this hypothesis may be inferred from the work of Sussman and colleagues (1986). Among thirteen Broca's aphasic subjects, it was found that reduced compensatory articulation, as studied acoustically from vowels produced under normal and bite-block conditions, was more related to oral apraxia than verbal apraxia scores.

Mateer and Kimura (1977) also reported that their most speech-impaired subjects, those being their nonfluent aphasic subjects, were also the most impaired for both the production of isolated oral movements and oral sequences. We would presume that those non-fluent subjects demonstrated apraxia of speech symptomatology but a definite diagnosis of AOS was not made by these researchers. Similar to Poeck and Kerschensteiner, Mateer and Kimura proposed that similar brain mechanisms underlie the production of oral nonverbal and verbal movements with one mechanism governing the production of gestures or phonemes and a second mechanism governing the transitionalization between oral verbal and nonverbal gestures.

LaPointe and Wertz (1974) specifically examined the relationship between AOS and OA. Of the thirteen patients whom they unequivocally considered to have apraxia of speech, ten (77 per cent) demonstrated a deficit for producing isolated oral movements and eleven (85 per cent) showed disabilities for sequencing oral motor gestures. Thus, a high proportion of verbally apractic patients also demonstrated oral apraxia but the relationship was not one to one.

Finally, Marquardt and Sussman (1984) studied fifteen Broca's aphasic subjects on tests of verbal, oral, and limb apraxia. While all demonstrated oral apraxia, only twelve demonstrated verbal apraxia and five limb apraxia. Thus, it would appear that among these particular LHD patients with verified lesions variably involving the frontal and/or temporal lobes and/or subcortical structures including the internal capsule, thalamus, and basal ganglia, the relationship between the occurrences of verbal and oral apraxia is high while that between verbal and limb, and oral and limb is much lower. In our laboratory, we are currently assessing consecutively referred patients, forty-eight of whom have left hemisphere damage and, fifteen with right-hemisphere damage, as well as ten normal geriatric subjects for the co-existence of unequivocally diagnosed verbal, oral, and limb apraxia. We anticipate that our investigations will help to clarify the issue of co–occurrences of the apraxias.

Symptomatology of the Apraxias

It is the purpose of this section of the chapter to review the commonalities and differences among the apraxias with regard to symptomatology. Specifically, we will examine disturbances of initiation of movement, spatial targeting, temporal coordination of subcomponents of movements, rate of movement, augmentations of motor behavior, omitted behaviors, perseverative behavior, and sequencing, *as traditionally defined in the literature.* The reader is cautioned that these traditional categories of error types are not mutually exclusive. In fact, identical behaviors have been interpreted as inferring different disordered mechanisms. In our laboratory, we are developing error notation systems for verbal, oral, and limb behaviors which explicitly describe the temporal course of motor behavior. Our movement notation systems are similar to those used in the study of dance (Benesh and Benesh, 1956; Ryman, Patla and Calvert, 1984) and facial expression (Ekman and Friesen, 1969), and we anticipate that their applications to the apraxias will result in more objective observations of praxis and better interpretations of the underlying mechanisms which are disrupted.

Several attempts have been made recently to examine apractic errors in a more systematic way (see Haaland and Flaherty, 1984; Rothi *et al.*, 1988; Roy *et al.*, 1985). In the systems developed in our laboratory (Roy *et al.*, 1985; Roy *et al.*, 1987b; Friesen *et al.*, 1987), several categories of errors have been identified for each of the three systems, i.e., limb, oral nonverbal, and speech, which involve spatial, temporal, postural, and action elements. The reliability of our limb system has been established, and the use of the system has revealed a predominance of *spatial*, i.e., location and orientation errors, and *postural*, i.e., hand posture errors, in limb and manual activity among subjects. In this section of our chapter, however, we will not present our mutually exclusive error categories. Instead, we will discuss error types as they have been traditionally presented in the literature. One intent of our discussion is to demonstrate that additional research must be undertaken before inferences regarding underlying disrupted mechanisms are made from the data collected using these traditional error categories.

Initiation of movement

Apraxia of speech

It was stated by Trost and Canter (1974) '... it is in the act of speech initiation that apraxia of speech poses its greatest hazard to motor speech' (p. 76). Disturbances of initiation of movement (speech) *might* possibly fall into two categories — silent pauses also known as delays or speech initiation latencies, and periods filled with oral nonverbal or oral verbal behavior. The incidence of 'delays' has been commented upon by many (Schuell, Jenkins and Jimenez-Pabon, 1964; Johns and Darley, 1970; Rosenbek, 1978; Wertz, LaPointe and Rosenbek, 1984), but empirically studied by few. Trost (1970), however, did specifically measure 'speech initiation latencies' in her study of *verbal apraxia among Broca's aphasic patients*. In repetition tasks, five of the ten subjects studied demonstrated such latencies. Trost speculated that the latencies may have reflected phoneme selection problems. Square, Darley and Sommers (1982; also Square, 1981) also studied the frequency of occurrence of pauses or silent periods perceived to be abnormally long and not marked by inaudible or audible struggle behavior, phoneme repetition or phoneme gropes, in repetition tasks. Among their *verbally apractic patients with no clinical evidence of aphasia*, i.e., 'pure' AOS subjects, the relative occurrence of such silent delays apparently was not as frequent as those difficult periods of 'speech initiation' which were marked by verbal and nonverbal oral behavior. While not specifically commenting on response delays in repetition tasks, Fromm *et al.*, (1982) did report the occurrence within their three apractic speakers of continuous undifferentiated EMG activity. The physiological occurrence of this phenomenon among the apractic speakers but not the normal speakers, may relate well to the hypothesis put forward by Kelso and Tuller (1981): motor pretuning may be aberrant among apractic subjects and, although purely speculative on our part, this, in turn, may relate to the incidence of response delays or latencies long identified as a feature of AOS though not thoroughly investigated.

Possible disturbances of initiation marked by verbal behavior in AOS have been identified and generally reviewed by Rosenbek (1978), Wertz, Lapointe and Rosenbek (1984) and Wertz (1985). Some of these which appear to fall into one and the same category have been variably termed as false starts and restarts (Kent and Rosenbek, 1983), groping behavior (Kent and Rosenbek, 1983), effortful groping and repetitive attempts (Rosenbek and Wertz, 1976), phonetic groping (Square, Darley and Sommers, 1982; also Square, 1981), phoneme reapproaches

(Trost and Canter, 1974), trial and error behavior (Rosenbek and Merson, 1971), sequences of phonemic approximations (Joanette, Keller and Lecours, 1980), phonologically oriented sequences (Kohn, 1984), and 'conduites d'approche phonemiques' (see Joanette, Keller and Lecours, 1980). Square, Darley and Sommers (1982; also, Square, 1981) reported that phonetic groping, operationally defined as attempts to produce target phonemes through trial and error production of other English phonemes, was the most prevalent initiation problem for their subcortical verbally apractic patient and among the three most prevalent for their two midparietal lesioned AOS patients. In her study of phoneme reapproaches among Broca's aphasic individual with apraxia of speech, Trost (1970) reported that 52 per cent of the reapproaches resulted in correct articulation while less than one-third resulted in responses which were further from the desired target. Joanette, Keller and Lecours (1980) studied sequences of phonemic approximations, a symptom thought by North Americans from the Mayo school (for example Darley, 1968; Rosenbek and Wertz, 1976; Wertz, Lapointe and Rosenbek, 1984) to represent apraxia of speech, among three aphasic groups. No subjects were said to have apraxia of speech, most probably because of philosophical and terminological differences in the study of aphasia among those from the Paris/Montreal/Boston schools (for example Lecours and Lhermitte, 1976; Lecours, Lhermitte and Bryans, 1983; Goodglass and Kaplan, 1972) and those from the Mayo/ Madison/Tokyo schools (for example, Darley, 1982; Rosenbek, 1978; Itoh, Sasanuma and Ushijima, 1979; Itoh *et al.*, 1980, 1982). Among the Broca's, conduction, and Wernicke's subjects studied, conduction aphasic subjects had the best ability for approaching the desired phonemic target for both consonants and vowels while Broca's subjects were more successful in approximating vowels as opposed to consonants during their reapproaches. Wernicke's patients were unsuccessful at both. Kohn (1984) studied the same subclassifications of aphasic patients and found that conduction aphasic subjects produced the most and the longest reapproaches. This finding was interpreted as evidence that this group of patients probably is more adept at recognizing their 'phonologic' errors; however, they were no more adept at correcting their errors than were the Broca's and Wernicke's patients. The conduction aphasia group was able to correct 45 per cent of their errors and did not differ significantly from the per cent corrected by the other two aphasic groups. Kohn (1984) further speculated that the mechanisms responsible for phonemic reapproaches among these aphasic groups are probably different. Pre-articulation programming, or the selection of sequences of phonological targets was implicated as the disrupted mechanism in conduction and Wernicke's aphasia, while it was speculated that articulation programming, i.e., the level of issue of motor commands, is most likely deviant in Broca's aphasia. Kent and Rosenbek (1983) speculated that initiation errors in verbal apraxia might be due to a disrupted spatial–temporal schema 'to specify motor commands, given the intended motor responses, the current state of the articulators, and motor experience in meeting similar demands' (p. 246). The issues of mechanism(s) underlying the behavior of phonetic groping among the various aphasic syndromes and those patients labelled as verbally apractic and the establishment of differential behavioral characteristics among these groups of patients, if indeed such differential characteristics exist, are areas certainly in need of further investigation.

Another type of initiation error reported to be characteristic of AOS is struggle behavior, both inaudible and audible. Square, Darley and Sommers (1982; also Square 1981) operationally defined these behaviors, respectively, as a silent period after a stimulus for repetition is presented which is characterized by facial grimacing and a period after a stimulus is presented for repetition in which sound(s) was produced which was perceived not to be phonemic in nature. Such struggle behaviors were observed to occur with notable frequency among the two AOS patients with left midparietal lesions. These behaviors were reminiscent of the struggle behavior associated with stuttering. It is interesting to note that Shtremel (1963) also identified stuttering-like symptoms in left parietal lobe syndrome and Rosenbek (1980) has noted some similarities between AOS and stuttering.

The final type of initiation disturbance observed in apraxia of speech is repetition, or the consecutive production of an unchanged phoneme, syllable(s), or word (Square, Darley and Sommers, 1982; also Square, 1981). This behavior was the most prevalent one observed among the midparietal lesioned 'pure' AOS subjects studied by Square and her colleagues. Among Trost's ten Broca's aphasic subjects, six presented with repetition behaviors (Trost, 1970). Further, these sub-jects repeated whole words with approximately the same frequency as single initial phonemes. Trost (1970) speculated that phoneme repeti-tions may have reflected motor perseveration and/or attempts to self-correct initial phonemes.

Oral apraxia

Disturbances of initiation of movement in oral apraxia have been considered an integral part of the disturbance in that error systems have acknowledged them frequently (DeRenzi, Pieczuro and Vignolo, 1966; LaPointe and Wertz, 1974; Poeck and Kerschensteiner, 1975; Tognolo and Vignolo, 1980). These disturbances have been viewed holistically in most cases and subcategories of initiation disturbances have not been presented in the above reports with the exception of that by Poeck and Kerschensteiner (1975) who examined oral apractic 'conduites d'approche' behavior. DeRenzi, Pieczuro and Vignolo (1966) and Tognolo and Vignolo (1980) defined oral apractic initiation errors as '...accurate performance (which) is preceded by protracted pauses, during which unsuccessful movements may be present' (DeRenzi, Pieczuro and Vignolo, 1966, p. 62) and LaPointe and Wertz (1974) used a similar definition. These researchers considered such performances to be the least impaired in oral apraxia. Poeck and Kerschensteiner (1975) did not attempt to infer severity of oral apraxia from incidence of 'conduites d'approche'. They did, however, look at frequency of occurrence of this behavior and found that, among all groups of aphasic subjects studied (amnesic, Broca, Wernicke, total and global) this behavior was the fifth most prevalent.

One of the major drawbacks of error systems used to study oral apraxia has been that they have been generally functional in nature. That is, they have indicated whether a goal has been reached but have not fully specified the unfolding movements and actions that led to achieving or not achieving the goal. As we mentioned previously, we have attempted, in our laboratory, to use motor notation systems which describe temporally the unfolding of action for the study of limb, oral, and verbal apraxia (Roy and Square, 1985b). More refined functional behavioral descriptors have evolved from our use of movement notation systems. In our naturalistic study, i.e., behavioral categories were not defined *a priori* but based upon assiduous transcription, of oral praxis function among eight LHD subjects and four normal control subjects, Qualizza, Square-Storer and Roy (1987) operationally defined nineteen types of behaviors which occurred, seven of which related to initiation. Delays occurred less than 1 per cent of the time among normal adults whereas they accounted for 9 per cent of all behaviors which were not rated as immediately correct for the LHD subjects. Step-wise excursion to the target and groping each accounted for 4 per cent of the behaviors recorded as not immediately correct among the LHD subjects, while step-wise excursions accounted for 6 per cent of the normal subjects' behaviors. Repeated behaviors accounted for 2 per cent of the pathological behaviors but only .003 per cent of the normal behaviors. Finally, repeated repaired (self-corrected) behaviors accounted for 3 per cent of the LHD subjects' responses which were not produced correctly immediately; self-corrections were not noted for the normal subjects, probably because they made significantly fewer errors overall than the LHD patients.

Limb apraxia

In considering limb apraxia problems, the initiation of movements *per se*, has not been very well studied. If we use the subcategorization outlined in our discussion of apraxia of speech, it is clear that patients with limb apraxia do experience difficulty with initiating movement. In reviewing the performance of patients we have observed in our laboratory (Roy *et al.*, 1987b; Friesen *et al.*, 1987) as well as the work of others, (e.g., Haaland and Flaherty, 1984; Lehmkuhl, Poeck and Willmes, 1983), these patients exhibit delays in the onset of movement which may be unfilled but more frequently are filled with a verbal response, often an echolalic repetition of the examiner's command. As well, these patients frequently make groping movements which reveal an attempt at approaching the spatial position and/or hand posture to accurately demonstrate the appropriate gesture. Haaland and Flaherty (1984) did not appear to have a specific category for this type of behavior. However, Lehmkuhl, Poeck and Willmes (1983) described fragmentary or augmentative errors in referring to this type of groping behavior. In our limb error system (Roy *et al.*, 1985), this behavior was referred to as movements of target (movements of the responding limb) and non target (movements of other body parts or verbalizations) effector structures. In our analyses of LHD subjects, these types of behaviors were one of the most frequently observed of all the categories (Friesen *et al.*, 1987).

Spatial targeting

Apraxia of speech

Articulatory errors of substitution and distortion of phonemes may be indicative, in part, of spatial targeting deficits due to a disrupted internal spatial coordinate system of the vocal tract (MacNeilage, 1970; Sussman, 1972). Early studies of AOS pointed to the predominance of articulatory errors of phoneme substitution (Johns and Darley, 1970; Trost and Canter, 1974; LaPointe and Johns, 1975). In addition, all of these reports implicated consonants as being more affected than vowels. The inconsistent and unpredictable occurrences of those substitutions was highlighted by Johns and Darley (1970), while Trost and Canter (1974) and LaPointe and Johns (1975) highlighted the relatedness of the 'substitution' to the target as being a salient feature of AOS behavior. In particular, Trost and Canter (1974) reported that more than 50 per cent of the 'substitutions' made by their subjects deviated from the target place (spatial target) of production by only one articulatory distance. In a later perceptual study of AOS speakers, Square, Darley and Sommers (1982) reported that, in their sample of apractic subjects with no clinical evidence of aphasia, distorted segments, both consonants and vowels, occurred more frequently than reported in previous studies. Evidence that at least some of the perceived AOS 'substitutions' and 'distortions' are attributable to errors of spatial targeting comes from more recent instrumental studies of apractic speech. The acoustic study by Kent and Rosenbek (1983) of thirteen apractic speakers verified that, in fact, vowel errors and some consonantal errors, particularly for /r/ and /l/, occurred and that these appeared to relate to spatial targeting deficits within the vocal tract. That is, the F1–F2 frequency value plots for vowels, at times, indicated gross inaccuracy of vocal tract positioning. Like the earlier perceptual reports, however, Kent and Rosenbek (1983) pointed to the variability within their patients for achieving specific targets within the vocal tract with the range of vocal tract positions being normal and only some productions being widely disparate. Ryalls (1981) also studied acoustically vowel production among eleven motor aphasic subjects. His subjects, like those of Kent and Rosenbek, were also found to be deviant and variable over time with regard to producing stable formant patterns.

Shinn and Blumstein (1983) reported on the results of a study specifically directed at determining aphasic subjects' abilities to reach static articulatory targets. Although subjects were not identified as 'verbally apractic' *per se*, four Broca's subjects were included. Whether or not any of these demonstrated symptoms consistent with a diagnosis of AOS is unknown. The spectral characteristics of the initial segment of stop-plosive consonants was studied using a template fitting procedure. Results indicated that the Broca's patients had a preserved ability to reach static targets. Further, it was concluded that the 'phonetic' deficit demonstrated by Broca's patients was primarily a 'dynamic' one and not primarily a 'static' one, i.e., spatial targeting. More will be said about the dynamics of speech production in verbal apraxia in a subsequent section.

Finally, results of an electropalatographic (EPG) study undertaken by Washino *et al.* (1981) with one AOS patient, indicated that groping behavior may, in fact, represent a spatial targeting disorder. EPG is a means of indirectly studying articulatory behavior, specifically lingua-palatal contact. A false palate, through which a small electrical current runs, is fitted intraorally. Linguapalatal contact, as measured by conduction of the electric current flow through the artificial palate, is recorded by a microcomputer. Washino and colleagues found that, within an utterance when some abnormal silent periods occurred, their apractic patient was groping for articulatory positions, specifically making lingua-alveolar contact as for /d/ in an attempt finally to produce /g/. These preliminary findings are of interest since they implicate the possibility of spatial targeting deficits underlying the phonetic groping behavior in AOS. Likewise, it has been proposed by Klich, Ireland, and Weidner (1979) that a disrupted internal representation of the vocal tract space coordinate system (MacNeilage, 1970) may underlie some AOS errors. Kent and Rosenbek (1983) more recently suggested that the disruption affects the spatiotemporal representation.

A study of velar activity using fiberoptics has also highlighted the variability of spatial targeting observed among apractic subjects. Itoh, Sasanuma and Ushijima (1979) studied velar raising and lowering among normal subjects and one apractic speaker. The subjects repeated the phrase, /dee nee desu/ five times. The normal subjects demonstrated regular oscillatory movements with peak velar raising for /d/ and lowering for /n/. The apractic subject, while demonstrating the same overall pattern of up and down movements, also demonstrated great variability in velar control. This variability for spatial targeting was so marked that one production of an intended /n/ resulted in a /d/.

In another EPG study of AOS, Hardcastle, Morgan and Clark (1985) reported that one subject demonstrated contact patterns for alveolar stops and nasals and palato-alveolar fricatives which were highly variable and frequently abnormal. For instance, in the production of alveolar stops and nasals, not only were normal closure patterns observed, but velar closure without alveolar contact and simultaneous anterior/posterior closure were also demonstrated. In the production of palato-alveolar fricatives, productions were marked by complete alveolar closure, an alveolar grooved onset, velar closure, and palatal grooving with asymmetrical contact patterns. It thus appears that AOS patients not only demonstrate spatial 'place of articulation' deficits but also deficits for achieving correct lingual postures. Further, extreme variability for achieving both of these components of movement — location (place) and posture — characterize the disorder. It would seem logical that many of the broadly perceived 'substitution' errors are actually distortion errors resulting from deviancies of place of articulation as well as lingual, labial, and facial posturing.

Oral apraxia

Even fewer studies of spatial targeting have been accomplished for oral apraxia. That spatial targeting deficits may be a component of the disorder can only be inferred from some of the definitions of error types presented in the literature. For instance, LaPointe and Wertz (1974) stated that some movements may be '... defective in amplitude, accuracy ...' (p. 42). In on-going work in our laboratory, we identified, two behaviors which *may* be indicative of spatial targeting deficits (Qualizza, Square-Storer and Roy, 1987). These behaviors, along with their proportion of occurrence among the fourteen behaviors which we defined as representative of actions not performed immediately correctly, were overexcursion of target effector oral structures (12 per cent) and insufficient excursion of target effector structures (2 per cent). Further investigations, especially instrumental ones, of spatial targeting performances among patients with OA are needed before definitive statements regarding the incidence and relevance of such kinematic disturbances to the disorder *per se*, can be made.

Limb apraxia

In limb apraxia we know that spatial factors play a role. More errors are observed in gestures requiring movements which are made toward the body in egocentric space, e.g., salute, comb hair, than in those which involve movements away from the body in allocentric space, e.g., wave goodbye, hammer a nail (Cermak, 1985; Roy, 1982). Indeed, Kimura (1977, 1979) has argued that apraxia in particular involves impairments in making transitions between postures and/or positions in body-centered space.

While these observations imply some disruption to spatial processing in apraxia, very few studies have examined spatial errors in the performance of apractic patients. In the study by Haaland and Flaherty (1984), two types of spatial errors, arm position and hand orientation, were identified. For various gestures, arm position errors occurred with a significantly greater frequency in left-hemisphere- than right-hemisphere-damaged patients. Roy *et al.* (1985) identified three types of spatial errors which were termed 'location', 'orientation', and 'plane of movement' errors. Examples were as follows: a 'location' error was noted when the patient correctly demonstrated how to comb the hair but the movements were made in the region of the face as opposed to on the head; a 'plane of movement' plus an 'orientation' error involved the patient demonstrating brushing the teeth with the movements at the wrist and elbow made in the horizontal plane as opposed to the vertical plane with the forearm oriented vertically at the mouth instead of in the horizontal position parallel to the patient's base of support. In preliminary analyses of a group of left-hemisphere-damaged patients, Friesen *et al.* (1987) found location and orientation errors to be two of the most frequently observed errors among the apractic patients.

Coordination of motor subsystems/subcomponents

Apraxia of speech

Instrumental studies of apraxia of speech point to disruptions of temporal coordination of speech subsystems, i.e., articulation with resonance, respiration, and/or phonation, or of speech muscles or muscle groups as prominent characteristics of the disorder. Square-Storer (1987) has thoroughly reviewed research from 1976 through 1985 regarding such errors in AOS. Readers should consult that review for a more indepth discussion of the topics presented here.

The coordination of voice onset time (VOT) with supralaryngeal articulation has been shown to be defective among speakers with apraxia of speech (Freeman, Sands and Harris, 1978; Fromm *et al.*, 1982; Itoh *et al.*, 1982; Kent and Rosenbek, 1983). While Kent and Rosenbek pointed to intrasubject variability for VOT productions, i.e., some productions being measured as normal while others being highly disparate, Freeman, Sands and Harris (1978) and Itoh and colleagues (1982) reported a compression of measured VOTs with marked overlap between cognate categories. Variability of production and overlap between cognate categories may well underlie the voicing errors perceived in apractic speech. For instance, Fromm and colleagues (1982), using a laryngeal accelerometer and movement transducers, demonstrated instances of articulatory movement without requisite laryngeal behavior (phonation). Such occurrences resulted in the perception of /p/ being produced rather than an intended /b/, and seemed to indicate that many of the cognate confusions (substitutions) perceived in apractic speech are the result of temporal discoordination of laryngeal behavior with articulation and not phoneme malselection. Itoh *et al.* (1982) also provided evidence that the VOT disorder in apraxia of speech reflected a phonetic disorder and not a phonemic one. It is of interest, however, to note that the VOT patterns observed by Freeman, Sands and Harris and Itoh *et al.* for verbally apractic patients, have also been identified for various groups of aphasic patients, specifically, Broca's (Blumstein *et al.*, 1977, 1980; Shewan, Leeper and Booth, 1984), a majority of patients with left anterior hemisphere lesions (Blumstein *et al.*, 1977) and some conduction patients (Shewan, Leeper and Booth 1984; Blumstein *et al.*, 1980). It would thus appear that temporal disorganization of motor speech production may be a hallmark of left-hemisphere-damage, especially to the frontal lobe, and may not reflect exclusively a characteristic of the disorder, 'apraxia of speech'. Further VOT research which thoroughly describes the perceived speech patterns of the aphasic patients being tested is needed.

Two studies have been undertaken which have examined specifically movements of several articulators simultaneously. Itoh *et al.* (1980), using lead pellets and an x-ray microbeam unit, tracked simultaneously the course of movements and their velocities of the lower lip, lower incisor, tongue dorsum, and lower surface of the velum. While the normal subjects demonstrated a temporal correspondence in movement among the structures in their repetitions of /ii deenee desu/, the apractic subject demonstrated an apparent disorganization of timing among several articulators. This temporal disorganization among the articulators was implicated as the source of inconsistent articulatory errors in AOS.

Fromm *et al.* (1982) added further evidence of discoordination among speech structures by simultaneously observing the upper and lower lips and jaw with transducers. Further, they demonstrated temporal discoordination of electrical activity among several speech muscles as apractic subjects attempted to repeat the sentence, 'Buy Bobbie a puppy'. By recording electromyographic (EMG) signals from the obicularis oris superior and inferior, depressor labii inferior, and mentalis muscles, the abnormal muscle innervation patterns of agonist −antagonist cocontraction, continuous undifferentiated EMG activity, and inappropriate muscle shutdown were noted. These observations led Fromm and her colleagues to conclude that neuromotor execution is disordered in apractic speakers in that temporal distortion among several articulators exists. Similar EMG results were reported for patients with 'phonetic disintegration', i.e., presumably patients with apraxia of speech, by Shankweiler, Harris and Taylor (1968). Further, Keller (1984), based upon his perceptual analysis of the speech of Broca's aphasic subjects presumably with coexisting apraxia of speech, concluded similarly to Fromm *et al.* that activation of agonist and antagonist neuronal pathways and/or the sequential rather than coactivation of some speech elements may underlie some of the observed speech errors.

Finally, the area of study of anticipatory coarticulation may shed some light on our understanding of temporal coordination of motor speech activity among apractic speakers. While Itoh, Sasanuma and Ushijima (1979), as a result of their velar fiberoptics study, concluded that some temporal aspects of speech production may be influenced by excessive anticipatory coarticulation, Ziegler and von Cramon, based upon perception by normals of acoustically gaited speech samples of an apractic speaker (1985) and from acoustically analyzed speech samples (1986), concluded that delayed onset of anticipatory coarticulation occurred and that it reflected confused articulatory time schedules in apraxia of speech. In our study of anticipatory coarticulation in one AOS subject with no clinical symptoms of aphasia, delays of onset towards articulatory targets were noted (Scholten, Square-Storer and Roy, 1988). It remains to be discerned whether the coarticulatory delays represent confused time schedules of neuromotor commands or a compensatory activity for achieving spatial targets.

Oral apraxia

To our knowledge, there have been no instrumental studies undertaken of oral praxis among normal or neurologically impaired individuals. Thus, inferences regarding deficits for the temporal integration of subcomponents of movements or individual muscles or muscle groups come solely from our observations and notations of behaviors. LaPointe and Wertz (1974) referred to 'crude' movements and characterized them similarly to DeRenzi, Pieczuro and Vignolo (1966) and Tognolo and Vignolo (1980). Such movements were said to be acceptable though defective in amplitude, accuracy, or speed. In our laboratory, based upon our assiduous naturalistic transcriptions of OA, we designated two error categories which might reflect disorders of temporal integration. These were inappropriate reciprocity of oral structures and uncoordinated facial and/or lingual symmetry not associated with hemiplegia (Qualizza, Square-Storer and Roy, 1987). Of the behaviors noted for all gestures which were not produced immediately and totally accurately, 5 per cent were due to an inappropriate reciprocity of oral structures. For instance, for the gesture 'tongue out', the mandible may have first been depressed and then the tongue protruded, rather than the subcomponents of the action being produced in a reciprocal simultaneous fashion. Uncoordinated symmetry apparently not due to hemiplegia, or the moving of the musculature of the right and left sides of the face to target positions in an asynchronous fashion, accounted for 1 per cent of all behaviors not characterized as immediately accurate. Both types of behaviors would appear to indicate difficulties in the temporal organization of motor commands. The behaviors of 'groping' and 'stepwise excursion' as well as 'under-excursion' and 'overexcursion' discussed above may have also reflected, in part or wholly, errors of temporal integration of muscle activity of the various effector structures.

Limb apraxia

In examining errors in apractic patients using the system developed by Roy *et al.* (1985), Friesen *et al.* (1987) noted a high incidence of hand posture errors. In one particular case Charlton *et al.* (1986) observed that, in demonstrating the salute gesture, the patient assumed the correct axial and proximal positioning of the body and arm, respect-ively, but used an incorrect hand posture (clenched fist). They argued that hand posture in gesturing involves a distal motor control system. This distal control must be coordinated with more proximal (arm, shoulder) and axial (whole body) control in order to effectively demonstrate a gesture. In observing this patient's limb praxis perform-ance, it appeared that he was able to control accurately the proximal and axial components of the gesture, but, as noted above, not the distal component as represented by hand posture.

In order to measure the coordination and control of these proximal and distal aspects in movement more accurately, this patient's limb behaviors in a reach and grasp task which had both proximal and distal control components were examined. The proximal component is represented by what Jeannerod (1984) referred to as the 'transport component' where the arm is directed toward the object to be grasped. The distal component is represented by what Jeannerod referred to as the 'manipulation component' involving the opening and closing of the fingers in the grasp of the object. Jeannerod (1984) has shown a clear temporal coordination between these two components in which key events in the distal or grasp component, e.g., initiation of hand opening and maximum hand aperture, are linked to phases in the proximal or transport component, e.g., peak velocity. Reaching, then, like gesturing, involves the temporal coordination between proximal and distal control components.

Using this logic, Charlton *et al.* (1986) compared the reaching performance of this apractic patient to a normal non-brain-damaged patient and found that the velocity profile for the transport or proximal component of reaching in the apractic patient was much like that observed in the normal patient. The distal or grasp component was different from the normal's in several respects, however. The opening of the grasp occurred much earlier, the maximum aperture was achieved much earlier, and the hand was opened much more widely. As in gesturing, then, an impairment in the distal postural component in reaching was observed. This distal grasp component seemed to be rather poorly coordinated with the proximal transport component and was spatially imprecise. This initial work provides some promising directions for understanding more clearly impairments in the spatiotemporal coordination of movements in limb apraxia much like those afforded through fiberoptic and x-ray microbeam analyses of movements in verbal apraxia (Itoh, Sasanuma and Ushijima, 1979; Itoh *et al.*, 1980).

Rate of movement

Apraxia of speech

A slow speaking rate, identified both perceptually and acoustically, is a notable characteristic of apraxia of speech (Wertz, 1985; Wertz, LaPointe and Rosenbek, 1984; Kent and Rosenbek, 1982, 1983). Articulatory prolongation of steady states and transitions, affecting both consonant and vowels, accounts partially for slow speaking rate. This phenomenon has been verified acoustically (Kent and Rosenbek, 1982, 1983; Collins, Rosenbek and Wertz, 1983; Caligiuri and Till, 1983; Lebrun, Buyssens and Henneaux, 1973). Also, use of EPG has highlighted prolonged articulatory contact times (Washino *et al.*, 1981). Finally, microbeam technology has highlighted reduced articulatory velocities (Itoh *et al.*, 1980) as has velar fiberoptics (Itoh, Sasanuma and Ushijima, 1979) and data obtained using movement transducers (Fromm *et al.*, 1982; Barlow, Cole and Abbs, 1983). Further, variability of articulatory rates over repetitions of an utterance has been highlighted (Itoh *et al.*, 1979, 1980; Kent and Rosenbek, 1983). Although most of our speech data indicates that articulatory prolongation is a hallmark of apraxia, there have been other reports which suggested that segments may be shorter in duration than normal; however, these results may have been due to the use of short stimuli, i.e., monosyllables (Duffy and Gawle, 1984) and/or interpretation of data (DiSimoni and Darley, 1977, see Kent and Rosenbek, 1983 for discussion; and Ryalls, 1981, see Rosenbek, Kent and LaPointe, 1984 for discussion).

Another source of slow speaking rate associated with AOS is the occurrence of articulatory hiatuses. These have been verified acoustically by Kent and Rosenbek (1982, 1983) and Square and Mlcoch

(1983). Kent and Rosenbek (1982, 1983) have defined two categories of behavior. Syllable segregation is characterized as '... a pattern of temporally isolated syllables' (Kent and Rosenbek, 1983, p. 233) in which voicing may or may not cease, whereas syllable dissociation gives the impression that speech is being programmed syllable by syllable in that there is not only syllable segregation but a lack of coherence of prosody, especially the lack of Fo dependencies.

Oral apraxia

There have been references to 'slow' movement as being one component of OA (DeRenzi, Pieczuro and Vignolo, 1966; LaPointe and Wertz, 1974; Tognola and Vignolo, 1980). However, this component of deviant oral praxis has been merely cited as one component of the error category, 'crude movement'. In our laboratory, we identified 'prolonged completion times' as characterizing 2 per cent of all the behaviors associated with oral gestures which were not produced accurately immediately among our eight LHD patients (Qualizza, Square-Storer and Roy, 1987). Certainly much more work in this area is needed and especially instrumental work aimed at defining the kinematics of oral apraxia.

Limb apraxia

Very little work has examined disruptions to rate of movement in the performance of gestures in LA, although some studies have investigated the relationship between apraxia and other motor impairments. Haaland, Porch and Delaney (1980), for example, compared apractic and non-apractic LHD patients in their performances on a range of motor tasks involving steadiness, finger tapping, grooved pegboard, and maze coordination. On the finger tapping task, a measure of speed or rate of fine motor control, the two groups did not differ. On the most complex tasks, grooved pegboard and maze coordination, however, the apractic patients were significantly slower. These findings suggested that, on complex tasks requiring the integration of sensory and motor information, apractic patients do demonstrate decreased rate of movement.

The only study which has specifically examined rate of movement in patients with LA is the one by Charlton et al., (1986) alluded to in the previous section. In that study the apractic patient performed a reach and grasp movement. Findings demonstrated that the apractic patient's reaching movements were slower than those of the normal control patient. Interestingly, though, the velocity profile for the apractic was very similar to the control patient's. This finding implied that, although the apractic patient was moving more slowly, the control dynamics of his movement as reflected in time to reach peak velocity were similar to those used by the control patient. A closer look at these dynamics as reflected in the acceleration profile, however, revealed this implication to be false. While both patients demonstrated a typical overall acceleration–deceleration profile, the apractic patient revealed many more oscillations involving acceleration–deceleration, particularly around the end of the movement. This observation suggested a much more intermittent type of control in the apractic patient in which there may be more reliance on feedback in controlling movement.

Additive or augmentative motor behavior

Appraxia of speech

Since the early studies of apraxia of speech, the occurrence of added articulatory movements aside from the repetitions and groping behaviors discussed above, have been cited as an error category, albeit a minor one. Both Trost (1970) and Johns (1969) investigated the occurrence of added segments in apractic speech. Johns and Darley (1970), in a subsequent report, revealed that 9 per cent of their patients' segmental errors involved the addition of phonemes. Such additions appeared to be one of two types — additions which resulted in more complex articulatory maneuvers such as /fl/ produced for /f/, and those which simplified articulation. An example of the latter is the insertion of the schwa between consonant members of a cluster. Keller (1984) has referred to such behavior as an example of 'gesture reduction'.

The studies cited above have all been based upon perceptual data. Several recent instrumental studies have also cited the occurrence of added articulatory movements in AOS. For instance, Kent and Rosenbek (1983) observed occasional intrusion errors in their acoustic analysis of apractic speech. Fromm *et al.* (1982), using movement transducers, and Washino *et al.* (1981) using EPG, reported the observation of additional movements of articulators which did not result in the perception of additional phonemes but which, indeed, were regarded as abnormal. It, thus, appears that the incidence of augmentative motor movements is a reality in AOS and that further investigations of these behaviors may increase our understanding of their underlying basis.

Oral apraxia

From the early reports of error types in OA, a category for augmentative behaviors was never established in such a way that these behaviors were notated as different from substitutive, irrelevant, or unique errors (DeRenzi, Pieczuro and Vignolo, 1966; LaPointe and Wertz, 1974; Mateer and Kimura, 1977; Tognolo and Vignolo, 1980). Poeck and Kerschensteiner (1975), however, did notate augmentative behaviors and subdivided them into oral, body, and additional noises which accounted for approximately 6 per cent, 5 per cent, and 3 per cent of all errors, respectively. In our laboratory, we designated a descriptive behavioral category as 'augmentative' behavior under which seven subtypes occurred including respiratory, facial, laryngeal, head, neck and torso movements, verbalizations, and others (Qualizza, Square-Storer and Roy, 1987). We found that 42 per cent of all gestures not produced as immediately correct ones were augmented in some way. However, we found that our normal subjects augmented 82 per cent of their gestures which were not produced correctly immediately. Thus, augmentation seems to be a preferred behavior among adult subjects when, for whatever reason, oral gestures are not produced correctly immediately. One reason 'augmentative' behaviors may have occurred among our LHD subjects more frequently than reported by Poeck and Kerschensteiner, is that we qualified even omitted and substituted behaviors as augmented in that we notated temporally the entire unfolding action. Poeck and Kerschensteiner notated a response holistically. Thus, what we may have termed as augmentation followed by an omission of some primary components of a target, Poeck and Kerschensteiner would have notated as a 'substitution' by denoting the augmentation the response. Thus, it would appear that our results and those of Poeck and Kerschensteiner (1975) are in accordance and that augmentation of attempted oral behaviors by LHD individuals as well as normal individuals, when they experience some difficulty, may be one of the most salient characteristics of oral praxis performances.

Limb apraxia

Augmentative or added movements have been the focus of some studies in LA. Lehmkuhl, Poeck and Willmes (1983) found that additional movements were made by patients with limb apraxia, although not with sufficiently increased frequency to be statistically significant. Rothi *et al.* (1988) also examined the performances of apractic patients and found that these types of added movements, termed 'occurrence errors', did occur much more frequently in patients with LA than in a group of normal controls. However, these errors occurred along with a number of other types of errors and Rothi *et al.* gave no indication of whether these 'occurrence' errors were more frequently observed than the other types.

Work by Roy and colleagues alluded to above (Friesen *et al.*, 1987; Roy *et al.*, 1985) also identified these types of added movement errors. In their work they described two basic types — added target effector movements (additional movements in the responding limb) and added nontarget effector movements (additional movements in other body parts or verbalizations). As an example of this latter type of error, the patient may repeat the command of the examiner in an echolalic fashion prior to or during the performance of the gesture. Alternately, the patient's verbal response, e.g., I don't know how; ask my grandson, he will show you; you use it in the kitchen, substitutes for the gesture requested. Each of these types was found to occur much more frequently in the apractic patients.

Omitted behaviors

Apraxia of speech

Errors of omission, like those of addition, are not considered to be a paramount characteristic of AOS, although they are consistently cited as a lesser symptom (Johns and Darley, 1970; Trost, 1970; Square, Darley and Sommers, 1982; Wertz, LaPointe and Rosenbek, 1984). Johns and Darley (1970) reported that only 1 per cent of the total responses made by their ten AOS subjects were errors of omission but we mention this error category here because it seems to be one which is salient for the other apraxias, particularly oral, and particularly with regard to only subcomponents of a movement. Also, if we reconsider the speech data, analogous behaviors do occur with relative frequency. That is the omission of articulatory *features* of manner, e.g., frication, or features of voicing, which subsequently result in perceived substitutions and distortions, is a paramount feature of apraxia. However, as discussed above, such errors appear to arise because of aberrantly generated spatial and/or temporal schemata for movement control. It may be that similar mechanisms underlie fragmented movements observed in oral and limb apraxia.

Oral apraxia

Partial responses, characterized as those in which some important part of the gesture was missing, was an error category used in the studies by DeRenzi, Pieczuro and Vignolo (1966), LaPointe and Wertz (1974) and Tognolo and Vignolo (1980). It cannot be discerned from these reports, however, the frequency with which this error category was applied to oral gesture production. Mateer (1978) used an error category called 'omission' but this referred to an entire gesture as well as an element of a gesture. Further, because this error type was applied to the analysis of sequences of oral gestures, we cannot interpolate from those data the occurrence of omissions, partial or full, for single gesture production. From the report of Poeck and Kerschensteiner (1975), however, it is conveyed that 'fragmented' gesture production was the second most common error to occur among all classifications of aphasic subjects with approximately 15 per cent of all errors being of this type. 'No reactions' or total omission of a response occurred with an overall frequency of 7 per cent but was most prominent among global and Wernicke aphasic subjects. Finally, in our laboratory, we found fragmented responses to account for only 1 per cent of our subjects' gesture productions which were not accurate immediately (Qualizza, Square-Storer and Roy, 1987). Our error categories of 'underexcursion' and 'overexcursion' discussed above, however, occurred with such frequencies as to account for the discrepancy between our results and those of Poeck and Kerschensteiner (1975). This error category seems particularly relevant to the understanding of OA and requires further research.

Limb apraxia

In LA, errors of omission have been referred to as a 'no response' (Rothi *et al.*, 1987; Roy *et al.*, 1985) or fragmentary response (Haaland and Flaherty, 1984; Lehmkuhl, Poeck and Willmes, 1983) category. Lehmkuhl, Poeck and Willmes (1983) had proposed that fragmentary errors reflecting the omission of particular elements of the gesture might be particularly apparent in patients with frontal brain damage and accompanying Broca's aphasia. Their results did support this hypothesis. Fragmentary errors were among the least frequently observed. Work by others (Haaland and Flaherty, 1984; Roy *et al.*, 1987a) has supported this finding that these types of omission errors occur very infrequently.

Disturbances of sequencing

Apraxia of speech

Errors of sequencing, both of muscle movements and phonemes, has been a symptom traditionally associated with the disorder (Darley, 1969; Johns and Darley, 1970; Trost and Canter, 1974). A thorough review of the literature, however, indicates that patients with apraxia of speech have more difficulty sequencing movements of the speech subsystems and individual muscles in a tight temporal pattern (see our discussion above) than they do sequencing actual phonemes or meaningful units of an action sequence.

LaPointe and Johns (1975) specifically studied the incidence of sequencing errors among thirteen patients with apraxia of speech. Metathetic, reiterative (perseverative), and anticipatory errors were investigated as they occurred on a modified version of a 141-item Templin-Darley Test for articulation (Templin and Darley, 1960). Thus, the stimuli upon which their analysis was based were self-formulated in response to pictorial stimuli and open-ended sentences. Results indicated that only four metathetic errors occurred in their entire sample of 1833 items. Further, only thirteen within-word reiterative (perseverative) errors occurred. (It is unknown from this study whether and/or how perseverative errors arising from preceeding stimuli influenced subsequent items.) Finally, seventy-eight within-word anticipatory errors occurred, thus exceeding reiterative errors in a ratio of 6 to 1. Sasanuma (1971) studied sequencing errors made by one apractic speaker during the task of reading prose. Her results differed markedly from those of LaPointe and Wertz. It was found that 71 per cent of all errors produced were due to sequencing difficulties including metathesis and backward and forward assimilation. The discrepancy of findings between these two reports may have been due to differential task demands and/or differential characteristics of the patients studied. (See our above discussion regarding different 'types' of apraxia of speech.)

Phonemic sequencing errors have been reported to be more characteristic of patients with posterior aphasia than anterior aphasia, the former group being less likely to have symptoms of AOS (Canter, Trost and Burns, 1985). Other researchers have reported phoneme sequencing errors, depending on task requirements, to occur with about an equal frequency among patients with anterior and posterior aphasia (Poncet *et al.*, 1972; Mateer and Kimura, 1977). The one conclusion which can be put forth with some degree of assurance is that patients with AOS have more difficulty with the phasing of movements, i.e., temporal coordination of subcomponents of meaningful units of movement, than the sequencing of phonemes. Further investigation is needed to determine whether difficulties of phoneme sequencing are an inherent part of apraxia of speech *per se*, or left-hemisphere damage in general, the latter of which gives rise to impairments of memory (Jason, 1983, 1985; Roy and Square, 1986) and/or disorders of transitionalization (Kimura, 1977, 1979, 1982).

Oral apraxia

Difficulties producing oral motor sequences is characteristic of LHD individuals (LaPointe and Wertz, 1974; Mateer and Kimura, 1977; Mateer, 1978). There is no evidence that patients with anterior lesions are more impaired than those with posterior lesions. The studies by Mateer and Kimura (1977) and Mateer (1978) did not evaluate thoroughly the performance of the nonfluent aphasic patients, (presumably anterior-lesioned) because of the high proportion of amorphous movements produced by those patients. Among the fluent aphasic subjects (presumably posterior-lesioned), omissions accounted for the highest proportion of sequencing errors with perseverative errors following. In fact, even among the left-hemisphere lesioned nonaphasic subjects, a high proportion of perseverative errors occurred. Finally, it is interesting to note that, while the anterior-lesioned patients had severe difficulties producing both isolated gestures and sequences of gestures, the fluent aphasic subjects had the greatest difficulty performing sequences. Further research is needed in order to establish better the relationship between deficits for oral praxis for the production of isolated gestures and oral sequences.

Limb apraxia

In limb apraxia, one of the commonest types of errors in sequencing involves performing elements of the sequence in the wrong order. For example, when asked to light a candle, the patient may put the match to the candle wick before having struck it on the match box to light it. Second, elements may be omitted. For example, in making a cup of instant coffee, the patient may omit putting the instant coffee in the cup. Finally, the patient may perseverate a previous action in the sequence and, thus, be unable to complete the action correctly. It is noteworthy that such sequencing disorders appear to be conceptual in nature in that meaningful units of behavior are out of sequence, omitted, or perseverated upon. Jason (1983, 1985) presented evidence that such errors were due to memory impairments. These limb apractic errors bear a strong resemblance to 'literal paraphasic' errors. Comparisons of these two areas of behavior may be fruitful.

Perseverative behavior

Verbal apraxia

We know from our studies of sequenced phoneme behavior among patients diagnosed as having verbal apraxia that few within-word perseverations occur. Recent studies of oral verbal perseveration among aphasic subjects have been undertaken by Santo Pietro and Rigrodsky (1982, 1986). These studies are of relevance here because one of the conclusions reached was that some perseverations occur due to an old 'motor program' being replayed. Specifically, it was found that some responses from previous items were repeated when a new target response required the same phoneme placement for its initial phoneme (Santo Pietro and Rigrodsky, 1986). This would seem to be an example in which the environment regulates the control of motor behavior; that is, bottom-up control prevails (Roy, 1978).

Oral apraxia

The incidence of perseverative behavior in oral apraxia has been reported in several studies. Poeck and Kerschensteiner (1975) reported a high incidence of perseverative errors among the performances of their aphasic subjects. Of the 1076 errors committed, 467 reflected partial perseverations. Further, perseverative behavior was characteristic of all aphasic subgroups and none was characterized by a particularly high or low incidence. Mateer and Kimura (1977) reported that nonfluent aphasic subjects demonstrated more perseverative behavior on the production of individual oral gestures than fluent aphasic patients; however, for sequence production, the fluent subjects demonstrated a high proportion of perseverations, ranking as the second most frequent error type out of the four used. In our laboratory, we found full perseverations to account for 9 per cent and partial perseverations 0.5 per cent, of the total errors made on the production of oral gestures of our eight patients (Qualizza, Square-Storer and Roy, 1987). Thus, perseveration appears to be more closely associated with oral apraxia than verbal apraxia.

Limb apraxia

In limb apraxia perseverations are also characteristic errors in which the patient repeats a previous action. Liepmann (1905) was the first to report those errors. Building upon some of the early work by Liepmann, Kimura (1977, 1979, 1982) has more recently emphasized the importance of perseverations in apraxia. She argued that these errors reflect a basic impairment in making transitions between postures or positions in egocentric space. Work by others (Haaland and Flaherty, 1984; Lehmkuhl, Poeck and Willmes, 1983; Rothi *et al.*, 1988) has subsequently supported the importance of perseverations in characterizing performance in limb apraxia.

Further insight into the nature of perseverative behavior may be afforded by the use of error notation systems such as the one developed by Roy *et al.*, (1985). Using such a system it will be possible to identify which aspects of the gesture the patient tends to perseverate, for example, the location in space in which the gesture is made, or the hand posture or action pattern used. Consistent with this proposal Poeck (1985) has demonstrated, using their movement transcription system (Poeck and Kerschensteiner, 1975), that, in apraxia, perseverations may frequently appear as repetitions of motor element, some of which may have been performed up to thirteen gestures before. Work by Roy (1981, 1983) on movement sequences has demonstrated that it is possible to identify the more specific nature of perseverations. For example, results of his work demonstrated that perseveration of a movement element in a sequence is not due to the persistence of an ideational set but rather appears due to the persistence of a particular postural set.

Conclusions

In this chapter, we have attempted to draw parallels between the apraxias from the standpoints of definitions, sites of neurologic damage, co-occurrence, and symptoms as traditionally defined in the literature. Our work has highlighted the commonalities among the apraxias especially when behaviours are observed perceptually. Adjunctively, at this point in time, we feel compelled to advocate kinematic investigations of movement in the three motor systems — limb, oral nonverbal, and oral verbal — among left-hemisphere-damaged individuals. It is our hope that our observations expressed herein will serve as the basis for future instrumental investigations related to AOS, OA, and LA, individually, but, more importantly, comparatively across the three motor systems.

Acknowledgments

Drs Square-Storer and Roy acknowledge the support of National Health and Welfare, Canada, for the project, 'Disruptions to Limb, Oral and Verbal Praxis: Assessment and Remediation'. The information presented in their chapter is an outgrowth of their supported research by that agency as well as Mount Sinai Hospital, Toronto Western Hospital, the Cummings Foundation, the Faculty of Medicine's Dean's Fund at the University of Toronto, and the Ontario District SPEBSQSA.

References

BARLOW, S., COLE, K. and ABBS, J. (1983) 'A new head-mounted lip-jaw movement transduction system for the study of motor speech disorders', *Journal of Speech and Hearing Research,* **26**, pp. 283–8.

BENESH, R. and BENESH, J. (1956) *'An Introduction to Benesh Dance Notation'*, London, A and C Black.

BLUMSTEIN, S., COOPER, W., ZURIF, E. and CARAMAZZA, A. (1977) 'The perception and production of voice-onset time in aphasia', *Neuropsychogia,* **15**, pp. 371–83.

BLUMSTEIN, S., COOPER, W., GOODGLASS, H., STATLENDER, S. and GOTTLIEB, J. (1980) 'Production deficits in aphasia: A voice onset time analysis', *Brain and Language,* **9**, pp. 153–70.

BUCKINGHAM, H. W. (1979) 'Explanation in apraxia with consequences for the concept of apraxia of speech', *Brain and Language,* **8**, pp. 202–26.

CALIGIURI, M. and TILL, J. (1983) 'Acoustic analysis of vowel duration in apraxia of speech', *Folia Phoniatrica,* **35**, pp. 226–34.

CANTER, G.J. (1969) 'The influence of primary and secondary verbal apraxia on output disturbances in aphasic syndromes'. Paper presented to the American Speech and Hearing Association, Chicago, Illinois (unpublished).

CANTER, G.J., TROST, J.E. and BURNS, M.S. (1985) 'Contrasting speech patterns in apraxia of speech and phonemic paraphasia', *Brain and Language,* **24**, pp. 204–22.

CERMAK, S. (1985) 'Developmental dyspraxia'. in ROY, E.A. (Ed.) *Neuro-*

psychological Studies of Apraxia and Related Disorders. Amsterdam: North-Holland, pp. 225–50.

CHARLTON, J., ROY, E.A., SQUARE, P.A. and MACKENZIE, C. (1986) 'Impairments to sequencing and motor control in apraxia'. Paper read at annual meeting of the Canadian Psychological Association, Toronto, 1986.

COLLINS, M., ROSENBEK, J. and WERTZ, R. (1983) 'Spectrographic analysis of vowel and word duration in apraxia of speech', *Journal of Speech and Hearing Research,* **26**, pp. 224–30.

DARLEY, F.L. (1968) 'Apraxia of speech: 107 years of terminological confusion'. Paper presented to the American Speech and Hearing association, Denver Colorado (unpublished).

DARLEY, F.L. (1982) *Aphasia,* Philadelphia, W.B. Saunders.

DARLEY, F.L., ARONSON, A.E. and BROWN, J. (1975) *Motor Speech Disorders,* New York, Saunders.

DERENZI, E. (1985) 'Methods of limb apraxia examination and their bearing on the interpretation of the disorder'. in ROY, E.A. (Ed.) *Advances in Psychology, Neuropsychological Studies of Apraxia,* **23**, Amsterdam, North-Holland Col., pp. 45–64.

DERENZI, E., PIECZURO, A. and VIGNOLO, L.A. (1966) 'Oral apraxia and aphasia', *Cortex,* **2**, pp. 50–73.

DEUTSCH, S.E. (1984) 'Prediction of site of lesion from speech apraxic error patterns', in ROSENBEK, J. C. *et al.* (Eds.) *Apraxia of Speech: Physiology, Acoustics, Linguistics and Management,* San Diego, College Hill Press, pp. 113–34.

DISIMONI, F. and DARLEY, F. (1977) 'Effects on phoneme duration control of three utterance-length conditions in an apractic patient', *Journal of Speech and Hearing Disorders,* **42**, pp. 257–64.

DUFFY, J. and GAWLE, C. (1984) 'Apraxic speakers' vowel durations in consonant-vowel-consonant syllables', in ROSENBEK, J. *et al.* (Eds.) *Apraxia of Speech: Physiology, Acoustics, Linguistics and Management,* San Diego, College Hill Press.

EKMAN, P. and FRIESEN, W. (1969) 'The repertoire of non-verbal behavior: categories, origins, usage and coding', *Semiotica,* **1**, pp. 49–298.

FREEMAN, F., SANDS, E. and HARRIS, K. (1978) 'Temporal coordination of phonation and articulation in a case of verbal apraxia', *Brain and Language,* **6**, 106–11.

FRIESEN, H., ROY, E.A., SQUARE-STORER, P.A. and ADAMS, S. (1987) 'Apraxia: Interrater reliability of a new error notation system for limb apraxia'. Poster presentation at annual meeting of the North American Society for the Psychology of Sport and Physical Activity, Vancouver, B.C.

FROMM, D., ABBS, J.H., MCNEIL, M.R. and ROSENBEK, J.C. (1982) 'Simultaneous perceptual-physiological method for studying apraxia of speech', in BROOKSHIRE, R. (Ed.) *Clinical Aphasiology Conference Proceedings,* Minneapolis, BRK Publishers, pp. 251–62.

GESCHWIND, N. (1965) 'Disconnection syndromes in animals and man', *Brain,* **88**, pp. 237–94, 585–644.

GOODGLASS, H. and KAPLAN, E. (1972) *The Assessment of Aphasia and Related Disorders,* Philadelphia, Lea and Febiger.

HAALAND, K.Y. and FLAHERTY, D. (1984) 'The different types of limb apraxia errors made by patients with left or right hemisphere damage'. *Brain and Cognition*, **3**, 370–84.

HAALAND, K.Y., PORCH, B.E. and DELANEY, H.D. (1980) Limb apraxia and motor performance. *Brain and Language, 9*, 315–23.

HARDCASTLE, W.J., MORGAN, R.A. and CLARK, C.J. (1985) 'Articulatory and voicing characteristics of adult dysarthric and verbal apraxic speakers', *British Journal of Disorders of Communication*, **20**, 249–70.

HEILMAN, K.M. (1975) 'A tapping test in apraxia', *Cortex*, **11**, pp. 259–63.

ITOH, M., SASANUMA, E. and USHIJIMA, T. (1979) 'Velar movements during speech in a patient with apraxia of speech', *Brain and Language, 7*, pp. 227–39.

ITOH, M., SASANUMA, S., HIROSE, H., YOSIOKA, H. and USHIJIMA, T. (1980) 'Abnormal articulatory dynamics in a patient with apraxia of speech', *Brain and Language, 11*, pp. 66–75.

ITOH, M., SASANUMA, S., TATSUMI, I., MURAKAMI, S., FUKUSAKO, Y. and SUZUKI, T. (1982) 'Voice onset time characteristics in apraxia of speech', *Brain and Language, 17*, pp. 193–210.

JACKSON, J.H. (1878) 'Remarks on nonprotrusion of the tongue in some cases of aphasia', in TAYLOR, J. (Ed.) *Selected Writings of John Hughlings Jackson, 2*, London, Hodder and Stoughton, 1932, pp. 153–4.

JASON, G. (1983) 'Hemispheric asymmetries in motor function: I. Left hemisphere specialization for memory but not performance', *Neuropsychologia, 21*, pp. 35–45.

JASON, G. (1985) 'Manual sequence learning after focal cortical lesions', *Neuropsychologia, 23*, pp. 483–96.

JEANNEROD, M. (1984) 'The timing of natural prehension movement', *Journal of Motor Behavior, 16*, pp. 235–54.

JOANETTE, Y., KELLER, E. and LECOURS, A.R. (1980) 'Sequences of phonemic approximations in aphasia', *Brain and Language, 11*, pp. 30–44.

JOHNS, D.F. (1969) 'A systematic study of phonemic variability in apraxia of speech'. Unpublished doctoral dissertation, Florida State University.

JOHNS, D.F. and DARLEY, F.L. (1970) 'Phonemic variability in apraxia of speech', *Journal of Speech and Hearing Research, 13*, pp. 556–83.

KELLER, E. (1984) 'Simplification and gesture reduction in apraxia and aphasia' in ROSENBEK, J.C. *et al.* (Eds.) *Apraxia of Speech: Physiology, Acoustics, Linguistics and Management*, San Diego, College Hill Press, pp. 221–56.

KELSO, J.A.S. and TULLER, B. (1981) 'Toward a theory of apractic syndromes', *Brain and Language, 12*, pp. 224–45.

KENT, R. and ROSENBEK, J. (1982) 'Prosodic disturbance and neurologic lesion', *Brain and Language, 15*, pp. 259–91.

KENT, R.D. and ROSENBEK, J.C. (1983) 'Acoustic patterns of apraxia of speech', *Journal of Speech and Hearing Research, 26*, pp. 231–49.

KERTESZ, A. (1984) 'Subcortical lesions and apraxia of speech', in ROSENBEK, J.C. *et al.* (Eds.) *Apraxia of Speech: Physiology, Acoustics, Linguistics and Management*, San Diego, College Hill Press, pp. 73–90.

KIMURA, D. (1977) 'Acquisition of a motor skill after left hemisphere damage', *Brain*, **100**, pp. 527–42.

KIMURA, D. (1979) 'Neuromotor mechanisms in the evolution of human communication', in STEKLIS, H.D. and RALEIGH, M.J. (Eds.) *Neurobiology of Social Communication in Primates*, New York, Academic Press.

KIMURA, D. (1982) 'Left-hemisphere control of oral and brachial movements and their relationship to communication', *Philosophical Transactions of the Royal Society of London*, **B298**, pp. 135–549.

KLICH, R., IRELAND, J. and WEIDNER, W. (1979) 'Articulatory and phonological aspects of consonant substitutions in apraxia of speech', *Cortex*, **15**, pp. 451–70.

KOHN, S.E. (1984) 'The nature of the phonological disorder in conduction aphasia', *Brain and Language*, **23**, pp. 97–115.

LAPOINTE, L.L. (1969) 'An investigation of isolated oral movements, oral motor sequencing abilities, and articulation of brain-injured adults', Unpublished doctoral dissertation, University of Colorado.

LAPOINTE, L.L. and JOHNS, D.F. (1975) 'Some phonemic characteristics in apraxia of speech', *Journal of Communication Disorders*, **8**, pp. 259–69.

LAPOINTE, L.L. and WERTZ, R.T. (1974) 'Oral movement abilities and articulatory characteristics of brain-injured adults', *Perceptual and Motor Skills*, **39**, pp. 39–46.

LEBRUN, Y., BUYSSENS, E. and HENNEAUX, J. (1973) 'Phonetic aspects of anarthria', *Cortex*, **9**, pp. 126–35.

LECOURS, A.R. and LHERMITTE, F. (1969) 'Phonemic paraphasia: Linguistic structures and tentative hypotheses', *Cortex*, **5**, pp. 193–228.

LECOURS, A.R. and LHERMITTE, F. (1976) 'The pure form of the phonetic disintegration syndrome (pure anarthria)', *Brain and Language*, **3**, pp. 88–113.

LECOURS, A.R., LHERMITTE, F., BRYANS, B. (1983) *Aphasiology*, London, Bailliere Tindall.

LEHMKUHL, G., POECK, K. and WILLMES, K. (1983) 'Ideomotor apraxia and aphasia. An examination of types and manifestations of apraxia symptoms'. *Neuropsychologia*, **21**, pp. 199–212.

LIEPMANN, H. (1905) *Uber Storungen des Handelns bei Ghirnkranken*, Berlin, Karger.

LIEPMANN, H. (1920) Apraxic. *Ergon der ges Med*, **1**, pp. 516–43.

LURIA, A.R. (1966) *Higher Cortical Functions in Man*. New York, Basic Books.

LURIA, A.R. (1976) *Basic Problems in Neurolinguistics*. The Hague, Moulton.

LURIA, A.R. (1980) *Higher Cortical Functions in Man*. New York: Basic Books.

MACNEILAGE, P.F. (1970) 'Motor control of the serial ordering of speech', *Psychological Review*, **77**, pp. 182–96.

MARIE, P. (1906) 'La troisieme circonvolution frontale gauche ne joue aucur role special dans la fonction du langage', *Semiaine Medicale*, **26**, pp. 241–7.

MARQUARDT, T.P. and SUSSMAN, H. (1984) 'The elusive lesion-apraxia of speech link in Broca's aphasia', in ROSENBEK, J.C. *et al.* (Eds.) *Apraxia of Speech: Physiology, Acoustics, Linguistics, and Management*, San Diego, College Hill Press, pp. 91–112.

MATEER, C. (1978) 'Impairments of nonverbal oral movements after left hemisphere damage: A follow-up analysis of errors', *Brain and Language*, **6**, pp. 334–41.

MATEER, C. and KIMURA, D. (1977) 'Impairments of nonverbal movements in aphasia', *Brain and Language*, **4**, pp. 262–76.

MAZZOCHI, F. and VIGNOLO, L.A. (1979) 'Localization of lesions in aphasia; Clinical-CT scan correlations in stroke patients', *Cortex,* **15**, pp. 627–54.

NAESER, M.A., ALEXANDER, M.P., HELM ESTABROOKS, N., LEVINE, H.L., LAUGHLIN, S.A. and GESCHWIND, N. (1982) 'Aphasia with predominately subcortical lesion sites', *Archives of Neurology,* **39**, pp. 2–14.

OJEMANN, G. and MATEER, C. (1979) 'Human language cortex: Localization of memory, syntax, and sequential motor-phoneme identification', *Science,* **205**, pp. 1401–3.

POECK, K. (1983) Ideational apraxia, *Journal of Neurology,* **230**, pp. 1–5.

POECK, K. (1985) 'Clues to the nature of disruptions in limb apraxia', in ROY, E. (Ed.) *Neuropsychological Studies of Apraxia and Related Disorders. Advances in Psychology,* Vol. 23, Amsterdam, North Holland.

POECK, K. and KERSCHENSTEINER, M. (1975) 'Analysis of sequential motor events in oral apraxia', in ZULCH, K.J. *et al.* (Eds.) *Cerebral Localization,* Berlin, Springer-Verlag, pp. 98–111.

PONCET, M., DEGOS, C., DELOCHE, G. and LECOURS, A.R. (1972) 'Phonetic and phonemic transformations in aphasia', *International Journal of Mental Health,* **1**, pp. 46–54.

QUALIZZA, L., SQUARE-STORER and P., ROY, E.A. (1987) 'Production of isolated and sequenced oral motor postures by left hemisphere damaged individuals', Working Paper, Neuropraxis Research Laboratory, Toronto (unpublished).

ROSENBEK, J.C. (1978) 'Treating apraxia of speech', in JOHNS, D.F. (Ed.) *Clinical Management of Communicative Disorders,* Boston, Little Brown, pp. 191–241.

ROSENBEK, J.C. (1980) 'Apraxia of speech-relationship to stuttering', *Journal of Fluency Disorder,* **5**, pp. 233–53.

ROSENBEK, J.C. and MERSON, R.M. (1971) 'Measurement and prediction of severity in apraxia of speech', Paper presented to the American Speech and Hearing Association, Chicago.

ROSENBEK, J.C. and WERTZ, R.T. (1976) 'Veterans' Administration Workshop on Motor speech Disorders', Madison, Wisconsin (unpublished).

ROSENBEK, J.C., WERTZ, R.T. and DARLEY, F.L. (1973) 'Oral sensation and perception in apraxia of speech and aphasia', *Journal of Speech and Hearing Research,* **16**, pp. 22–36.

ROSENBEK, J., KENT, R. and LAPOINTE, L. (1984) 'Apraxia of speech: An overview and some perspectives', in ROSENBEK, J. *et al.* (Eds.) *Apraxia of Speech: Physiology, Acoustic, Linguistics and Management,* San Diego, College Hill Press.

ROTHI, L.J.G., HEILMAN, K.M., MALK, L., VERFAELLIE, M. and BROWN, P. (1987) 'Ideomotor apraxia: Error pattern analysis'. Paper presented to the annual meeting of the International Neuropsychological Society, Atlanta.

ROY, E.A. (1978) 'Apraxia: A new look at an old syndrome', *Journal of Human Movement Studies,* **4**, pp. 191–210.

ROY, E.A. (1981) Action sequencing and lateralized cerebral damage: Evidence for asymmetries in control. in LONG, J. and BADDELEY, A. (Eds.) *Attention and Performance,* **IX**. New Jersey, L. Erlbaum.

ROY, E.A. (1982) 'Action and performance'. in ELLIS, A. (Ed.) *Normality and Pathology in Cognitive Function.* New York, Academic Press.

ROY, E.A. (1983) 'Neuropsychological perspectives on apraxia and related action disorders'. in MAGILL, R.A. (Ed.) *Advances in Psychology*, **12**, pp. 293–320 *Memory and Control of Action*. Amsterdam: North-Holland Co.

ROY, E.A. (1985) *Advances in Psychology, Neuropsychological Studies of Apraxia and Related Disorders*, **23**, Amsterdam, North Holland Co.

ROY, E.A. and SQUARE, P.A. (1985a) 'Common considerations in the study of limb, oral, and verbal apraxia'. in ROY, E.A. (Ed.) *Neuropsychological Studies of Apraxia and Related Disorders*. Amsterdam: North Holland, pp. 111–62.

ROY, E.A. and SQUARE, P.A. (1985b) 'Error/movement notation systems in apraxia', *Recherches Semiotiques/Semiotics Inquiry*, **5**, pp. 402–12.

ROY, E.A. and SQUARE, P.A. (1986) 'Sequencing disorders in the apraxias', Working Paper, Neuropraxis Research Laboratory, Toronto (unpublished).

ROY, E.A., SQUARE, P.A., ADAMS, S. and FRIESEN, H. (1985) 'Error/movement notation systems in apraxia', *Semiotic Inquiry*, **5**, pp. 402–12.

ROY, E.A., SQUARE-STORER, P.A., ADAMS, S. and FRIESEN, H. (1987a) Disruptions to sequencing of limb, oral and verbal movements: Effects of sequence length and presentation modality'. Poster presentation at annual meeting of the North American Society for the Psychology of Sport and Physical Activity, Vancouver, B.C.

ROY, E.A., SQUARE-STORER, P.A., PATLA, A., MACKENZIE, C. and CHARLTON, J. (1987b) 'Developing systems for describing apraxic performance: Comparisons between normal and brain-damaged adults'. *Canadian Psychology*, **28**, p. 522.

RYALLS, J.H. (1981) 'Motor aphasia: acoustic correlates of phonetic disintegration in vowels', *Neuropsychologia*, **19**, 365–74.

RYMAN, R., PATLA, A.E. and CALVERT, T.W. (1984) 'Adaptation of labanotation for the clinical analysis of kinematics of human gait', *Dance Notation*, **2**, pp. 12–31.

SANTO PIETRO, M. and RIGRODSKY, S. (1982) 'The effects of temporal and semantic conditions on the occurrence of the error response of perseveration in adult aphasics', *Journal of Speech and Hearing Research*, **26**, pp. 184–92.

SANTO PIETRO, M. and RIGRODSKY, S. (1986) 'Patterns of oral-verbal perseveration in adult aphasics', *Brain and Language*, **29**, pp. 1–17.

SASANUMA, S. (1971) 'Speech characteristics of a patient with apraxia of speech', *Annual Bulletin, Research Institute of Logopedics and Phoniatrics*, University of Tokyo, **5**, 85–89.

SCHIFF, H.B., ALEXANDER, M.P., NAESER, M.A. and GALABURDA, A.M. (1983) 'Aphemia: Clinical-anatomic correlations', *Archives of Neurology*, **40**, pp. 720–7.

SCHOLTEN, L., SQUARE-STORER, P. ROY, E.A. (1988) 'Coarticulation within CV syllables in an apractic patient', Working Paper, Neuropraxis Research Laboratory, Toronto (unpublished).

SCHUELL, H., JENKINS, J.H. and JIMENEZ-PABON, E. (1964) *Aphasia in Adults: Diagnosis, Prognosis, and Treatment*, New York, Harper and Row.

SHANKWEILER, D., HARRIS, K. and TAYLOR, M.S. (1968) 'Electromyographic studies of articulation in aphasia', *Archives of Physical Medicine and Rehabilitation,* **49**, pp. 1–8.

SHEWAN, C., LEEPER, H.A. and BOOTH, J.C. (1984) 'An analysis of voice onset time (VOT) in aphasic and normal subjects', in ROSENBEK, J.C. *et al.* (Eds.) *Apraxia of Speech: Physiology, Acoustics, Linguistics, and Management*, San Diego, College Hill Press, pp. 197–220.

SHINN, P. and BLUMSTEIN, S.E. (1983) 'Phonetic disintegration in aphasia: Acoustic analysis of spectral characteristics for place of articulation', *Brain and Language,* **20**, pp. 90–114.

SHTREMEL, A.K. (1963) 'Stuttering in left parietal lobe syndrome', *Zhurnal nevropathologii i psikhiatrii imeni S.S. Zorsakova,* **63**, pp. 823–32.

SQUARE, P.A. (1981) 'Apraxia of speech in adults: Speech perception and production', Unpublished doctoral dissertation, Kent State University.

SQUARE-STORER, P.A. (1987) 'Acquired apraxia of speech', in WINITZ, H. (Ed.) *Human Communication and its Disorders: A Review*, Norwood, New Jersey, Ablex, pp. 88–159.

SQUARE, P.A. and MLCOCH, A.G. (1983) 'The syndrome of subcortical apraxia of speech: An acoustic analysis', in BROOKSHIRE, R. (Ed.) *Clinical Aphasiology Conference Proceedings*, BRK Publishers, Minneapolis, pp. 239–43.

SQUARE, P.A., DARLEY, F.L. and SOMMERS, R.K. (1982) 'An analysis of the productive errors made by pure apractic speakers with differing loci of lesions', in BROOKSHIRE, R. (Ed.) *Clinical Aphasiology Conference Proceedings*, BRK Publishers, Minneapolis, pp. 245–50.

SQUARE-STORER, P.A., DARLEY, F.L. and SOMMERS, R.K. (1988) 'Speech processing abilities in patients with aphasia and apraxia of speech', *Brain and Language,* **33**, pp. 65–85.

SUSSMAN, H. (1972) 'What the tongue tells the brain', *Psychological Bulletin,* **77**, pp. 262–72.

SUSSMAN, H., MARQUARDT, T., HUTCHINSON, J. and MACNEILAGE, P. (1986) 'Compensatory articulation in Broca's aphasia', *Brain and Language,* **27**, pp. 56–74.

TEMPLIN, M. and DARLEY, F. (1960) *The Templin Darley Tests of Articulation.* Iowa City, Bureau of Educational Research and Service, Extension Division, State University of Iowa.

TOGNOLO, G. and VIGNOLO, L.A. (1980) 'Brain lesions associated with oral apraxia in stroke patients: A clinico-neuroradiological investigation with the CT scan', *Neuropsychologia,* **18**, pp. 257–72.

TROST, J.E. (1970) 'Patterns of articulatory deficits in patients with Broca's aphasia', Unpublished doctoral dissertation, Northwestern University.

TROST, J.E. and CANTER, G.J. (1974) 'Apraxia of speech in patients with Broca's Aphasia', *Brain and Language,* **1**, pp. 63–79.

WASHINO, K., KASAI, Y., UCHIDA, Y. and TAKEDA, K. (1981) 'Tongue movements during speech in a patient with apraxia of speech', *Current Issues in Neurolinguistics: A Japanese Contribution* (Supplement to *Language Sciences*), Tokyo, International Christian University.

WATAMORI, T., ITOH, M., FUSHUSAKO, Y. and SASANUMA, S. (1981) 'Oral apraxia and aphasia, *Annual Bulletin, RI LP,* **15**, pp. 129–46.

WERNICKE, K. (1885) 'Die neueren Arbeiten uber Aphasie', *Forschritte der Medizine*, **3**, pp. 824–30.

WERTZ, R.T. (1985) 'Neuropathologies of speech and language: An introduction to patient management', in JOHNS, D.F. (Ed.) *Clinical Management of Neurogenic Communicative Disorders*, Boston, Little Brown, pp. 1–96.

WERTZ, R.T., LaPOINTE, L.L. and ROSENBEK, J.C. (1984) *Apraxia of Speech in Adults: The Disorder and Its Management*, New York, Grune and Stratton.

WILSON, S.A.K. (1908) 'A contribution to the study of apraxia', *Brain*, **31**, pp. 164–216.

ZIEGLER, W. and VON CRAMON, D. (1985) 'Anticipatory coarticulation in a patient with apraxia of speech', *Brain and Language*, **26**, pp. 117–30.

ZIEGLER, W. and VON CRAMON, D. (1986) 'Disturbed coarticulation in apraxia of speech: Acoustic evidence', *Brain and Language*, **29**, pp. 34–47.

Chapter 3

Articulatory Variability

Kevin G. Munhall

In this chapter I make no attempt to bridge the considerable gap between pathology and normal speech processes in any comprehensive manner. Rather, I discuss an issue that is so fundamental to the phenomenon of spoken language, that it must be a primary concern of clinicians and basic scientists alike. As a result, the issue is open to insights from both applied and basic science research communities. I am referring to articulatory variability.

Variability is ubiquitous in nature and seems especially evident in behavioral phenomena. In speech we see variability in any dependent variable we measure from acoustic durations to movement amplitudes or velocities. People speak at different rates, move their articulators different amounts, and speak with more or less precision. Clinicians have correctly focused on this articulatory variability as a potential window into the nature of illness and health in speech processes. They assume that differences in the amount and kind of variability in certain disorders will indicate their etiology. But, while variability is of primary concern in clinical assessment, the measures used to assess variability are often unsophisticated and sometimes inappropriately used. Further, comparisons of variability between clinical and normal populations are frequently made without the aid of good normative data. A common diagnostic conclusion is that a clinical sample exhibits more variability than normal. In articulatory studies statements such as this are often based on comparison to a single normal control subject, e.g., Itoh and Sasanuma (1984); McGarr and Löfqvist (1982). A primary focus of this paper will be on how we characteristically assess variability and what other options are open to us.

A second reason for addressing variability in this chapter has to do with the nature of the behavioral units of speech. This is particularly appropriate for a volume on apraxia of speech since many phonetic studies suggest that intrasegment deterioration is a key feature of this disorder.

Behavioral units are not structures like solid objects that exhibit a fairly rigid form. Rather they are organizations that are defined by their goal-directedness and the 'correlated variability' they exhibit. Correlated variability is an old notion in the study of natural variation (see Cowles, 1988, for an historical perspective) and is described by Darwin (1861/1896) in the *Origin of Species* in this manner: 'I mean by this expression that the whole organization is so tied together, during its growth and development, that when slight variations in any one part occur and are accumulated through natural selection, other parts become modified' (p. 128). From an articulatory perspective our definitions of units are often simply bounds on such correlated variability. We identify as units those parts of the articulatory system that co-vary to achieve a phonetic goal.

Phonology has traditionally defined units in a quite different way. Phonological units have been defined in a static manner that owes its form to the mathematical theory of information. Most clinicians have been influenced by this representational format and have adopted it as a primary assessment tool. In spite of the proven utility of this transcription scheme, a reconsideration of the nature of these units is timely for clinicians given the state of the art in theorizing about 'segmental structure'. In the last fifteen to twenty years phonological theory has undergone considerable change and there is much less certainty about the existence of the segment let alone the 'geometry of the features' (see Clements, 1985). One of the more promising approaches is articulatory phonology (Browman and Goldstein, 1986) which attempts to capture the facts of languages with representations of the motion or gestures. (See also Chapter 4 for a brief description of Square-Storer and colleagues' articulatory-error system.) Ultimately, this gestural approach requires that phonology come to grips with natural variation.

The Combination of Observations

In the nineteenth century, mathematical statistics was frequently referred to as 'the combination of observations' (Stigler, 1986). All the techniques centered on managing the different values from repeated observations. This simple phrase still summarizes the most important aspects of behavioral research. First, at all levels of the nervous system and thus at all behavioral levels there is variation. A series of observations will thus yield a scatter of measurement values. Secondly, as researchers we are faced with the task of economically describing this variation, particularly the systematic variation. We must combine the scores in some meaningful way to aid interpretation. Traditionally, measures of central tendency in a data set, e.g., mean or median, and measures of dispersion, e.g., variance, are reported. It is the latter, how we measure dispersion of scores and the interpretation of these measures, upon which I want to focus.

I will begin by discussing the more commonly used summary statistics for discrete measures of speech movements such as amplitude, durations, and velocity measures. In describing variation of such measures there are two things that are important: magnitude or amount of variation and the form or type of variation. By and large the former has been emphasized in speech research but as I will point out neither the amount nor type of variation should be considered independently.

Static magnitude estimates of variability

While variability is everywhere in our world it is not uniformly everywhere. Some behaviors, some individuals, some situations seem to produce more variable observations than others. We associate these relative differences in variation with differences in skill, development, stability, creativity, speed/accuracy demands, health, etc.

The simplest and perhaps oldest measure of the magnitude of such variation of a measure is its range. If the difference between the highest and lowest value is very large, then the scores are more variable than if the range is small. However, this simple logic fails for a number of reasons. First, the extreme values in a sample depend on the sample size, and secondly, the measure is too sensitive to the two extreme observations rather than the dispersion of the observations as a whole (see Yablokov, 1974). Finally, because the range as an index has a dimension, comparisons cannot be made between measures having different units, e.g., between the amplitude and duration of a speech movement. The first two of these problems are addressed by the familiar standard deviation, σ, (or its square variance) and the final problem is addressed by the coefficient of variation, cv.

The standard deviation takes into account the size of the sample[1] as well as characterizing the contribution of the variation of all of the measurements. The cv does this and, in addition, is a dimensionless index that in principle allows measures of different sizes and units to be compared (see Yablokov, 1974). Equipped with these indices (σ and cv) we can compare the variability of populations (normal vs apractic, adult vs child), segment types (consonant vs vowel), languages (Japanese vs English), or dimensions (amplitude vs duration) and make inferences about the nature of speech control. In fact comparisons of exactly this type are frequently made.

For example Caruso, Abbs, and Gracco (1987) compared the variability of lip and jaw movements of stutterers and normals. To remove any influence of the size of the movement, coefficients of variation were calculated for the peak amplitude of the oral closing movements of the upper lip, lower lip, jaw, and oral aperture (combined signal) for both stutterers and normals. The cv allowed Caruso and his colleagues to make direct comparisons across articulator and population. In this instance they found no consistent differences between stutterers and normals on this measure of variability (see Folkins and Brown, 1987, for a critique of this study).

Two major issues make these obviously important comparisons sometimes difficult to interpret. The first of these is the general relation between size of the mean and variance. Secondly, differences in the shape of distributions complicate comparisons (see the subsequent section, 'Characterizing Distributions').

For as long as variance and standard deviation have been a part of biometrics an increase in variance as the mean increases has been noted. For example, the height of a larger species like an elephant is more variable in absolute terms than the height of a smaller species like a mouse. This co-scaling of the absolute variance and the mean is so common as to seem trivial yet it surely reveals something basic about the processes involved in behavior and morphology. In many cases, however, researchers have been interested in the *relative* variability between groups or individuals independent of differences in their means. Thus, adjustments for the effect of scale or size of the mean are needed. For years it has been common practice to normalize the variance by dividing the standard deviation by the mean, i.e., the coefficient of variation. This practice assumes that any change in variance is proportional to the change in the square of the mean. As Day and Fisher (1937) comment, this proportionality is by no means a logical necessity. In fact in some biological phenomena the increase in the variance is proportional to the mean not to the square of the mean (Bryant, 1986). In the study of movement, Carleton and Newell (1988) have recently pointed out that the assumption of strict proportionality between the forces produced and the force variability does not hold over a wide range of conditions. Thus, if relative variability is at issue, it is essential to understand the mean/variance relationship for the phenomena or population you are interested in. As Fisher (1937) said, the allowances that are to be made for the effect of the mean should be derived from the data themselves, i.e., from the covariance of the means and standard deviations.

In speech research this is rarely done. This is unfortunate for a number of reasons. First, comparisons are frequently made between clinical populations and normal speakers and one facet of many speech disorders is a change in speaking rate. For example a decrease in speaking rate has been reported for apraxia of speech (Kent and Rosenbek, 1983; but cf. Duffy and Gawle, 1984). With the longer speech durations exhibited by apractic speakers greater variance should be expected than for faster talking normals. But are apractic speakers relatively more variable than normals, other things being equal? This is difficult to tell. There is little research examining the articulatory properties of slow speech in normals. Some preliminary work by Robin Story (Story, Alphonso and Munhall, 1987) is suggestive, however.

Gracco and Abbs (1986) have recently reported that in oral closing movements, the upper lip, lower lip, and jaw peak velocities are sequenced in that order in approximately 98 per cent of the measured trials produced by normal speakers. What Story has done is to measure normal speakers at various rates including slower than normal. While she replicated the pattern reported by Gracco and Abbs (1986) for the fast and normal rates of speaking, the slow rate of speaking produced a far less consistent ordering. Thus, slowing down seems to produce a different pattern of articulatory data than speeding up. It is clear that in clinical studies, if the relative variability of articulation with respect to normals is of interest, attempts must be made to match the clinical population and normal controls on speaking rates. Optimally, data should be collected at various rates for both groups so that comparisons of the absolute articulatory variation and also comparisons of the mean/variance functions for the two groups can be carried out. Without directly comparable rate data some *post hoc* computational solution can be attempted. Unfortunately, without knowing the variance–scaling relationship, choosing the appropriate computational adjustment is not straight forward.

A second reason that it is unfortunate that no comprehensive program exists for understanding mean/variance scaling in speech, is that such information provides insight into the underlying probabilistic structure of the behavior. If the system responsible for speech coordination can be characterized as a certain class of mathematical structure then this can be revealed in the data patterns (see below.) One of the ways this is revealed is the shape of the distribution of scores. As will be shown below, the relationship between the mean and the variance is not independent of the shape of the distribution.

Let me summarize. For the kinds of discrete measures we usually make in speech research, the standard deviation and coefficient of variation are the standard tools used to assess dispersion. The use of these indices for comparisons between populations is complicated by the correlation between the size of the mean and the size of the variance and a related problem owing to the relationship between the shape of the distribution and the variance. When we compare variances we want to separate differences due to the processes responsible for changes in scale, i.e., size or rate of movement, and differences due to the form of the underlying distribution from differences due to pathology, skill, or development. No simple rule of thumb has yet emerged for speech research in this regard.

Functional descriptions of variation

The measures discussed up to this point have been point estimates of speech movements and acoustics. The gestures producing the speech sounds are usually summarized by scalar measures of their durations, amplitudes, and peak or average velocities. These measures give an incomplete description of the actual movement. In recent years there has been a growing recognition that movement data are derived from what are, in fact, continuous response functions. This means that the underlying function has some degree of smoothness such that the data at point t are related to the data at point $t - 1$ in a specifiable way (see Besse and Ramsay, 1986). It is felt that movement analyses should take this continuity into account and describe the variation of movements in functional terms. For example, in simple harmonic motion the movement amplitude/time plot can be described by a sinusoidal *function*. It makes little sense to analyze the time series of measurements of this motion as if they were a series of independent points. I will describe two different approaches to this more continuous view of articulatory variability.

Georgopolous, Kalaska and Massey (1981) and more recently Darling and Cooke (1987) have described the variability in individual limb movements by calculating the variability at various points in the movement trajectory. In the Darling and Cooke analysis, movements measured on successive trials were averaged and the variability in displacement and velocity were calculated at 10 ms intervals. Using radii equal to one standard deviation in position and one standard deviation in velocity, variability ellipses could be calculated throughout the movement. This technique provides a striking graphical display of the variability over the course of a single movement as well as a quantitative measure of variability at any point in the movement, i.e., area of the ellipse. Darling and Cooke (1987) have found using this technique that, in simple limb movements, variability increases quite rapidly during the acceleratory phase of movements but the rate of increase of variability slows down or variability even decreases in the deceleratory phase of movement. They interpret this finding to indicate that the entire trajectory of limb movement is controlled with variation in acceleration forces being compensated by variations in deceleration forces. Interestingly, they found that this acceleration/deceleration relationship is refined with practice with an overall decrease in variability with increased skill.

Ramsay (1982; Besse and Ramsay, 1986) has taken a somewhat different approach. He and his colleagues have been trying to express the traditional multivariate analyses such as principal components analysis in functional analytic terms. Ramsay has demonstrated the utility of this approach by analysing tongue movements in speech as well as three-dimensional limb movement. Interested readers are directed to Ramsay's (1982) presidential address to the Psychometric Society.

Briefly, the technique takes advantage of the characteristics of spline functions. The sampled data are first interpolated with some optimal spline. Then the functional variation in the data is partitioned into independent components. In general this involves partitioning the data into predictable and residual variance components and then the known or predictable functions can be removed from the data. This isolation of the so-called residual components allows the opportunity for new patterns to be discovered in the remaining variation in the data set. The important point here is that the variance components that are identified are functions. The modes of variation of trajectories are thus expressed in a form similar to the trajectories themselves.

Both of these more functional approaches to variability (Ramsay, 1982; Darling and Cooke, 1987) have clear advantages. They reflect the underlying continuity of the physiological system generating the behavior. They demonstrate temporal dependencies in the data owing to this continuity. Finally, they provide methodologies to deal quantitatively with the complexities of time series data like those collected in speech experiments. I believe analyses of this type will prove to be indispensable to future kinematic research. Particularly promising are extensions of Ramsay's work to multivariate analyses that may be appropriate for the study of interarticulator control. Such a tool could provide convenient descriptions of the differences in interarticulator variability, for example between apractic and normal speakers.

The form of variation: distributional descriptions

One of the most informative ways of examining any data set is to construct classes (quantitative or qualitative) into which the data could fall and then tally the number of observations in each class. This combination of measurement class and frequency is known as a frequency distribution. When displayed graphically in any of the common formats, e.g., cumulative or relative frequency plots, frequency distributions provide an immediately graspable summary of the dispersion and concentration of the data set.

Independent of this role as a descriptive tool for empirical data, distributional analysis is also an important technique for showing the expected behavior of theoretical models. Mathematical structures can be differentiated by the patterns of data they produce. For example, a Bernoulli process is one in which we have a sequence of independent trials and, on each trial, an event either occurs or does not. Bernoulli processes produce characteristic theoretical distributions with known shapes and relative probabilities, e.g., the binomial distribution used in statistical analyses. There exist a large number of such theoretical distributions with well-known mathematical properties, ranging from the familiar Gaussian or normal distribution to the less common Gumbel and Pareto distributions. (For a graphical display of common distributions see Rothschild and Logothetis, 1986.)

Figure 3.1 shows two distributions (binomial and Poisson distributions) that differ in their shape and therefore the relative dispersion of the scores.[2] Such differences in form of the underlying distribution are extremely important to data analysis and modeling. For example, the variance and the mean in normal distributions are, in principle, independent. This is not true of the Poisson distribution. In Poisson distributions the mean equals the variance and thus the relative variability is necessarily influenced by the mean. It is important, then, to describe the full distribution of scores in such a way that the shape of the distribution can be discerned. The aim is to be able to hypothesize about the underlying mathematical structure or generating function for the data as well as to provide a good description of experimental results.

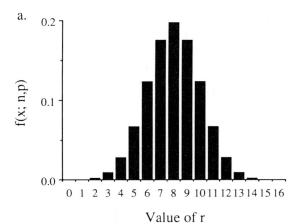

Figure 3.1a   Binomial distribution: $f(x; n, p) = \binom{n}{r} p^r q^{n-r}$, $p = .5$

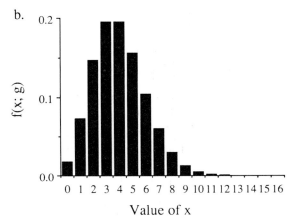

Figure 3.1b   Poisson distribution: $f(x; g) = g^x e^{-g}/x!$, $g = 4$

As with variance magnitude estimates there are discrete and more continuous measures of distributions.

Characterizing distributions

There are many statistics that can be used to describe distributions, though the static measures of variance magnitude mentioned above are by far the most common. As should be apparent, measures like the standard deviation by themselves cannot unequivocally distinguish between distributions like those depicted in Figure 3.1 that differ in overall shape. These distributions differ in symmetry and could differ in relative flatness or peakedness. Each of these characteristics, degree of asymmetry and degree of peakedness, can be indexed by relatively simple statistics.[3]

Measures of skew and kurtosis, as asymmetry and peakedness are called respectively, are rarely reported in the speech literature. There are a couple of possible reasons for this. Most prominent among these reasons is the belief that the underlying populations, or at least the sampling distributions, approximate the normal curve. (In this case, the skew index equals zero and the measure of kurtosis equals three.) Thus, the distribution is seen as symmetrical with a medium degree of kurtosis. As will be shown below, this assumption of normality is an unjustified and perhaps incorrect assumption about speech data.

The second reason for the rarity of skew and kurtosis measures lies in the nature of the indices themselves. As Newell and Hancock (1984) point out, in a cleverly titled paper, skewness and kurtosis estimates become increasingly less stable as the sample size decreases. That is, the standard error of these measures becomes quite large with small sample sizes. While this is indeed a problem, the sample size in some speech studies is sufficiently large to provide good parameter estimates. It is unfortunate that this information is not usually available.

Simple graphical techniques are becoming more popular tools in descriptive and inferential statistics (Turkey, 1977; Wainer and Thissen, 1981). While quantification is not stressed, the richness of the information available makes frequency plots essential for exploratory data analysis and general descriptive statistics. A more sophisticated approach is to match the experimental distribution to the best fit theoretical distribution. Here, we try to match a mathematical expression to a set of scores. Ideally, we are searching for a mathematical structure that shares properties and behavior with the data set. There is no single way to carry out this model identification. At one extreme a class of model could be chosen for theoretical reasons independent of the data. At the other extreme we have curve fitting or empirical model identification. In both cases the match between the model and data is expressed in terms of some goodness of fit criteria. (See Crystal and House (1988a) for a description of Markov modeling of speech distributions.)

Distributional data of any kind are rare in the speech literature but there are notable exceptions. In particular Crystal and House (1982, 1986, 1988a, b) have recently provided an extensive analysis of various acoustic durations from passages read by a number of speakers. The results of this research point to a common property of speech. The data consistently show a positive skew. This skewness is independent of the natural speaking rate of the subjects and of the type of acoustic event being measured. Overall, the shape of the distribution is quite similar to a Poisson distribution. To the extent that the data approximate a Poisson distribution, the variance (and standard deviation) will be dependent on the mean (see above).

As Crystal and House (1986) point out, this has important implications. Much clinical and developmental work has suggested that children or patients exhibit greater variability in their articulation. Given that children and many clinical populations have slower rates of speaking, the higher standard deviation could be a statistical phenomenon rather than any indication of maturation or health.

Eric Vatikiotis-Bateson (1987) found similar results in the analysis of speech movements. In a large study of lip and jaw movements in speakers of three languages (Japanese, French, and English) he found that the variance of the Japanese data was less than the other two languages. However the distributions of the movement durations were positively skewed much like the Crystal and House data. Given that the Japanese speakers as a group spoke faster than the French and English, the possibility exists that the often reported differences in temporal variability between languages might, in part, be statistical (Vatikiotis-Bateson, 1987).

The earliest and perhaps most extensive use of distributional analysis for speech movements was carried out by R.H. Stetson (1928/1988). Stetson was interested in how changes in speaking rate influenced the pattern of speech. For example, in one experimental series Stetson examined the behavior of the consonants in closed syllables when they were forced together by increasing rate. One question was whether the linking of two identical consonants ('doubling') as in *bad day* was the same phenomena as linking two different consonants ('abutting') as in *bad boy*. Stetson answered this question not by examining the average durations but by looking at the distribution of the duration measures. Figure 3.2 shows one of Stetson's figures for these data. Stetson concluded that the distributions were practically identical having similar modes and limits.[4] Thus, in his view, doubling and abutting were the same phenomenon. Distributional similarity indicated to him the underlying identity. It is worth noting the marked positive skew in these data and much of the other data reported in Stetson's monograph.

In summary, the existing data suggest that speech movements derive from a markedly non-Gaussian distribution. The distributions reported in the literature are in fact positively skewed. This fact has important implications for comparisons of variability between different populations. It suggests that the variance may scale with the mean for

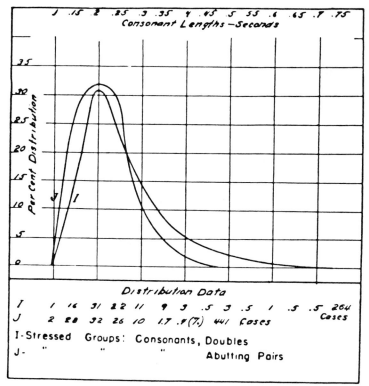

Figure 3.2 R.H. Stetson's distributional data showing the durations of consonants for doubles (curve I) and abutting pairs (curve J)

statistical reasons quite independent of any mean/variance scaling in the underlying processes that produce speech. It is suggested that caution be exercised when comparing variation if the different groups are not matched on movement rate and magnitude.

Units

What characteristics should the units of speech possess? It would seem that they have to be able to do at least two things. First, they must capture the articulatory regularities of a given linguistic community. Secondly, in doing so they must embody the bounds of natural variation in articulation. This is necessary to define the equivalence classes for pattern recognition in speech perception and to enable coordination in speech production. Traditional feature inventories are deficient on both counts.

In phonology prior to the early 1970s the representation of a spoken word was in a sense 'orthographic'. For example the word 'bag' was represented by the concatenation of the three sound units /b/, /æ/, and /g/. Within these units there was a minimum of internal structure. The segments were composed solely of feature columns or feature matrices. Segments of this type have a number of points in common (see Browman and Goldstein, 1986; Lisker, 1974). First, the segments are timeless or, at the very least, of equal duration where every column of feature values acts as a temporal place holder. For example, the segments in 'bag' are temporally undifferentiated even though they come from different classes of sounds (stops versus vowel). Second, the features in a segment are unorganized. There is no specification of any timing relationship between features in a column. They are depicted as being simultaneously present with no onset staggering or development over time. Further, there is no representation of closeness or cohesion between features in a segment. Thus, there is no internal hierarchy of features. Finally, the mode of sequencing is almost universally concatenation and thus there is no mechanism for temporal overlap at the phonological level. Overlap observed at the surface level was thought to be due to the process of phonetic implementation.

As a tool for the description of speech this scheme has great utility. But, at least since the mid 1970s, there has been concern about how well this approach captures the ontological basis of speech units. Phonologists, following John Goldsmith's (1976) dissertation, began to find these strictly linear, nonoverlapping segments too restrictive to describe certain phenomena, e.g., vowel harmonies, tonal patterns following vowel deletion, etc. Further, they wanted to express the fact that some groups of features within a segment cohere more than others. Phoneticians, on the other hand, have long argued that the detailed temporal structure of speech is relevant linguistically and that overlap and interleaving are basic to serial order in speech (see Lisker 1974).

Two solutions to the problems of traditional segments have been proposed (see Browman and Goldstein, 1986; Fowler, 1987). The first is to put the explanatory burden for the observed articulatory patterns on 'implementation rules'. These are hypothesized translation programs which convert the binary features into the continuous motion of real articulation. The second solution has been to reconceptualize the nature of the sound unit or representation. Choice of the latter solution has resulted in a proliferation of new phonologies, e.g., dependency phonology (Ewen, 1982), autosegmental phonology (Goldsmith, 1976), CV phonology (Clements and Keyser, 1983), metrical phonology (Liberman and Prince, 1977). I want to briefly describe one of these new developments, articulatory phonology, because it makes an important first step towards incorporating articulation and its associated variability into linguistic representation (Browman and Goldstein, 1986; Fowler, *et al.*, 1980; Saltzman and Munhall, 1988). The basic assumption of articulatory phonology is that both the internal components of speech units and the manner in which these components are organized are constrained by the process of articulation. Unlike the representations of speech that have dominated the field for the better part of this century, articulatory phonology views speech in a dynamical manner.

The primitives of this approach are gestures defined explicitly with the aid of a model of coordinated movement developed by Elliot Saltzman (1986). Saltzman's model, called the task–dynamic model, represents speech in a multileveled fashion. In addition to the articulators themselves, the model defines goals in an abstract task space and a tract-variable space. In the task space, the qualitative characteristics of a given utterance, e.g., discrete or repetitive motion, are represented by dynamical equations, i.e., equations with inertial, damping, and stiffness coefficients. In the tract-variable space the time course of changes in the local constrictions in the vocal tract such as oral aperture, laryngeal aperture, etc. is also represented dynamically. The act of speaking involves the transformation between these levels of representation. Speech sounds are thus represented at different levels of abstraction as spatiotemporal relationships within and between articulators.

There are many advantages to a gestural description of speech, such as the inclusion of time in the representation. As Browman and Goldstein (1986) point out, this not only allows the description of many cross-linguistic temporal phenomena but it increases the resolution of the representation. From the present perspective, though, the most attractive aspect of the approach is the potential for representing some of the variability we observe in fluent speech.

For many of the constrictions produced in the vocal tract during speech, more than a single articulator is involved. In the control of the opening and closing of the mouth, the upper lip, lower lip, and jaw are simultaneously active. The movements produced by the individual articulators when controlling these constrictions are not stereotyped. On any given movement the amount each articulator contributes to the oral closing or opening varies. For example, Sussman, MacNeilage and Hanson (1973) found that the jaw contributes less to an oral closing movement if the bilabial closure precedes a low vowel than if it precedes a high vowel. Similarly, it has been reported that when the jaw is unexpectedly perturbed and mechanically prevented from moving up to contribute to the oral closure in a bilabial stop, there is a compensatory response produced by the lips so that closure is achieved (Folkins and Abbs, 1975). Behavior of this sort can be reproduced by Saltzman's model. The tract-variable goal is achieved in the face of different gestures by individual articulators because the model articulators act together. The 'correlated variability' of the articulators in the model is a consequence of a synergistic coupling for a *specific* phonetic goal. The model, thus, provides a formalism for representing linguistic goals in the presence of surface variability.

This is clearly a preliminary model that undoubtedly will be incorrect in many of its details. However, the attempt to instantiate units in the phonology, that involve bounds on the variation of articulation, is important. What the model and the field, in general, need now is more data to constrain the details of our hypotheses about speech. In particular, research that is aimed at describing the range of natural variation in speech would help specify the tolerances that speech units must exhibit.

Implications for the Study of Apraxia of Speech

In closing I would like to make some brief comments about the implications of what I have said for the study of AOS. Variability is one of the key features of speech, even of precise, fluent speech. Speech movements vary in their overall size and duration as well as their trajectories. This variability is not constant but depends on conversational style, speaking rate, etc. Apractic speech will share this natural variation and will presumably have, in addition, another source of variation. The task that faces us is how to partition the variation we see in apractic speech so as to isolate the variability specific to the disorder. First, we must carry out studies with this specific aim. Many existing studies of apraxia provide no opportunity to collect good within-subject variance. Collins, Rosenbek and Wertz (1983), for example, had their subjects produce only a single repetition of each test utterance. Many of the instrumental studies, likewise, have a small number of repetitions per test utterance. Itoh and Sasanuma (1984), for example, in an experiment on velar movement had their apractic speaker say the speech material only three to five times. Clearly, studies that test many repetitions of a small corpus would be useful. As Rosenbek, Kent and LaPointe (1984) point out, stability of production is best assessed with within-subject measures.

Second, we need to examine apractic speech in relation to comparable control data. This means that speaking rate and movement amplitude should be controlled. There is some indication that apractic speakers have different conversational speaking rates. Collins, Rosenbek and Wertz (1983) and Kent and Rosenbek (1983) report a decrease in speaking rate while Duffy and Gawle (1984) found an increase in speaking rate. Given these reported changes in speaking rate, experiments that attempt to show the mean/variance functions for normals and apractic speakers across a wide range of speaking rates would be useful. Such experiments would require tight control of speaking rate. This is admittedly difficult but the potential benefits warrant the effort. As noted above the direct comparison of the standard deviation or coefficients of variation between apractic and normal speakers has many potential pitfalls. Itoh and Sasanuma (1984) report that the velar movements of their apractic speaker were more variable than normal. However, it is evident in the displayed movement traces that the apractic speaker had a much slower speaking rate than the normal speaker. It is impossible to determine what role the slower speaking rate played in the observed patterns in these data. Mean/variance functions for normals and apractic speakers would be helpful in this regard.

Finally, we should begin to explore more continuous measures of speech. Interarticulator coordination must involve fine temporal and spatial adjustments over time and techniques are emerging that will allow these patterns to be summarized, e.g., Ramsay (1982). The emphasis on continuous measures should also be extended to phonological units. There is considerable uncertainty about the nature of segments yet in the study of apraxia the traditional segments have become reified in the explanation of the disorder. Rosenbek, Kent and LaPointe (1984), for example, point out the dangers of letting our 'phonetic habits' bias our transcriptions. In fact, a number of authors (Square, Darley, and Sommers, 1982; Kent and Rosenbek, 1983; Itoh and Sasanuma, 1984) suggest that distortions occur much more frequently in apractic speech than is reported in the literature because there is a transcription bias to report the errors as substitutions of features or segments. Some of the new phonological approaches, e.g., Browman and Goldstein (1986), are particularly attractive for the study of apraxia of speech in terms of such spatiotemporal distortions (see Kent and Rosenbek (1983) and Chapter 2).

In conclusion, increased variability has long been seen as an important property of apraxia of speech, e.g., Johns and Darley (1970), and there seems to be a consensus that the variability in a data set provides useful information about the nature of speech in general. It is hoped that this valuable source of information can be more frequently and effectually tapped in future research.

Notes

1 It should be noted that the standard deviation is susceptible to outliers and as Newell and Hancock (1984) point out the standard deviation provides a markedly less stable estimate of the population parameters for small ns.
2 See Hays (1973) for a demonstration that the Poisson distribution is a special case of the binomial distribution.
3 Asymmetry or skew is measured with reference to the third moment about the mean of the distribution,

$$\sum_{i=1}^{n} (X_i - \bar{X})^3 \ /n/S_x^3$$

Peakedness or kurtosis is measured with reference to the fourth moment about the mean of the distribution,

$$\sum_{i=1}^{n} (X_i - \bar{X})^4 /n/S_x^4$$

4 Some readers may find the measure of similarity used by Stetson to be a bit crude.

Acknowledgments

Dr Munhall acknowledges that partial support for the preparation of his chapter was derived from a grant from Atkinson College, York University, Toronto. Drs David Ostry, Randy Flanagan, and Paula Square-Storer provided valuable comments on earlier versions of this manuscript.

References

BESSE, P. and RAMSAY, J. (1986) 'Principle components analysis of sampled functions', *Psychometrika*, **51**, pp. 285–311.
BROWMAN, C. and GOLDSTEIN, L. (1986) 'Towards an articulatory phonology', *Phonology Yearbook*, **3**, pp. 219–52.
BRYANT, E. (1986) 'On the use of logarithms to accommodate scale', *Systematic Zoology*, **35**, pp. 552–9.

CARLETON, L. and NEWELL, K. (1988) 'Force variability and movement accuracy in space-time', *Journal Experimental Psychology HPP*, **14**, pp. 24–36.

CARUSO, A., ABBS, J. and GRACCO, V. (1987) 'Kinematic analysis of speech multiple movement coordination in stutterers', *SMCL Preprints*, Spring-Summer, pp. 31–51.

CLEMENTS, G. (1985) 'The geometry of phonological features', *Phonology Yearbook*, **2**, pp. 225–52.

CLEMENTS, G. and KEYSER, S. (1983) *CV Phonology: A Generative Theory of the Syllable*, Cambridge, MA, MIT Press.

COLLINS, M., ROSENBEK, J. and WERTZ, R. (1983) 'Spectrographic analysis of vowel and word duration in apraxia of speech', *Journal Speech and Hearing Research*, **26**, pp. 224–30.

COWLES, M. (1988) *Statistics in Psychology: A Historical Perspective*, Unpublished manuscript, York University.

CRYSTAL, T. and HOUSE, A. (1982) 'Segmental durations in connected speech signals: Preliminary results', *Journal Acoustical Society America*, **72**, pp. 705–16.

CRYSTAL, T. and HOUSE, A. (1986) 'Variability of timing control. Maturational or statistical?' Paper presented at the meeting of the Acoustical Society of America, Cleveland, Ohio.

CRYSTAL, T. and HOUSE, A. (1988a) 'Segmental durations in connected-speech signals: Current results', *Journal Acoustical Society America*, **83**, pp. 1553–73.

CRYSTAL, T. and HOUSE, A. (1988b) 'Segmental durations in connected-speech signals: Syllabic stress', *Journal Acoustical Society America*, **83**, pp. 1574–85.

DARLING, W. and COOKE, J.D. (1987) 'Changes in the variability of movement trajectories with practice', *Journal of Motor Behavior*, **19**, pp. 291–309.

DARWIN, C. (1896) *The Origin of Species*, New York, Caldwell.

DAY, B. and FISHER, R. (1937) 'The comparison of variability in populations having unequal means. An example of the analysis of covariance with multiple dependent and independent variates', *Annals of Eugenics*, **7**, pp. 333–48.

DUFFY, J. and GAWLE, C. (1984) 'Apraxic speakers' vowel duration in consonant-vowel syllables', in ROSENBEK, J., MCNEIL, M. and ARONSON, A. (Eds.), *Apraxia of Speech: Physiology, Acoustics, Linguistics and Management*, San Diego, College-Hill Press.

EWAN, C. (1982) 'The internal structure of complex segments', in VAN DER HULST, H. and SMITH, N., (Eds.), *The Structure of Phonological Representations*, **2**, Dordrecht, Foris.

FISHER, R. (1937) 'The relation between variability and abundance shown by the measurement of the eggs of British nesting birds', *Proceedings of the Royal Society of London*, B, **122**, pp. 1–26.

FOLKINS, J. and ABBS, J. (1975) 'Lip and jaw motor control: Responses to resistive loading of the jaw', *Journal Speech and Hearing Research*, **18**, pp. 207–20.

FOLKINS, J. and BROWN, C. (1987) 'Upper lip, lower lip, and jaw interactions during speech: Comments on evidence from repetition-to-repetition variability', *Journal Acoustical Society America*, **82**, pp. 1919–24.

FOWLER, C. (1987) 'Perceivers as realists, talkers too: Commentary on papers by Strange, Diehl *et al.*, and Rakerd and Verbrugge', *Journal of Memory and Language*, **26**, pp. 574–87.

FOWLER, C., RUBIN, P., REMEZ, R. and TURVEY, M. (1980) 'Implications for speech production of a general theory of action', in BUTTERWORTH, B. (Ed.) *Language Production*, New York, Academic.

GEORGOPOLOUS, A., KALASKA, J. and MASSEY, J. (1981) 'Spatial trajectories and reaction times of aimed movements: Effects of practice, uncertainty and change in target location', *Journal of Neurophysiology*, **46**, pp. 725–43.

GOLDSMITH, J. (1976) *Autosegmental Phonology*, Indiana University Linguistics Club.

GRACCO, V. and ABBS, J. (1986) 'Variant and invariant characteristics of speech movements', *Experimental Brain Research*, **65**, pp. 156–66.

HAYS, W. (1973) *Statistics for the Social Sciences*, New York, Holt, Rinehart, and Winston.

ITOH, M. and SASANUMA, S. (1984) 'Articulatory movements in apraxia of speech', in ROSENBEK, J., MCNEIL, M. and ARONSON, A. (Eds.), *Apraxia of Speech: Physiology, Acoustics, Linguistics and Management*, San Diego, College-Hill.

JOHNS, D. and DARLEY, F. (1970) 'Phonemic variability in apraxia of speech', *Journal of Speech and Hearing Disorders*, **13**, pp. 556–83.

KENT, R. and ROSENBEK, J. (1983) 'Acoustic patterns of apraxia of speech', *Journal of Speech and Hearing Research*, **26**, pp. 231–48.

LIBERMAN, M. and PRINCE, A. (1977) 'On stress and linguistic rhythm', *Linguistic Inquiry*, **8**, pp. 249–336.

LISKER, L. (1974) 'On time and timing in speech', in Sebeok, T., (Ed.), *Current Trends in Linguistics*, **12**, The Hague, Mouton.

MCGARR, N. and LÖFQVIST, A. (1982) 'Obstruent production in hearing-impaired speakers: Interarticulator timing and acoustics', *Journal Acoustical Society America*, **72**, pp. 34–42.

NEWELL, K. and HANCOCK, P. (1984) 'Forgotten moments: A note on skewness and kurtosis as influential factors in inferences extrapolated from response distributions', *Journal of Motor Behavior*, **16**, pp. 320–35.

RAMSAY, J. (1982) 'When data are functions', *Psychometrika*, **47**, pp. 379–96.

ROSENBEK, J., KENT, R. and LAPOINTE, L. (1984) 'Apraxia of speech: An overview and some perspectives', in ROSENBEK, J., MCNEIL, M. and ARONSON, A. (Eds.), *Apraxia of Speech: Physiology, Acoustics, Linguistics and Management*, San Diego, College-Hill Press.

ROTHSCHILD, V. and LOGOTHETIS, N. (1986) *Probability Distributions*, New York, Wiley.

SALTZMAN, E. (1986) 'Task dynamic coordination of the speech articulators: A preliminary model' in HEUER, H. and FROMM, C. (eds.), *Generation and Modulation of Action Patterns (Experimental Brain Research Series 15)*, pp. 129–44, New York, Springer-Verlag.

SALTZMAN, E. and MUNHALL, K. (1988) 'A dynamical approach to gestural patterning in speech production', unpublished manuscript.

SQUARE, P., DARLEY, F. and SOMMERS, R. (1982) 'An analysis of the productive errors made by pure apractic speakers with differing loci of lesions', in BROOKSHIRE, R. (Ed.), *Clinical Aphasiology Conference Proceedings*, Minneapolis, BRK Publishers.

STETSON, R.H. (1988) in KELSO, J. and MUNHALL, K., (Eds.) *R.H. Stetson's Motor Phonetics*, Boston, College-Hill Press.

STIGLER, S. (1986) *The History of Statistics*, Cambridge, MA, Belknap.

STORY, R., ALPHONSO, P. and MUNHALL, K. (1987) 'Lip and jaw kinematics at various speaking rates', Paper presented at the meeting of the American Speech and Hearing Association. New Orleans, Louisiana.

SUSSMAN, H., MCNEILAGE, P. and HANSON, R. (1973) 'Labial and mandibular dynamics during the production of bilbial consonants', *Journal of Speech and Hearing Research*, **16**, pp. 397–420.

TUKEY, J. (1977) *Exploratory Data Analysis*, Reading, MA, Addison-Wesley.

VATIKIOTIS-BATESON, E. (1987) *Linguistic Structure and Articulatory Dynamics: A Cross-Language Study*, Unpublished doctoral dissertation, Indiana University.

WAINER, H. and THISSEN, D. (1981) 'Graphical data analysis', in ROSENZWEIG, M. and PORTER, L., (Eds.), *Annual Review of Psychology*, **32**, Palo Alto, CA, Annual Reviews.

YABLOKOV, A. (1974) *Variability in Mammals*, New Delhi, Amerind.

PART TWO
Clinical Issues

Chapter 4

Differential Diagnosis of Aphasic Syndromes and Apraxia of Speech

Michael J. Collins

Apraxia of speech, Broca's aphasia, and conduction aphasia theoretically represent independent clusters of identifiable and classifiable speech and language behaviors. Unfortunately, these clusters are, and have been perceived differently with resulting semantic polarization. The terms 'apraxia of speech', 'conduction aphasia', 'Broca's aphasia', and 'literal paraphasia' frequently elicit a cacophony of alternatives, including 'phonetic disintegration', 'motor aphasia', and 'sensory aphasia'. In this chapter, we try to avoid this terminological morass, but do not suggest that the semantic differences are trivial. The purpose of this chapter is to present a pragmatic, clinical discussion of the three disorders' characteristics and present typical clinical and standardized assessment profiles of each syndrome.

Broca's Aphasia

Goodglass and Kaplan (1983) tell us that Broca's aphasia most commonly results from a lesion or lesions involving the third frontal convolution of the left hemisphere, the subcortical white matter, and extends posteriorly to the inferior portion of the motor strip, or precentral gyrus. Its essential characteristics are awkward articulation, restricted vocabulary, restriction of grammar to its simplest, most overlearned forms, and relative preservation of auditory comprehension. Writing is usually impaired at least as severely as speech, and reading is only mildly affected. This profile is typical, but not invariant. Mohr *et al.* (1978), for example, suggest that there may be both a 'big' and 'little' Broca's aphasia, which depend upon an interaction of size and location of lesion. They have suggested that lesions restricted to the inferior frontal cortical areas of the left hemisphere yield fairly rapidly to a picture of mild impairment of language with 'speech apraxia' as the principal distinguishing characteristic. He suggests that a true Broca's aphasia results when lesions extend far beyond Broca's area into the operculum, insula, and adjacent cerebral regions. The typical picture resulting from this extensive lesion is one of global aphasia initially, which over time evolves to a Broca's aphasia.

Conduction Aphasia

Geschwind (1965) attributes conduction aphasia to a lesion in the arcuate fasciculus, the fiber pathways believed to carry information from Wernicke's area to Broca's area. Goodglass and Kaplan (1983) apply this term to the syndrome in which repetition is dispropor-tionately and severely impaired in relation to the level of fluency in spontaneous speech and to the near normal level of auditory com-prehension. It is considered a 'fluent' aphasia because the patients usually produce well-articulated sequences of English phonemes with normal intonation, and initiate a variety of syntactic patterns. This is contrasted with the awkward articulation and paucity of grammatical form and restricted vocabulary seen in Broca's aphasia. And yet, according to Goodglass and Kaplan, spoken output may range from fluent to nonfluent. Thus, there may be a fine line between the nonfluent speech of the Broca's aphasic and the nonfluent conduction aphasic.

Apraxia of Speech

The lesion responsible for apraxia of speech is generally thought to involve the left frontal lobe but may result from lesions far removed from Broca's area. Wertz, Rosenbek and Deal (1970) for example, found that apraxia of speech may result from lesions involving the frontal, parietal, or the temporal lobes. Deutsch (1984) and Square, Darley and Sommers (1981, 1982) seem to support the notion of a primary or efferent apraxia, and a secondary or afferent kinesthetic speech apraxia (Canter, 1969; Luria, 1966). These reports imply that type of apraxia of speech may be lesion-dependent.

Despite the more narrow focus of symptoms and lesions in recent years, there are several generally accepted behaviors typically seen in AOS. Darley (1982) summarized them:

1 Articulatory errors increase as the complexity of motor-adjustments required of the articulators increases

2 Consonants in the initial position may be misarticulated more often than consonant phonemes in other positions

3 Patients with apraxia of speech demonstrate a consistency effect on repeated readings of the same material, and they tend to make fewer errors on successive readings of the same passage

4 There is some evidence that phonemes with a higher frequency of occurrence may be more accurately articulated than phonemes which occur less frequently

5 Errors are variably related to the target sounds, with the percentage of the errors differing by one or two distinctive features

6 The most common types of sequencing errors observed are anticipatory, reiterative, and metathetic

7 Performance on automatic and reactive speech production is relatively better than performance on volitional purposive speech production. Imitative responses frequently contain more articulatory errors than spontaneous production

8 As words increase in length, so do articulation errors

9 Articulatory errors in oral reading are not random — they are more frequent on words that carry linguistic or psychologic 'weight' and that are more essential for communication

10 Articulation is more accurate when speech stimuli are presented by a visible examiner than when presented via tape recorder or read aloud from a printed stimulus

11 Articulation is facilitated more by repeated trials of a word than by an increase in the number of stimulus presentations

12 Accuracy of articulation is not influenced by a number of auditory, visual, and psychological variables, including visual feedback, masking noise, delayed response, instructional set, or the imposition of an external auditory rhythm.

These rules have guided us in our diagnosis and treatment for nearly 20 years. They will continue to be our foundation while our notions and our techniques undergo refinement.

Paraphasias in Neurogenic Motor Programming Disorders

This brief discussion of paraphasias in motor speech disorders is intended as a modest guide for the readers of this chapter. The nature of literal paraphasias is discussed from a different perspective in Chapter 2.

Goodglass and Kaplan (1983) define paraphasia as '...the production of unintended syllables, words, or phrases during the effort to speak' (p. 8). In their view, paraphasia is characteristic of patients whose speech sounds are uttered fluently. They do not include the distorted pronunciation of patients with 'poor articulation'. This exclusion may signal a crucial distinction.

Goodglass and Kaplan list four specific varieties of paraphasias. *Literal (or phonemic) paraphasia* refers to a paraphasia in which, in spite of 'easy' articulation of individual sounds, the patient produces syllables in the wrong word order or embellishes his words with unintended sounds. For example 'pipe' may become 'hike ... no, pike ... pipe'. Some phonemic features of the intended word are usually preserved. *Neologistic distortions* are words which are gross, literal paraphasias, or 'extreme' literal paraphasias. *Verbal paraphasias* are real words used inadvertently in place of another. *Paragrammatism*, or extended paraphasia, refers to running speech which is logically incoherent either because the phrases do not make sense together or because of intrusions of misused words, neologisms, or all of these features.

For a review of the fairly distinct differences between apraxia of speech and dysarthria, the reader is referred to Darley, Aronson and Brown (1975), Kent (1976) and Kent and Rosenbek (1983). The difference between literal paraphasias and apraxia of speech are less distinct as the following section will illustrate.

Errors resulting from apraxia of speech may frequently resemble literal paraphasias, and literal paraphasias may frequently resemble errors attributable to apraxia of speech. Indeed, the two often coexist. Blumstein, Cooper and Zurif (1977), for example, found that Broca's, conduction, and Wernicke's aphasic patients demonstrated both phonetic (motoric) and phonemic (linguistic) errors. Blumstein's analyses were instrumentally based, as were those of Itoh *et al.* (1982). However, Itoh and his colleagues reported that neither conduction nor Wernicke's patients demonstrated evidence of a motor speech disorder. Similarly, perceptual analyses, particularly those of MacNeilage (1981) suggest that the sound substitutions of anterior lesion patients result primarily from difficulty with motor production of speech, but the same was not true for posterior lesion patients.

Kent (1976) defines apraxia of speech as disturbed motor programming directly due to impairment of motor association systems, manifested as disturbances in initiation, transitionalization, repertoire, and selection of articulatory gestures. Literal paraphasias, he believes, reflect disturbed motor programming secondary to impairment of sensory association systems or their frontal projections. The speech characteristics of apraxia of speech are predominantly errors of phoneme substitution, at least as we perceive them (Kent and Rosenbek, 1983), but prosody is affected, and initiation of speech is particularly difficult. In contrast, literal paraphasias are most frequently errors of phoneme substitution, as measured by both perceptual and acoustic analysis (Blumstein, Cooper and Zurif, 1982; Itoh *et al.*, 1980; Square-Storer, 1987). These errors are frequently much less predictable than in apraxia of speech. Phoneme additions and errors in phoneme sequences are common, speech is normally prosodic and fluent, and there is no impairment of phonation, resonation, or respiration. Unfortunately, many aphasic patients are unclassifiable by any means even with careful testing and confirmed sites of lesion.

Considerations in the Evaluation of Apraxia of Speech

An adequate evaluation should allow the clinician to determine severity, provide some information about site of lesion, establish a prognosis, and focus treatment. No single test for aphasia or apraxia allows one to perform all these tests, and exhaustive testing does not guarantee accurate diagnosis. Accurate diagnosis requires discriminating testing. Discriminating testing requires care in the selection of tests to be administered, in the precision of analysis of the information these tests provide, and critical, insightful, and thoughtful interpretation of the data. The first requirement for discriminating testing is an adequate scoring system.

Traditional speech and language testing has relied on a useful and simple system to record the adequacy of responses, the plus–minus scoring system. Implicit in the use of this system is the notion that a behavior is either right or it is wrong. While we recognize that the notion is in some ways absurd, its simplicity perpetuates its use. We need to know not only that a patient was right or wrong but why he was right or wrong, and in what ways that performance differs from other patients or from normals. Several scoring systems have evolved to serve one or more of these purposes. A brief description of the more common and/or more useful scoring systems follows.

The seven-point equal-appearing interval scoring system represents a response to the recognition that most behaviors cannot be adequately described by plus-minus scoring. It is also efficient. The scoring system is used to rate adequacy of performance from mild involvement, or '1', to severe involvement, '7'. In the speech and language literature, perhaps the most common use has been to rate the severity of dysarthria, for example in the dysarthria studies of Darley, Aronson and Brown (1969). More recently, Wertz *et al.* (1981) used a seven-point scale to rate the severity of dysarthria and apraxia. Dabul (1979) utilizes a three-point version of that scale to rate apraxia.

The usefulness of the seven-point rating scale is limited because it is unidimensional. It provides no information about other parameters of the response, such as delay, self-correction, or relatedness of the response to the target. A more useful scoring system for determining not only the adequacy of the response but the potentially revealing nuances of the response is Porch's (1967) binary choice, multi-dimensional scoring system. Nominally a 16-point scale (the infrequently used score of sixteen indicates a complex response to the stimulus), scores range from '1', no response and no apparent awareness of the tester or test stimulus, to '15', indicating an accurate, responsive, complete, prompt, and efficient response.

An earlier version of the scoring system (Porch, 1967), shown in Table 4.1, provided for several scores which were useful in quantifying efficiency of verbal production, and by inference, behaviors which suggested the presence or absence of apraxia of speech. A score of '14', for example, suggested a verbal production which was distorted and produced slowly and awkwardly; a score of '10' documented self-corrections for example 'cigarette...no, cigelette...no, cigarette'; a score of '7' suggested either a verbal paraphasia, for example 'match' for 'cigarette' or a literal paraphasia, in which the majority of the response corresponded to the target response, for example 'cigerlette'; and a score of '4', which encompassed several behaviors — a distorted, unintelligible response, a response which may resemble the target but differ by more than one-half of the intended phonemes, or neologistic jargon. The scoring system and the test it was designed to be used with, the Porch Index of Communicative Ability (PICA) (Porch, 1967) is useful in identifying apraxia of speech. Wertz, Rosenbek and Collins (1972) found that by using the four verbal subtests (object description, object naming, sentence completion, and repetition) judges agreed with the diagnosis of apraxia of speech 74 per cent of the time.

A potentially more useful version of that scoring system has recently appeared (Porch, 1983). The use of diacritics, for example the 'boxed' score to indicate a motorically inefficient response, and serial scoring, in which the sequence of scores produced by a patient in attempting to respond to each item are recorded, are at least potentially powerful tools in the differential diagnosis of apraxia of speech and aphasia. It should be noted that this scale is not truly a scale of goodness, and only superficially represents a continuum of response adequacy.

Collins *et al.* (1980) developed a fourteen-point scale that rates severity of apraxia of speech and permits quantification of delay, prosodic disturbance, distortion, self-correction, groping, and such errors as substitutions, omissions, and additions. This scale, shown in Table 4.2, has face validity, and interjudge reliability in the ordering of behaviors is high. With the exception of the plus–minus system, the systems described permit quantitative assessment.

Recently, Roy and Square (1985) developed qualitative alpha-numeric scoring systems for the appraisal of limb, verbal, and oral apraxia. Basically, these systems allow the user to note both type of error and the order in which they occur during the temporal unfolding of an action. All three notation systems (limb, oral, and verbal praxis) are comprised of ten categories, and can be elaborated by diacritical marks. In the case of the verbal system, over 130 diacritics are used.

The scoring system the clinician uses to describe and quantify behaviors should be reliable, valid, and efficient, and applied to formal

Table 4.1: Scoring System for the Porch Index of Communicative Ability

Score	Category	Dimensional Characteristics
16	COMPLEX	Accurate, responsive, complex, prompt, efficient
15	COMPLETE	Accurate, responsive, complete, prompt, efficient
14	DISTORTED	Accurate, responsive, complete or complex, prompt, distorted.
13	COMPLETE-DELAYED	Accurate, responsive, complete or complex, delayed
12	INCOMPLETE	Accurate, responsive, incomplete, prompt
11	INCOMPLETE-DELAYED	Accurate, responsive, incomplete, delayed
10	CORRECTED	Accurate, self-corrected
9	REPEATED	Accurate, after instructions are repeated
8	CUED	Accurate, after cue is given
7	RELATED	Inaccurate, almost accurate
6	ERROR	Inaccurate attempt at the task item
5	INTELLIGIBLE	Comprehensible but not an attempt at the task item
4	UNINTELLIGIBLE	Incomprehensible but differentiated
3	MINIMAL	Incomprehensible and undifferentiated
2	ATTENTION	No response, but patient attends to the tester
1	NO RESPONSE	No response, no awareness of task

Table 4.2: Scoring System for Rating Apraxia of Speech

16	Normal
15	Normal except slow because of changes in articulation and/or pause time
14	Normal except for prosodic disturbance (pitch, loudness, stress, effort)
13	Distortion
12	Distortion and prosodic disturbance
11	Self-correction
10	Self-correction except for prosodic disturbance
9	Self-correction except for distortion
8	Groping which does not cross phoneme boundaries and which is followed by the correct response
7	Sound substitution(s), omission(s), or addition(s), without sound distortion(s) or prosodic disturbances, but may have mild to moderate changes in articulation and/or pause time. Word remains recognizable
6	Sound substitution(s), omission(s), or addition(s) with distortion(s) or prosodic disturbances. Word remains recognizable
5	As in 7 above except word is unrecognizable
4	As in 6 above except word is unrecognizable
3	Verbal paraphasia, self-corrected
2	Verbal paraphasia
1	No response, or rejection, or unintelligible, undifferentiated response

and informal speech, non-speech, and language tests. The following section describes what to us is an adequate sampling of these behaviors.

The Evaluation

Aphasia testing is essential to efficacious management of these patients. Patients with conduction aphasia, and patients with apraxia of speech and significant aphasia, do not profit from the same treatment, and recover in different ways and at different rates than patients with mild aphasia. Comprehensive testing for aphasia should allow the clinician to determine severity, type of aphasia, prognosis, and focus treatment, but not all tests do. Type of aphasia, for example, is best determined with the Boston Diagnostic Aphasia Examination (BDAE) (Goodglass and Kaplan, 1983) or the Western Aphasia Battery (WAB) (Kertesz, 1982), but both are weak in predictive validity and treatment focus. They are reliable and valid, but the psychometric soundness of the BDAE is questionable (McNeil, 1988) and their scoring systems lack sensitivity for detailed analysis of individual responses.

The PICA is one of the most efficient and comprehensive commercially available tests for the evaluation of aphasia. The scoring system is powerful, it is valid and reliable, it permits the determination of severity and prognosis, and it is extremely useful for focusing treatment. With appropriate interpretation, the test allows for determination of type of aphasia (Wertz *et al.*, 1981). The test is, however, of limited usefulness with profoundly impaired or very mildly involved patients.

A comprehensive examination for aphasia and apraxia should include a wide range of communicative difficulty. It should include supplementary tests for assessment of auditory comprehension, reading comprehension, nonverbal intelligence, oral nonverbal and limb praxis, and speech production in a variety of contexts. Our choice of components for such an examination is described below and has been influenced by our training, setting, needs, and biases.

Auditory comprehension

The Token Test (DeRenzi and Vignolo, 1962) is a sixty-one-item test of auditory comprehension. It is not well-standardized but appears to be sensitive and valid. Normative data for patients with left-hemisphere lesions and aphasia, right-hemisphere lesions, and normals are unpublished but available (Wertz, Keith and Custer, 1971).

The Revised Token Test (McNeil and Prescott, 1978) consists of ten subtests of ten items each. Responses are scored with a fifteen-point scoring system which requires extensive training to use but is sensitive to small changes in behavior. The test is standardized, reliable, and valid, and normative data are available for left-hemisphere aphasic, right-hemisphere damaged, and normal adults.

Reading comprehension

The only commercially available test which was designed specifically to assess reading ability in aphasic patients is the Reading Comprehension Battery for Aphasia (LaPointe and Horner, 1979). Nicholas, MacLennan and Brookshire (1985) have suggested an alternative, the Nelson Reading Skills Test (Hanna, Schell and Schreiner, 1977).

Nonverbal intelligence

Tests of nonverbal intelligence may be of limited value in aphasia assessment, and no such test specifically designed for testing of aphasic patients is commercially available. Perhaps the most widely used test is the Colored Progressive Matrices (Raven, 1962). A particular advantage to this test is that it has been used extensively in aphasia research, and normative data are available (Wertz, Keith and Custer, 1971).

Word fluency

The form of the Word Fluency Measure most commonly used (Borkowski, Benton and Spreen, 1967) requires the patient to produce as many words as possible, in one minute, beginning with each of four letters — 'S', 'T', 'P', and 'C'. Normative data for right-hemisphere damaged patients, left-hemisphere damaged patients with aphasia, and normal subjects are available (Wertz, Keith and Custer, 1971).

A standard speech sample

Finally, the evaluation should include an adequate sample of the patient's speech and nonspeech abilities in a variety of contexts. It may include standardized, commercially available tests not specifically designed for aphasic patients, for example the Deep Test of Articulation (MacDonald, 1964); a sample constructed from parts of several tests or a combination of the two. An argument against using nonstandardized tests is that, until they become standardized, even for a single clinician or a single clinic, our perceptions are at a disadvantage because they lack a stable memory of what other patients sound like on the same tasks. Standardized tests let us listen to our memories as we listen to our patients.

Tests for apraxia of speech

The embryonic state of our clinical evaluation of apraxia of speech is perhaps best reflected by the dearth of commercially available tests to assess it. The only commercially available test, developed by Dabul (1979) is the Apraxia Battery for Adults (ABA). The purpose of this test is to verify the presence of apraxia in the adult patient, and provide for assessment of progress through periodic retesting. There are six subtests, each designed to assess a specific parameter: diadochokinetic rate, words of increasing length, limb and oral praxis, latency and utterance time for polysyllabic words, a repeated trials test, and an inventory of articulation characteristics of apraxia. Severity is rated on a three-point scale (0, 1, 2). When the scores are summed and averaged, they yield an overall rating of mild to profound involvement. These scores and profiles may be compared to Dabul's normative sample, consisting of forty aphasic subjects, seventeen of whom were apractic as well. The test is not standardized, and contains serious deficiencies in reliability and validity. It does provide a more secure anchor for our perceptions.

The tasks required in the Apraxia Battery for Adults reflect much traditional wisdom about the nature of apraxia of speech. They are discriminating, and suggest that clinician's intuitions are in general agreement. If we know anything about apractic patients, we know they have trouble talking. The more talking they do, in structured, systematic tasks varying in difficulty, the more likely they are to reveal the frailties of their articulatory systems.

The evaluation we use was adapted from Rosenbek and Wertz (1976). We use it to elicit speech in a variety of contexts: spontaneous speech in picture description and in conversation; vowel prolongation; diadochokinetic rate on at least three syllables (/pʌ/, /tʌ/, and /kʌ/) separately and sequentially; repetition of monosyllabic and polysyllabic words; repetition of sentences; repetition of words of increasing length, for example flat, flatter, flattering; counting to twenty; an oral reading task; picture description, for example the 'Cookie Thief' picture from the Boston Diagnostic Aphasia Examination (Goodglass and Kaplan, 1983); and imitation of several sentences generated by that patient in the picture description task. The evaluation is recorded on audio tape for subsequent and, if necessary, more fine-grained analysis. Variations may include a repeated trials task to assess variability of performance. Clinicians may find it useful to request repeated trials of polysyllabic words. Several authorities, including Johns and Darley (1970) and Deutsch (1984) have found the imitation of polysyllabic words to be powerful in differentiating apractic errors from other types.

Oral nonverbal and limb apraxia

Nonspeech apraxias, particularly oral and limb apraxias, may not be of particular significance in differentiating type of aphasia. Nevertheless, we include, as part of our standard assessment, tests of oral nonverbal and limb apraxia, for such information is useful for selecting appropriate treatment (see Chapter 6). A sampling of those tasks appears in Table 4.3. Typically, we ask patients to perform these tasks in three conditions: to request, to repeat the task, and to imitate it.

Table 4.3: Tasks for Assessing Oral and Verbal Apraxia

1 Spontaneous speech in picture description and in conversation
2 Vowel prolongation
3 Diadochokinetic rate on at least three syllables (/pʌ/, /tʌ/, and /kʌ/) separately and sequentially at rates of 1, 2, 3, and 4 per second, and as rapidly as possible
4 Repetition of monosyllabic and polysyllabic words
5 Repetition of sentences
6 Repetition of words of increasing length, for example flat, flatter, flattering.
7 Counting to 20
8 Oral reading task, for example the Grandfather Passage
9 Picture description, for example the 'Cookie Thief' picture from the Boston Diagnostic Aphasia Examination
10 Imitation of several sentences generated by that patient in the picture description task (Record the evaluation on audio tape for subsequent and, if necessary, more fine-grained analysis. Variations may include a repeated trials task to assess variability of performance. Clinicians may find it useful to request repeated trials of polysyllabic words.)

Special tests

The human ear is the ultimate arbitrator of the acceptability of speech. Nevertheless, instruments have begun to assume a prominent position in the management of speech and language disorders. They have the potential to demystify and to demythologize when combined with sensitive perceptual analyses. Many of the more sophisticated techniques are beyond the skills and resources of most clinical facilities. They are discussed briefly in the next section because they reflect the breadth and depth of analysis possible, and because, in some cases, their revelations may help guide us in our treatment.

Acoustic analysis

Interest in acoustic analysis and its potentially powerful contribution to differentiation among speech and language disorders has undergone a recent resurgence. Some recent and important acoustic studies were reviewed in Chapter 2. Kent and Rosenbek's (1983) analyses, however, deserve special consideration because of their compelling evidence of the power of spectrographic analyses in the detection of measurable, acoustic events in dysarthric and apraxic speakers. Their composite description of the apraxic speaker is presented succinctly in Table 4.4.

Electromyography

Electromyographic analysis in the investigation of apraxia of speech appears to be undergoing a resurgence in popularity since Shankweiler, Harris and Taylor's (1968) study of two apraxic patients. Fromm *et al.*

Table 4.4. Composite Description of Apraxic Speakers

1 Slow speaking rate with prolongations of transitions and steady states as well as intersyllable pauses
2 Restricted variation in relative peak intensity across syllables
3 Slow and inaccurate movements of the articulators to spatial targets for both consonants and vowels
4 Frequent mistiming or dyscoordination of voicing with other articulations
5 Occasional errors of segment selection or sequencing including intrusion, metathesis, and omission
6 Initiation difficulties often characterized by false starts and restarts
7 Complex sound sequences associated with prolongations, interruptions, and inappropriate phonetic variations

(1982), for example, studied the temporal and spatial organization of apraxic speech. Their results led them to suggest that any definition of apraxia must include discoordination of multiple speech muscles and speech movements.

Aerodynamic studies

Dyscoordination, which is seen so prominently in the acoustic and physiological studies, seems to be revealed in aerodynamic parameters, particularly those which require coordination of two or more structures. Keatley and Pike (1976), for example, found that peak expiratory flow was a sensitive measure of pulmonary function. It was lower than that for normals for four of their subjects, and was related to severity of apraxia of speech.

Summary

We have undergone a period of exhaustive perceptual analysis best exemplified by the work of Darley and his coauthors. This work was followed by a succession of acoustic studies for example by Blumstein *et al.* (1977), and physiological studies of apraxia of speech, such as those of Fromm *et al.* (1982) and by Malcolm McNeil and his associates at the University of Wisconsin (personal correspondence, 1988).

These studies, and the studies that will surely follow, promise to provide us with a clearer focus on the nature of articulatory behaviors following brain insult. The practising clinician should be aware of these studies. The clinician's responsibility, of course, is to make the best possible use of the available data. Those data are in most cases perceptual. In the following section, test profiles of three more or less 'typical' patients will be presented. In all cases, the data was perceptual, and clinical decisions were made on this basis alone. These patient profiles conform in a general sense to profiles of 'typical' patients. They were selected not because they fit these profiles precisely, but because they are representative of a diversity of behaviors confronting the clinician. We believe their behaviors are illustrative of, and consistent with: Broca's aphasia, conduction aphasia, and apraxia of speech.

Clinical Profiles

Broca's aphasia

Patient DF, a patient with Broca's aphasia, was seen in our speech clinic eight years after suffering a gunshot wound to the left frontal-parietal area. He was 33 years old, married with two children, and employed full-time. He had a dense right hemiplegia, a right homonymous hemianopsia, and severe aphasia. He received speech and language treatment almost continuously for nearly four years at a clinic near his home. He made significant gains during that time, although his communicative skills remained severely impaired. He requested, and we consented to, a 30-day trial of intensive speech and language treatment.

Our initial evaluation revealed a moderate to severe aphasia crossing all modalities but demonstrably more severe in expressive modalities. Performance on the PICA was at the 49th percentile. Gestural performance, which included reading, pantomime, and auditory comprehension, was at the 47th percentile; verbal performance was at the 48th percentile, and writing at the 51st percentile. The mean of his performance on his nine 'best' subtests was 13.11, and the mean of his nine lowest subtest scores was 7.82, yielding a performance gap of 5.30. His poorest performance was on the writing and speaking tasks, and his best performance on copying, reading, listening, and gestural tasks. Performance on the Word Fluency Measure yielded a total score of 2, well below the 10th percentile for aphasic adults. On the Colored Progressive Matrices, he achieved a score of 27 correct of 36 possible, placing him at the 60th percentile for aphasic adults and between the 20th and 30th percentiles for normal males his age. He had inordinate difficulty with the Token Test, scoring 5 of a possible 61, yet made no errors on subtests 6 and 10 of the PICA, yielding an average score for these two subtests of 12.85. His profile on the Boston Diagnostic Aphasia Examination is shown in Figure 4.1. On the Standard Speech Sample, vowel prolongation was within normal limits; rapid alternating movements were somewhat slow and distorted (3.9

RATING SCALE PROFILE OF SPEECH CHARACTERISTICS

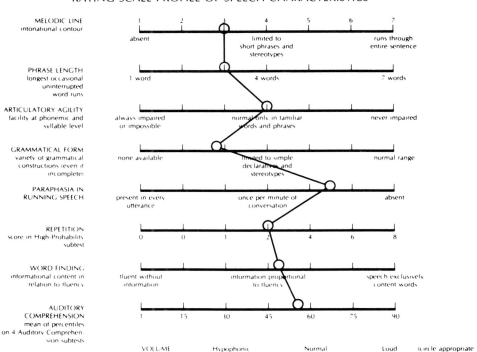

Figure 4.1   *BDAE profile for the patient with Broca's aphasia*

per second) and he was unable to produce /pʌ/, /tʌ/, or /kʌ/ in combination. Polysyllabic words were inordinately difficult for him, and more difficult phrases, such as 'Methodist Episcopal Church' were impossible. Monosyllabic words were produced accurately and intelligibly with occasional slight distortions. Picture description and reading aloud elicited distorted, telegraphic, and awkwardly articulated phrases. Most single word productions, except the few he was able to revise or correct, were scored as boxed 7 or distorted, i.e., 14. He was unable to repeat or generate an entire sentence, and scores on subtest 1 of the PICA, object description, reflected this, often yielding scores of boxed 12, reflecting distorted productions of incomplete sentences. The tests of oral, nonverbal and limb apraxia revealed severe deficits in planning and sequencing movements. Performance improved significantly with imitation but was never perfect.

Our evaluation revealed moderate deficits in auditory processing, a moderate to severe apraxia of speech, and severe deficits in the formulation of oral-verbal output. His speech was strikingly telegraphic, with inconsistent omission of pronouns, verbs, and adjectives. His primary mode of communication at that time was oral, but syntax and grammar were grossly impaired, and verbal communication was only minimally functional, often quite delayed, and only approximated his intended communication. Writing was also grossly impaired, and did not provide an adequate means of communication. His profile, we feel, is most comparable to that of a 'big' Broca's aphasia (Mohr *et al.*, 1978). Despite his chronic aphasia, we felt he was a good treatment candidate. We initiated a program of intensive speech and language treatment with an emphasis on oral production of phrases and sentences. His performance justified our optimism. He improved an average of 41 per cent on all treatment tasks, and his last PICA, given one month after we initiated treatment, improved 16 percentile units, i.e., to the 65th percentile. Additionally, his wife reported at follow-up that he was using the phone more, spoke in more complete sentences, responded more quickly and more appropriately, and seemed pleased with his gains. The intent that clinical gains translate into functional gains seems to have been at least partially realized. The real test of those gains was in his ability to retain them over time.

Apraxia of speech

Patient GF was 53 years old when he suffered a left frontal CVA. On initial evaluation, approximately three weeks post onset, his speech and language deficits were moderate. Overall performance on the PICA was at the 59th percentile, 65th on gestural, 51st on verbal, and 61st in graphic modalities. He was ambulatory and oriented, and he described his communication problems at that time as forgetting some words and not being able to say what he wanted. He denied problems understanding and, in fact, only when material was long or complex did his deficits emerge. His score of 18 of 61 correct on the Token Test was below the 10th percentile for males his age. Reading comprehension was intact for single words and simple sentences but poor for paragraph-length material. Speech was hesitant and effortful, with revisions and substitutions predominating. He scored 23 on the Colored Progressive Matrices and 5 on the Word Fluency Measure. Oral, nonverbal movements were moderately compromised. Several productions were augmented by inappropriate accompanying sounds or words, e.g., 'whistle' on attempts to whistle. Most attempts were initially wrong

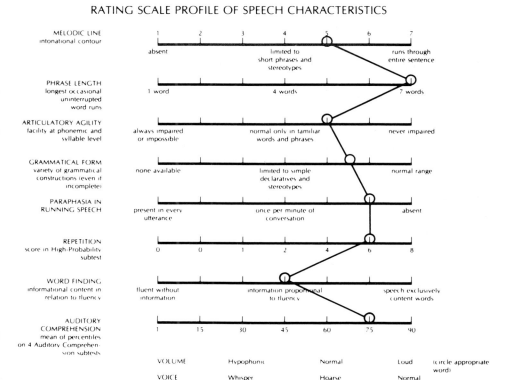

RATING SCALE PROFILE OF SPEECH CHARACTERISTICS

Figure 4.2   BDAE profile for the patient with apraxia of speech

and marked by repeated, awkward and groping attempts, only two of which approximated the intended gesture. Performance on the BDAE, shown in Figure 4.2, was within the range for mild Broca's aphasia, and is probably consistent with a diagnosis of 'little' Broca's aphasia (Mohr *et al.*, 1978).

A conservative prognosis, based on his general good health, relative youth, and recency of onset, told us that this man would probably improve substantially. This behavioral profile approach to prediction of recovery was corroborated by Porch's (1973) High Overall Prediction (HOAP) and was confirmed by the patient's recovery. Therapy was directed toward:

1 Expanding length of utterance
2 Improving auditory comprehension for complex materials
3 Recognition of errors

4 Improving ability to generate written sentences spontaneously
5 Improving referential reading comprehension
6 Improving word-finding
7 Stabilizing initial sibilants and fricatives.

At two months post onset his overall performance on the PICA was at the 88th percentile. Word fluency improved to 30, Token Test performance to 43 of 61, and Colored Progressive Matrices performance to 28. His most prominent residual deficit was in speech. No longer telegraphic, he spoke in full, complete sentences which were marked by initiation difficulty, and very occasional revisions, distortions, and substitutions. He consistently recognized his errors, and was generally able to correct them with one or two attempts. Despite his excellent recovery, he returned to work only temporarily. His work was stressful and demanding, and he found the lure of an early, comfortable retirement more appealing. At last test, he had held his gains.

Conduction aphasia

Patient EG was a 60-year-old retired United States Army Sergeant who suffered a left parietal lobe lesion. At our initial evaluation, one week post onset, he was globally aphasic or nearly so. He was unable to point to pictures or follow simple commands involving body parts or objects in the room. Observation of conversation with his wife suggested that he recognized some familiar, key words such as his daughter's name, but there was no evidence to suggest that he could understand the details or complexities of the discussion. He was unable at that time to match single words to pictures or point to words when named. More complex reading was impossible, and he could not copy single words or letters. Speech was limited but what speech he did have suggested that he would not remain globally aphasic. He used some phrases consistently, such as 'I don't know what happened'. Most of his replies to questions were neologistic jargon, and ended in frustrated silence. Although he seemed to recognize his errors, his attempts to correct them were excruciating for him and his listeners. He was unable to follow enough commands to take part in formal testing for oral, nonverbal and limb apraxia, but imitated several oral and limb gestures accurately and promptly. He was not hemiplegic, and manual strength tested several days post onset was nearly within normal limits.

His medical condition improved and, at approximately one month post onset, we were able to complete much of our evaluation. Overall

performance on the PICA was at the 21st percentile, gestural performance at the 18th, verbal performance at the 22nd, and graphic performance at the 39th. He rejected naming and object description tasks, and
without exception produced literal paraphasic responses or neologisms
regardless of the task, for example 'helicaliper' for 'helicopter', 'opticus'
for 'octopus', and 'caluna' for 'canoe'. He rejected the more difficult
reading subtests, but was correct on 8 of 10 items on the easier reading
tasks. Auditory comprehension scores averaged 10.25. He was unable
to write spontaneously, but copied 4 of 10 words correctly, and 7 of 10
geometric shapes and letters correctly. Most oral, nonverbal, and limb
praxis responses were prompt and accurate. His tolerance for testing
and for his deficits was minimal, and testing proceeded slowly.

At two months post onset, objective test scores had nearly
doubled, to the 41st percentile. Writing was still impossible for him,
but he could copy accurately. Responses to the auditory and reading
comprehension subtests were prompt and accurate, and scores on the
pantomime subtests improved significantly. The verbal subtests continued to be difficult for him. Responses to confrontation naming were
fluently produced, with fewer neologisms. Literal paraphasias continued to predominate, but were closer approximations of the target.
Repetition of monosyllabic words was now generally accurate, but
longer words were much more difficult. At six months post onset,
overall performance on the PICA approached the 50th percentile.
Performance on the auditory comprehension portion of the BDAE had
improved dramatically — of 119 points possible, he obtained a score of
107, and no z-score fell into the negative range. His performance on the
BDAE yielded a profile of speech characteristics which was typical of
that seen for conduction aphasia. His most recent profile is shown in
Figure 4.3. His literal paraphasias were prominent in connected speech
and naming, but his struggles were less effortful, and often several
attempts would yield an accurate response. His life is apparently
rewarding and fulfilling. He is a volunteer at the hospital, and communicates functionally with hospital personnel and patients.

Patient comparisons

Several important factors differentiated these three patients; they are
summarized in Table 4.5. Some of these factors were identifiable close
to onset, and several did not emerge until months after onset. One or
two only emerged retrospectively and with more fine-grained analysis.

RATING SCALE PROFILE OF SPEECH CHARACTERISTICS

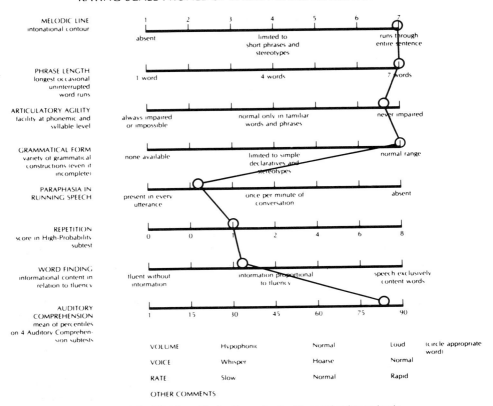

Figure 4.3   BDAE profile for the patient with conduction aphasia

Auditory comprehension

Auditory comprehension scores for most of our patients with Broca's aphasia have been near or above the 30th percentile initially. They improve with physiological recovery and that recovery is enhanced by treatment. Some improve more than others. Auditory comprehension for patient DF improved from the 29th to the 40th percentile as measured by the PICA, suggesting a more moderate to severe aphasia. Auditory comprehension has remained near that level at revaluations over several years. His failure to improve more substantially is in all likelihood related to his more extensive lesion. The relationship of size of lesion and recovery from aphasia is, however, beyond the scope of this chapter.

Auditory comprehension in apraxia of speech was impaired but

Table 4.5: *Summary of Features Differentiating Conduction Aphasia, Apraxia of Speech, and Broca's Aphasia*

	Broca's	Conduction	AOS
Auditory comprehension	5	5	1
Reading comprehension	5	6	2
Writing	6	6	2
Oral, nonverbal apraxia	5	0	3
Limb apraxia	4	3	1
Naming	4	6	1
Literal paraphasia	3	6	3
Verbal paraphasia	2	2	2
Neologisms		5	1

0 = absence of symptom
1 = mild
7 = severe

functional initially, and improved rapidly in several weeks to near normal levels.

Auditory comprehension in conduction aphasia was severely impaired initially, possibly because of the proximity of the lesion to the temporal lobe, unobserved infiltration into the temporal lobe, or long-reaching metabolic effects on the temporal lobe. Auditory comprehension resolved slowly, but eventually reached near-normal levels of performance.

In general, initial auditory comprehension scores did not differentiate among these patients as clearly as they did several months post onset. The clearest distinctions were between conduction aphasia and Broca's aphasia, and apraxia of speech.

Reading comprehension

Reading comprehension for DF, our Broca's aphasic patient, was at the 44th percentile initially as measured by the PICA and reached the 62nd percentile when we last tested him. The PICA reading comprehension subtests yielded a percentile of 65 at approximately three weeks post onset for our apraxia of speech patient. When we assessed those abilities near the end of treatment, at ten months post onset, performance was at the 99th percentile.

Reading comprehension for our patient with conduction aphasia was severely impaired initially, at the 22nd percentile, and resolved slowly and gradually. When last tested formally, performance had reached the 66th percentile.

Writing

Writing for our Broca's aphasic patient was severely impaired initially. Even incomplete sentences were virtually impossible for him, and he either rejected writing the task or produced one word, usually a noun. When last tested, writing had improved. As Figure 4.4 shows, his writing communicates despite the severity of his deficit. Written performance in apraxia of speech was moderately impaired initially, but became functional rapidly. At three weeks post onset, responses were telegraphic and related semantically ('knife it' for knife) but nearly unintelligible. They suggested, however, that with even minor improvement these responses would move into the 'correct' range. They did. At just over a month post onset he could write an occasional, grammatically incorrect sentence ('Used to quarter to spend it') in which the majority of letters were intelligible. At two months post onset he wrote 'The quarter I can spend with it', and at six months post onset wrote, 'I use a quarter to buy things'. Responses by then were somewhat distorted motorically, but intelligible.

Writing for our conduction aphasic patient was severely impaired

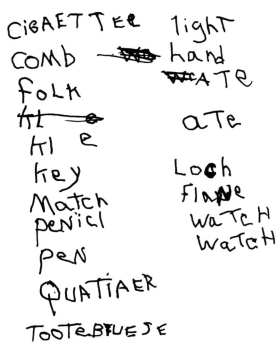

Figure 4.4 Writing sample for the patient with Broca's aphasia

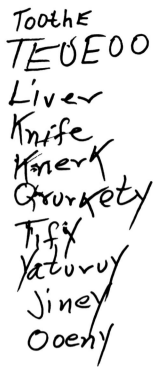

Figure 4.5 Writing sample for the patient with conduction aphasia

initially. Because of his severe deficit, our patient rejected most difficult writing tasks. He could copy five of five simple words correctly at five weeks post onset, and at two months post onset could copy the same words flawlessly, but he was unable to write even simple words to dictation. It was not until nearly a year post onset that he was able to write some simple words and phrases to dictation and produce a few words spontaneously. Writing was never distorted motorically. His writing never became functional. When last tested, he produced the examples shown in Figure 4.5.

Verbal expression

Intonational contours, grammatical form, and phrase length in our Broca's aphasia patient were severely reduced, and speech was telegraphic. Paraphasias were present, but infrequently, and, when they were produced, they were frequently self-corrected. Repetition was impaired but performance on these tasks was superior to spontaneous productions. Articulatory agility was normal only in familiar words and phrases, and word-finding was severely impaired, as evidenced by performance on the Word Fluency Measure and in naming tasks. The patient demonstrated a severe, oral nonverbal apraxia, and limb praxis was only slightly better. This performance was not significantly related to weakness or slowness of the peripheral musculature.

The patient with apraxia of speech produced a modest repertoire of intonational contours and grammatical forms. Phrase length was very close to normal, but interrupted by groping and self-correction. Speech was dysprosodic and marked by a damping of the intonational contour and frequent distortion of initial phonemes and, somewhat less frequently, vowels. Literal paraphasias were rare. When they occurred they were close approximations which were, with few exceptions, corrected. This patient successfully employed a 'conduite d'approche', or zeroing in, in which with repeated attempts at a target, he achieved closer and closer approximations. (See Chapter 2 for discussion of 'conduite d'approche'.) Word finding ability did not reach normal levels of performance, but nearly so. Naming was rarely inaccurate. Generally, PICA scores ranged from '7', a close approximation to the target, to '14', indicating some distortion of the response, to a normal response, '15'.

The patient with conduction aphasia had a normal variety of intonational contours and grammatical forms available. Phrase lengths were normal. Speech was marked by extended neologistic jargon in the early stages of recovery. In later stages, speech was frequently fluent and error-free. When errors did occur, they were most frequently literal paraphasias and, rarely, neologistic jargon. Examples of neologisms included 'nobly' for door, 'lale' for bike, and 'beeon' for blanket. Examples of literal paraphasias included 'razlr' for razor, 'legr' for leg, 'watchli' for watch, and 'skop' for stop. The patient was frequently unable to correct these literal paraphasias. Repetition was frequently impossible, although greater success on familiar words and phrases was achieved. Speech was also marked by a greater number of verbal paraphasias than for the apraxia of speech patient or the Broca's aphasia patient, including 'soup' for soap, 'coughing' for smoking, or, in more extended contexts, 'I got one from home' for 'I got home from work'.

Perhaps the single most striking feature of his speech was the seeming inability to profit from either a model or his own off-target productions of the target. If the initial response was a close approximation to the target, the target was achieved in the next several attempts. If not, he was as likely to move away from the target as he was to move toward it. (This observed behavior is not in agreement with the literature reviewed in Chapter 2.) For 'eraser', for example, he produced 'eraner', 'encra', 'enca', and then 'enaple'. Nevertheless, responses were seldom perseverative, and the variety of phonemes produced revealed a phoneme pool which was undiminished. Frequency of occurrence was not a good predictor of repetition performance. Performances on oral, nonverbal and limb tasks, whether requested or initiated, were within normal limits.

Conclusion

These critical factors allowed us to differentiate these patients. Differences were camouflaged initially by severity, but became increasingly prominent. Repetition was inordinately impaired for the patient with conduction aphasia, less so for the Broca's patient, and least for the apraxia of speech patient. Oral, nonverbal and limb apraxia was severe in the Broca's patient, mild in the apraxia of speech patient and in the conduction aphasia patient. Auditory comprehension was most impaired in the Broca's patient, less impaired in the conduction aphasia patient, and essentially normal in the apraxia of speech patient.

With the possible exception of the patient with apraxia of speech, the syndromes these patients presented were not readily identifiable initially, but revealed themselves with the passage of time. We are reluctant to say that their diagnoses were apparent, or that all would agree with our conclusions. We feel strongly, however, that their diagnoses dictated individualized approaches to treatment. That is the most compelling reason for accurate, differential diagnoses. Selection of treatment approaches for patients with coexisting apraxia of speech and aphasia is the topic addressed in the next chapter by Tonkovich and Peach.

References

BLUMSTEIN, S.E., COOPER, W.E. and ZURIF, E.B. (1977) 'The perception and production of voice-onset time in aphasia', *Neuropsychologia,* **15**, pp. 871–82.

BORKOWSKI, J.G., BENTON, A.L. and SPREEN, O. (1967) 'Word fluency and brain damage', *Neuropsychologia,* **5**, pp. 135–40.

CANTER, G.J. (1969) 'The influence of primary and secondary verbal apraxia on output disturbances in aphasic syndromes'. Paper presented to the American Speech and Hearing Association in Chicago, Illinois, (unpublished).

COLLINS, M., CARISKI, D., LONGSTRETH, D. and ROSENBEK, J. (1980) 'Patterns of articulatory behavior in selected motor speech programming disorders', in BROOKSHIRE, R. (Ed.) *Clinical Aphasiology: Conference Proceedings*, Minneapolis, BRK Publishers, pp. 196–208.

DABUL, B. (1979) *Apraxia Battery for Adults*, Tigard, OR: CC Publications.

DARLEY, F.L. (1982) *Aphasia*. Philadelphia, W.B. Saunders.

DARLEY, F.L., ARONSON, A.E. and BROWN, J.R. (1975) *Motor Speech Disorders*. Philadelphia, W.B. Saunders Company.

DERENZI, E. and VIGNOLO, L.A. (1962) 'The Token Test: A sensitive test to detect disturbances in aphasia', *Brain*, **85**, pp. 665–78.

DEUTSCH, S. (1984) 'Prediction of site of lesion from speech apraxic error patterns', in ROSENBEK, J., MCNEIL, M. and ARONSON, A. (Eds.) *Apraxia of Speech: Physiology-Acoustic-Linguistics-Management*, San Diego, College-Hill Press.

FROMM, D., ABBS, J., MCNEIL, M. and ROSENBEK, J. (1982) 'Simultaneous perceptual–physiological method for studying apraxia of speech', in BROOKSHIRE, R. (Ed.) *Clinical Aphasiology: Conference Proceedings*, Minneapolis, BRK Publishers, pp. 251–62.

GESCHWIND, N. (1965) 'Disconnection syndromes in animals and man', *Brain*, **33**, pp. 237–94.

GOODGLASS, H. and KAPLAN, E. (1983) *The Assessment of Aphasia and Related Disorders*, Philadelphia, Lea and Febiger.

HANNA, G., SCHELL, L.M. and SCHREINER, R. (1977) *The Nelson Reading Skills Test*. Chicago: Riverside Publishing.

ITOH, M., SASANUMA, S., HIROSE, H., YOSHIOKA, H. and USHIJIMA, T. (1980) 'Abnormal articulatory dynamics in a patient with apraxia of speech: X-ray microbeam observation', *Brain and Language*, **11**, pp. 66–75.

ITOH, M., SASANUMA, S., TATSUMA, I.F., MURAKAMI, S., FUKASAKI, Y. and SUZUKI, T. (1982) 'Voice onset time characteristics in apraxia of speech', *Brain and Language*, **17**, pp. 193–8.

JOHNS, D. and DARLEY, F.L. (1970) 'Phonemic variability in apraxia of speech', *Journal of Speech and Hearing Research*, **13**, pp. 556–83.

KEATLEY, M. and PIKE, P. (1976) 'An automated pulmonary function laboratory: Clinical use in determining respiratory variations in apraxia', in BROOKSHIRE, R. (Ed.) *Clinical Aphasiology: Conference Proceedings*. Minneapolis: BRK Publishers, pp. 98–109.

KENT, R.D. (1976) 'Models of speech production', in LASS, N. (Ed.) *Contemporary Issues in Experimental Phonetics*. New York: Academic Press.

KENT, R and ROSENBEK, J. (1983) 'Acoustic patterns of apraxia of speech', *Journal of Speech and Hearing Research*, **26**, pp. 231–49.

KERTESZ, A. (1982) *Western Aphasia Battery*. New York: Grune and Stratton.

LaPOINTE, L.L. and HORNER, J. (1979) *Reading Comprehension Battery for Aphasia*. Tigard, OR: CC Publications.

LURIA, A.R. (1966) *Higher Cortical Functions in Man*, New York, Basic Books.

MacDONALD, E.T. (1964) *A Deep Test of Articulation: Sentence Form*, Pittsburgh, Stanwix House.

McNEIL, M. (1988) 'Review of Boston Diagnostic Aphasia Examination (BDAE)', in *Tenth Mental Measurements Yearbook*, Buros Institute of Mental Measurements, Lincoln, NE (in press).

MCNEIL, M.R. and PRESCOTT, T.E. (1978) *Revised Token Test*, Baltimore, University Park Press.

MACNEILAGE, P.F. (1981) 'Speech production mechanisms in aphasia', in GRILLNER, S., LINDBLOOM, B., LUBKER, J. and PERRSON, A. (Eds.) *Speech Motor Control*, London, Pergamon.

MOHR, J., PESSIN, M., FINKELSTEIN, S., FUNKENSTEIN, H., DUNCAN, G. and DAVIS, K. (1978) 'Broca aphasia: Pathologic and clinical aspects', *Neurology*, **28**, pp. 311–24.

NICHOLAS, L., MACLENNAN, D. and BROOKSHIRE, R. (1985) 'Validity of multi-sentence reading comprehension subtests in aphasia tests', in BROOKSHIRE, R. (Ed.) *Clinical Aphasiology: Conference Proceedings*, Minneapolis, BRK Publishers, pp. 196–208.

PORCH, B. (1967) *The Porch Index of Communicative Ability*, Palo Alto, CA, Consulting Psychologists Press.

PORCH, B. (1973) PICA Workshop, Albuquerque, NM.

PORCH, B. (1983) *The Porch Index of Communicative Ability*, Palo Alto, CA, Consulting Psychologists Press.

RAVEN, J.C. (1962) *Colored Progressive Matrices*, London, H.K. Lewis.

ROSENBEK, J.C. and WERTZ, R.T. (1976) 'Treatment of apraxia of speech in adults', in WERTZ, R.T. and COLLINS, M.J. (Eds.) *Clinical Aphasiology: Conference Proceedings*, Madison, Wis., BRK Publishers, pp. 83–8.

ROY, E. and SQUARE, P. (1985) 'Error/movement notation systems in apraxia', *Semiotic Inquiry*, **5**, pp. 402–12.

SHANKWEILER, D., HARRIS, K.S. and TAYLOR, M.L. (1968) 'Electromyographic studies of articulation in aphasia', *Archives of Physical Medicine and Rehabilitation*, **49**, pp. 1–8.

SQUARE, P., DARLEY, F.L. and SOMMERS, R.I. (1981) 'Speech perception among patients demonstrating apraxia of speech, aphasia, and both disorders', in BROOKSHIRE, R. (Ed.) *Clinical Aphasiology: Conference Proceedings*, Minneapolis, BRK Publishers, pp. 83–8.

SQUARE, P., DARLEY, F.L. and SOMMERS, R.I. (1982) 'An analysis of the productive errors made by pure apractic speakers with differing loci of lesions', in BROOKSHIRE, R. (Ed.) *Clinical Aphasiology: Conference Proceedings*, Minneapolis, BRK Publishers, pp. 245–50.

SQUARE-STORER, P.A. (1987) 'Acquired apraxia of speech', in WINITZ, H. (Ed.) *Human Communication: A Review*, New York, Ablex Publishing, pp. 88–165.

WERTZ, R.T., KEITH, R. and CUSTER, D.D. (1971) 'Normal and aphasic behavior on a measure of auditory input and a measure of verbal output'. Paper presented to the American Speech and Hearing Association, Chicago, Il.

WERTZ, R.T., ROSENBEK, J. and COLLINS, M. (1972) 'Identification of apraxia of speech from PICA verbal tests and selected oral-verbal apraxia tests', in BROOKSHIRE, R. (Ed.) *Clinical Aphasiology: Collected Conference Proceedings, 1972–1976*, Minneapolis, BRK Publishers, pp. 119–23.

WERTZ, R., ROSENBEK, J. and DEAL, J. (1970) 'A review of 228 cases of apraxia of speech: Classification, etiology, and localization'. Paper presented to the American Speech and Hearing Association, New York.

WERTZ, R.T., COLLINS, M., WEISS, D., KURTZKE, J., FRIDEN, T., BROOKSHIRE,

R., PIERCE, J., HOLTZAPPLE, P., HUBBARD, D., PORCH, B., WEST, J., DAVIS, L., MATOVICH, V., MORLEY, G. and RESURRECCION, E. (1981) 'Veterans Administration cooperative study on aphasia: A comparison of individual and group treatment', *Journal of Speech and Hearing Research,* **24,** pp. 580–94.

Chapter 5

What to Treat: Apraxia of Speech, Aphasia, or Both

John Tonkovich and Richard Peach

For the past decade or so, clinicians developing treatment programs for apraxia of speech have been confronted with an array of unresolved conflicts regarding the description of the disorder, its underlying mechanisms, and influencing variables. For instance, when sampling the contemporary as well as historical (see Chapter 1) literature related to apraxia of speech, one finds a diversity of terms including among others aphemia, anarthria, apraxia, apraxic dysarthria, cortical dysarthria, motor aphasia, verbal aphasia, and little Broca aphasia which have been attributed to essentially the same phenomenon (Darley, 1967; Johns and Darley, 1970; Johns and LaPointe, 1976; Mohr *et al.* 1978; Schiff *et al.* 1983; Rosenbek, Kent and LaPointe, 1984; Wertz, LaPointe and Rosenbek, 1984). Considering the apparent confusion created by these disparate labels referring to articulatory deficits of a seemingly common basis, confusion in the clinical treatment of the disorder has also existed.

Liberal usage of the term, 'apraxia of speech' to refer to all surface articulatory disorders resulting from motor speech programming deficits (Canter, 1969; Wertz, Rosenbek and Deal, 1970; Buckingham, 1979; Deutsch, 1984) also has been as misleading to the clinician and others as have been denials of the existence of apraxia of speech in favor of a general notion of aphasic phonological impairment. One attempt to clarify this issue is represented by Canter's (1973) description of apraxia of speech as a primary verbal apraxia while another articulatory disturbance, literal paraphasia, is alternately described as a secondary verbal apraxia. Yet these distinctions are obscured in recent findings which document the existence of these separate forms of articulatory deficits but characterize these phenomena as a unitary disorder, i.e., apraxia of speech (Deutsch, 1984) (see also Chapter 2).

Some have argued that the misarticulations observed in apractic speech occur only as a function of disrupted motor programming (e.g.,

Darley, 1968; Darley, Aronson and Brown, 1975). Others maintain that while the symptom itself reflects poor motor programming for speech, the misarticulations are influenced to a large extent by linguistic variables (e.g. Deal and Darley, 1972; Hardison, Marquardt and Peterson, 1977). Still others deny the existence of apraxia of speech and attempt to account for the prototypical misarticulations by attributing them to a more central aphasic impairment (Martin, 1974; Martin and Rigrodsky, 1974).

In this chapter, we attempt to reconcile some of these differences insofar as they relate to treatment programs for the apractic/aphasic patient. The neuropsychological mechanisms underlying speech production are reviewed with special reference to the conditions which result in apraxia of speech. Language variables that interact with apractic speech production are discussed to demonstrate how the selection of treatment stimuli may facilitate or impede successful speech production. Guidelines for treatment decisions and clinical methodologies are presented for patients with concomitant apraxia of speech and aphasia.

Neuropsychological Mechanisms

Neuroanatomical models

The key principles in models of speech production remain largely derived from the work of Flechsig (1901). More recent descriptions of speech and language syndromes based upon Flechsig's work have been provided by Geschwind (1965a, b). Classifying cortical regions according to their chronological stages of myelinization, Flechsig identified three groups and described them as follows: early developing regions called primordial zones, intermediate developing regions called intermediate zones, and late developing regions called terminal zones. In more contemporary terminology, the primordial, intermediate, and terminal zones have been described as primary, secondary association, and tertiary cortical areas, respectively. Two groups of white matter fibers, projection and association, were also identified. The primary areas are characterized by numerous long projection fibers leading to and from areas outside the cortex. Short association fibers are found projecting to secondary association areas contiguous to the earlier developing primary areas. Areas said to be further apart are connected by long association fibers. From these observations Flechsig inferred that:

1 Primary zones neither send nor receive long connections to other parts of the cortex, their only connections being to secondary zones
2 Secondary zones receive input from several cortical areas and transmit information to areas farther away.

With regard to speech and language functions, sensory inputs from auditory, visual, and tactile stimuli are received by the cortex in the dominant hemisphere at their respective primary areas. These areas correspond to the transverse gyrus of the temporal lobe (Heschl's gyrus) for audition, the postcentral gyrus of the parietal lobe for somesthesia, and the calcarine cortex of the occipital lobe for vision. Since primary areas have secondary association areas as their only cortical connections, the sensory input is transmitted to these secondary association areas for interpretation and elaboration. Included here are the posterior, superior temporal lobe (Wernicke's area) for auditory association, the superior parietal lobule for somesthetic association, and the cuneus and lingual gyrus of the occipital lobe for visual association.

Language, being essentially an auditory event, requires the participation of Wernicke's area to provide information relevant to the interpretation of stimulus meaning for understanding and the guidance of other cortical regions for expression. When cross–modal associations are required for language formulation, as in naming an object which is seen or felt or reading a word aloud, secondary association areas transmit their distinct information to tertiary cortex to integrate these sensory impressions. The inferior parietal lobule, composed of the supramarginal gyrus and the angular gyrus, constitute this region of cortex which, because of these functions, has been called an 'association area of association areas' (Geschwind, 1965a).

As a pivotal region responsible for sensory integration, it has also been noted that the inferior parietal lobule acts as the center for 'the conversion of meaningful content into language for exteriorization' (Darley, Aronson and Brown, 1975). In this respect, the inferior parietal lobule uses its access to the auditory, visual, and tactile association areas to formulate appropriate sensory representations which will provide the basis for subsequent oral and written expression.

For expression, the sensory information is forwarded over the arcuate fasciculus, a long association fiber pathway, to secondary association areas in the frontal lobe responsible for motor encoding of language output. These regions are recognized as Broca's area and Exner's area for speech and writing, respectively. To Broca's area falls the function of transducing these sensory impulses to a series of motor impulses which will program the musculature for the intended speech movements of a given output. This task is carried out over the upper motor neuron system of the primary motor area which in turn provides input to the lower motor neurons of the oral–facial masculature.

In essence then, language requires conceptualization and sensory representation of the intended output in posterior areas, forwarded transmission of the sensory information by means of association pathways to anterior regions for motor programming, and projection of the commands from anterior areas to the musculature for execution of the output (Canter, 1973). The language mechanisms which subsume the functions delegated here to specific cortical regions for language conceptualization and representation have been designated the central language processor and the auditory speech processing systems while the select programming of neural directions for motor execution has been called the motor speech programmer (Darley, Aronson and Brown 1975).

Neurofunctional systems and apraxia of speech

Intracortical approaches

As one views the process of speech and language production, it is evident that a failure in the transmission of information required for normal output can occur due to disruptions at one of several stages in the sequence. Damage to particular cortical regions which underlie critical functions will result in deterioration of those functions, while impairment of an association pathway due to cortical lesion, will prevent adequate transmission of information between cortical regions. While faulty motor programming of speech may occur in either situation, some writers have argued that apraxia of speech, as a true disorder of volitional movement, only occurs following damage to the specific cortical region responsible for motor speech programming, i.e. Broca's area. Others have claimed that articulatory errors resulting from disruption of fiber pathways or posterior regions providing guidance to anterior regions via association fiber pathways, are also apractic in nature. These two positions have been referred to as the center lesion and disconnection approaches (Buckingham, 1979). One need only reflect on the qualitatively different neurological deficits which contribute to types of phoneme production errors to conclude that *apraxia of speech results from impairment of specific mechanisms, anteriorly located, which perform the requirements of transducing sensory information to motor impulses for phoneme production.* Phonemic errors which result from deficient sensory guidance of motor programming due to association pathway disruption or auditory association impairment are not equivalent to apraxia of speech and as such are considered separate from apraxia of speech. We believe that these phoneme errors are best termed 'literal paraphasias'.

Integrative accounts

Apraxia of speech resulting from infarction limited to deep white matter and basal ganglia structures has been demonstrated based upon the more sophisticated localization techniques provided by CT scanning. Square and Mlcoch (1983), Peach and Tonkovich (1983, 1984), and Kertesz (1984) have presented cases in which apraxia and/or apraxia of speech with aphasia have been documented without cortical extension of these lesions. Kertesz (1984) has proposed an explanation for these findings. The putamen and the caudate nucleus comprise the striatum and receive input over projections arising from virtually all cortical regions, the substantia nigra, the intralaminar nuclei of the thalamus and the raphe nuclei of the midline brainstem (Brodal, 1981). Output projections of the striatum are primarily to the globus pallidus and the substantia nigra. Fibers from the globus pallidus project to the thalamus which has numerous reciprocal connections with the cortex. As a central structure in the integration of afferent and efferent impulses associated with skilled motor movements, the striatum is also said to integrate intention and perception into movement (Hassler, 1978 as cited by Kertesz, 1984). According to Kertesz, the basal ganglia '...can be assumed to play a special role in the sequential integration of the complex activity of speech' (p. 89). Damage to these subcortical nuclei therefore effectively inhibits performance of these integrative functions while damage to white matter structures interrupts the pathways over which articulatory information is transmitted.

Sensory-perceptual descriptions

Speech output is continuously monitored for accuracy by analyses of sensory information derived from auditory, tactile, and proprioceptive sources (Mlcoch and Noll, 1980). Deficits in motor speech production might logically derive, therefore, from reduced or altered feedback of impaired sensory systems. As such, this component has been invest- igated to determine whether sensory disturbances significantly con- tribute to the speech production deficits in apractic speakers and if so, to characterize the nature of those disturbances.

Auditory perceptual processing among apractic patients has been studied by Aten, Johns and Darley (1971), Square-Storer, Darley and Sommers (1988), and Hoit-Dalgaard, Murry and Kopp (1983). In the Aten, Johns and Darley study, phoneme discrimination was assessed by requiring patients to point to pictures corresponding to auditory sequences of two- and three-word lengths with minimal phoneme variations. Two general performance patterns emerged from the results: patients who demonstrated at most mild disturbances, if any, and patients who performed significantly worse than other apractic patients. Based upon the observations that some apractic patients showed little difficulty on this phoneme discrimination task, the authors concluded that auditory feedback deficits cannot be associated to any large degree with the phoneme production difficulties of apractic patients. Square- Storer, Darley and Sommers (1988) presented an extensive battery of auditory and speech perceptual tests to four groups of subjects: pure apractic speakers, aphasic patients without apraxia, aphasic patients with apraxia, and normal subjects. The major content areas of these tests included auditory and speech sequencing tasks, speech discrimina- tion tasks, recognition and sequencing tasks, and internal speech discrimination tasks. The results suggested that apractic patients with no aphasia process auditory information similarly to normal speakers, at least insofar as the types of processing assessed in this study. The aphasic patients performed at a level significantly below that of apractic and normal speakers. Further support for the conclusions of Aten, Johns and Darley were therefore provided by this investigation but with the stronger evidence of a more comprehensive test battery. Hoit-Dalgaard, Murray and Kopp (1983) assessed apractic subjects' perception of voice onset time (VOT). Synthetic speech stimuli con- taining 38 VOT variants representing the voicing continuum for the cognates 'bees-peas' were used in this study. Subjects pointed to pictures (either 'bees' or 'peas') to indicate which initial consonant had been perceived. Of the five subjects performing this task, perceptual boundaries between the cognates were established for only three subjects. The relationship between perception and production was directly examined for these three subjects by comparing their percep- tual judgments with VOT productions for the same cognates. The results demonstrated the normal pattern of VOT productions within the corresponding perceptual region for only one of the three subjects.

These authors concluded that 'VOT perception and production in apractic speakers are neither congruent nor predictable' (p. 337). Generally, therefore, these studies cumulatively suggest that apraxia of speech is not related to sensory disturbances of auditory processing.

Oral sensation and perception in apractic patients was investigated by Rosenbek, Wertz and Darley (1973) to determine the occurrence of tactile-kinesthetic impairment and its relationship to apraxia of speech. The test battery included oral form identification, two-point discrimination, and mandibular kinesthesia. Three groups of subjects were tested: apractic patients with aphasia, aphasic patients without apraxia, and normal subjects. Collectively, apractic patients demonstrated more errors on these sensory-perceptual tasks than did aphasic or normal subjects. However, the apractic subjects actually comprised two separate groups: one with oral sensory-perceptual deficit and one with normal oral sensation and perception. These findings were related to the overall severity of apractic impairment: the more severe the apraxia, the more poorly the patient performed on these tasks. It was concluded that sensory deficits underlie the errors made by apractic speakers and may characterize specific kinds of errors such as phoneme distortions.

Apparently, what is more at issue in these findings is the interpretation of group trends at the expense of individual differences within apractic patients. That apractic patients are observed without oral sensory-perceptual deficits should be viewed strongly as evidence for arguments which maintain a classically motoric basis for the disorder. It is not surprising that the tactile-kinesthetic deficits of these apractic speakers varied with the severity of their impairment. Severity of involvement is commonly associated with the size or extent of lesion. More severely apractic speech likely resulted from larger lesions of motor association cortex relative to that of the less severely apractic patients. Given these larger lesions, it is likely that more posterior extension of the lesion into postcentral sensory areas could account for these patients' accompanying perceptual deficits. The distinction recognizes oral sensory-perceptual deficits as a reasonable *coexisting* impairment with apraxia of speech without attributing a partial basis for the apractic disorder to sensory difficulties. The investigators did qualify that sensory deficits cannot account for the phoneme selection and sequencing problems characteristic of apraxia of speech. Also, their particular reference to phoneme distortions, a relatively less frequently occurring variant of perceived apractic errors, as the type of error most likely associated with sensory deficits, seemed to retain emphasis upon apraxia as a disorder of motor speech programming. These results can therefore support the classical perspectives of the disorder regarding its motoric basis without diminishing the role of sensory modulation in the speech of apractic patients.

Mlcoch and Noll (1980) cited evidence in their paper to suggest that deficient production of fricatives, affricates, and consonant clusters may be due to a disruption of afferent modulation for complex motor patterns which results from postcentral gyrus destruction. They speculated in turn, that apractic patients who demonstrate a preponderance of these types of errors might also have a sensory–perceptual deficit. Such reasoning requires closer examination in light of the preceding discussion. The relationship between severity and extent of lesion has been described. In apractic patients, postcentral gyrus involvement would be expected with larger lesions which reasonably would be associated with more severe symptoms. Yet these classes of sounds are also the targets which present the greatest difficulty for less severe apractic patients who presumably exhibit cortical damage limited to anterior motor association areas. Patients with milder apraxia of speech demonstrate no significant oral-sensory impairment (Rosenbek *et al.*, 1973). One might therefore conclude that the difficulties with these sounds lies in the complexity of their motor programming rather than because of disturbed sensation. Whereas Mlcoch and Noll (1980) proposed two distinct categories of articulatory errors (motor preprogramming and sensory), the validity of this dichotomy seems questionable. Perhaps articulatory programming is best viewed as a more unitary process.

Clinical considerations

Several features at the level of speech output can be associated with apraxia of speech due to the nature of the neuropsychological deficits in this disorder. A major factor is the fluency of speech production (Canter, Trost and Burns, 1985). Following damage to anterior regions resulting in apraxia of speech, motor association areas become deficient in programming articulatory features, speech initiation, and articulatory transition, all of which are necessary for effortless speech. With posterior damage, motor association areas remain intact to program aberrant information which has been fed forward. These factors contribute to the prosodic alterations which are observed in apraxia of speech but are absent in instances of literal paraphasia. The struggle approximating that of apraxia of speech observed in cases with posterior lesions, as in the conduit d'approche of conduction aphasia, appears distinct due to the underlying neuropathologies of sensory guidance versus motor speech programming. Cautions regarding confusion of impaired speech initiation as a result of apraxia versus word-finding difficulties in posterior aphasic patients (Buckingham, 1979) have been advanced, but discrimination is assisted by patients' verbal reports.

Another factor which distinguishes apraxia of speech from other types of articulatory errors is the nature of the phoneme sequencing deficit. Two forms of sequencing errors have been observed: those related to transitionalization (ability to make smooth transitions between articulatory movements; see Kent and Rosenbek, 1983) and those characterized by transposition of phonemes (metathesis). Patients with anterior brain damage resulting in apraxia of speech demonstrate relatively greater transitionalization difficulties; patients with posterior damage and literal paraphasias are typified by errors of metathesis (Canter, 1973). When phoneme sequencing errors do occur in apraxia of speech, the majority are characterized by substitution of a phoneme with one that occurs later in the word (anticipatory) (LaPointe and Johns, 1975). Errors characterized by substitution of a phoneme occurring earlier in the word (reiterative) or the transposition of two phonemes (metathesis) occur much less frequently, or, as in the case of metathetic errors, rarely at all. Generally, LaPointe and Johns (1975) reported that sequential errors accounted for a rather small percentage (7 per cent) of the total errors made by their group of patients with apraxia of speech. On the other hand, Burns and Canter (1977) found that 31 per cent of the errors made by posteriorly involved patients were due to phoneme or syllable sequencing errors. Collectively, these findings support the differentiation of these two patient groups based upon the nature of sequencing difficulties (Canter, Trost and Burns 1985). Buckingham (1979) has described these problems in anterior patients as one of sequential flow whereas the problem for posterior patients is one of sequential ordering. Kent (1983), cited in Kent and Rosenbek (1983), uses the terms 'phasing errors' and 'sequencing errors' to describe these phenomena. However, Kent and Rosenbek (1983) proposed that substitution errors which are not related to other elements in a word, i.e., are not anticipatory, reiterative, or metathetic in nature, might also be considered 'sequential' based upon impairment of preceding functions 'that might be disturbed in apraxia of speech' (p. 45). This argument sounds precariously close to positions which characterize all motor programming deficits, whether secondary to motor selection or sensory guidance impairment, as 'apraxia of speech.' Within this chapter, we adopt a framework in which errors related to the context in which they are produced are considered phoneme sequencing errors, and errors unrelated to the linguistic context (whether substitution, omission, or addition) are thought of as phoneme selection errors. Such clinical distinctions, aided by assessments of fluency, will aid the clinician in determining whether that articulatory deviation is representative of apraxia of speech or literal paraphasia. (See Chapters 1, 3, and 4 for further and differing discussions of apractic and literal paraphasic errors).

In treatment planning, the necessity for determining the type of articulatory disturbance is not of only superficial consequence. To the contrary, as in most diagnostic algorithms, the accurate identification of the disorder will dictate to a large degree the approach which will be used for remediation. This point cannot be made too strongly for it is not lost even in nosological arguments which reject the concept of an independent apraxia of speech (Buckingham, 1979). For instance, recognition of an articulatory deficit as an apraxia of speech might suggest utilization of techniques (as described in Chapter 6) which rely upon repetitious drill of a stimulus in conditions of varying feedback (Deal, 1974). Alternatively, stimulation procedures which strengthen the sensory representation of a concept might be recommended to decrease literal paraphasic errors in an utterance at the point of its surface realization. These decisions, quite obviously, require precision in arriving at the conclusion which best represents the exact nature of the disorder.

Clinical judgments regarding apraxia of speech are also influenced in almost all cases by the presence of an accompanying aphasia, i.e. Broca's or global aphasia. The bases for these coexisting disorders may be found in the cerebral blood supply to the responsible regions. In patients demonstrating Broca's-area infarction, Mohr (1976) observed focal infarction affecting the left third frontal convolution either alone or in combination with surrounding anatomical areas which are supplied by the anterior branches of the upper division of the left middle cerebral artery. Broca's area is supplied by one of these branches, the inferior lateral frontal branch. Mohr has characterized Broca's area infarction as an embolic event. This precise definition may be assumed to be based upon two factors. First, occlusion of blood vessels due to thrombosis most commonly occurs at the origins of the internal carotid and vertebral arteries. Thrombosis of intracranial vessels such as the middle cerebral artery tends to be more generalized due to the more frequent branching of these vessels. Second, emboli leaving the left ventricle of the heart frequently enter the left common carotid artery where they lodge in the middle cerebral artery and its branches. Emboli may also be released from ulcerated plaques in cervical vessels with similar neurological consequences (Gilroy and Meyer, 1975). That

Broca's area infarction is assumed to be of embolic origin is important, for the likelihood of an embolic infarction is only one in seven when compared to those due to thrombosis (Kurtzke and Kurland, 1983; Merritt, 1979). Clinically, therefore, there is significantly increased likelihood that apraxia of speech will appear in the context of a more extensive thrombotic opercular syndrome resulting from infarction of the larger upper branch of the middle cerebral artery (Mohr, 1976). In other words, the isolated existence of apraxia of speech without associated linguistic deficits due to a cortical insult is apparently an infrequently occurring, although not unreal, phenomenon (see Dunlop and Marquardt, 1977). This is not to suggest that all articulatory errors due to cortical lesions are necessarily aphasic in nature (Buckingham, 1979). It does suggest that motor speech programming deficits resulting from lesions of motor association regions may often be influenced or exacerbated by linguistic deficits which occur with these more extensive lesions. As such, in treatment planning, greater attention may need to be given to the combined effects of both motor programming and linguistic variables than previously acknowledged. Treatment considerations of this type follow from similar conclusions which have recent experimental foundations (Kent and Rosenbek, 1983).

Treating the Deficits

Given the nature of the lesions associated with apraxia of speech, most often the concomitant aphasia will be the Broca's variety (Goodglass and Kaplan, 1972; Trost and Canter, 1974). Patients with this type of aphasia have generally well-preserved auditory comprehension and telegraphic speech output characterized chiefly by reduced syntax and diminished use of functors. While it is not unlikely that some apractic speakers will have additional communicative deficits in auditory and reading comprehension and writing, emphasis in this section of the chapter will be on examining those methodologies which facilitate speech production in patients with Broca's aphasia *and* apraxia of speech.

A review of recent developments in intervention strategies for individuals with Broca's aphasia *and* apraxia of speech reveals three primary types of procedures:

1 Those which promote reacquisition of syntactic form only
2 Those which promote articulatory precision only
3 Those which purport to do both.

While it is beyond the scope of this chapter to discuss in depth the treatment of agrammatism, this area must be broached since grammatical formulation and motor speech programming deficits often coexist and interact unfavorably. Thus, a discussion of those methods which facilitate grammatical form and motor speech programming will be the emphasis of this section. If these treatment approaches do not facilitate verbal expression, considerations must be given to providing nonvocal communicative options or adjuncts as discussed by Yorkston and Waugh in Chapter 11.

Methods which promote reacquisition of syntactic form

A number of treatment approaches have been applied to remediate syntactic form in patients with Broca's aphasia, including operant conditioning techniques (Goldfarb, 1981) and the Language Assessment, Remediation and Screening Procedure (LARSP) described by Crystal, Fletcher and Garman (1976). The two most recent methods of choice have been the Helm Elicited Language Program for Syntax Stimulation (Helm-Estabrooks, 1981) and the matrix training procedure. Both focus on expanding the agrammatic aphasic patient's repertoire of syntactic structures, and both have been demonstrated to accomplish this goal effectively in some patients. Adequate comprehension skills, both visual and auditory, are prerequisite for both procedures. Further, both may be considered appropriate options for addressing not only spoken syntactic form, but also written expression.

Helm Elicited Language Program for Syntax Stimulation

The HELPSS (Helm-Estabrooks, 1981) was developed to parallel the hierarchy of difficulty of syntactic structures observed among Broca's aphasic patients (Gleason *et al.*, 1975). Each construction in the HELPSS has multiple exemplars, trained in a story completion format at two levels of difficulty: Level A and Level B. The patient must respond in delayed imitation of the clinician in Level A. For instance:

> Clinician: 'When people ask what my friend does at the park I tell them "He plays baseball." What do I tell them?'
> Patient   'He plays baseball.'

A spontaneous (self-retrieved) target response is required for Level B items, such as:

Clinician: 'John can't reach the light, but Paul can. Why?'
Patient   'He's taller.'

The verbal prestimulation in the HELPSS is accompanied by simple line drawings which are presented just prior to the patient's verbal response.

Matrix training

Another paradigm for retraining syntactic skills in agrammatic aphasic patients is the notion of miniature linguistic systems or matrix training procedures. By using such training tactics, the agrammatic patient's ability to produce new, generalized, i.e., not directly trained, syntactic combinations is enhanced.

Matrix training procedures are attributable to Esper (1925), who used them to study the transfer of novel verbal behavior in nonaphasic individuals relative to color and shape attributes. The matrix training paradigm is typified by stimuli that vary along two dimensions. These stimuli are presented to the patient for labeling. Each required response consists of a portion from one dimension (or syntactic class) and a second from another dimension (or syntactic class). An example of a response matrix for training noun phrase + verb phrase combinations is presented in Figure 5.1.

Results of matrix training investigations with aphasic subjects generally have shown the same trend (Thompson, McReynolds and Vance, 1982; Tonkovich and Loverso, 1982). Learners tend to produce untrained stimulus sequences within the matrix following training on several exemplary sequences. For example, a clinician interested in training the noun phrase + verb phrase combinations in the matrix of

	DIMENSION 2 (VP)			
	ate bread.	drank wine.	spent money.	smoked cigars.
Those women	Those women ate bread.	Those women drank wine.	Those women spent money.	Those women smoked cigars.
Some girls	Some girls ate bread.	Some girls drank wine.	Some girls spent money.	Some girls smoked cigars.
A boy	A boy ate bread.	A boy drank wine.	A boy spent money.	A boy smoked cigars.
The man	The man ate bread.	The man drank wine.	The man spent money.	The man smoked cigars.

DIMENSION 1 (NP)

Figure 5.1 A sample 4 × 4 matrix for training noun phrase (NP) + verb phrase (VP) constructions

Figure 5.1, may arbitrarily decide to train only four exemplars:

Those women ate bread.
Some girls drank wine.
A boy spent money.
The man smoked cigars.

During training of these exemplars, the patient would be exposed to stimuli representing the other twelve target responses within the matrix, and any generalization effects would be noted. If the matrix training procedures are successful, the patient will produce untrained noun phrase + verb phrase combinations inside the matrix.

While the HELPSS and matrix training procedures have not been promoted as methodologies for facilitating articulatory precision or motor speech programming, it is interesting to speculate how they might. Kean (1977, 1980) argued that the omitted elements in Broca's aphasia represented phonological rather than syntactic ones. She distinguished the class of phonological clitics, e.g., free-standing grammatical morphemes, inflectional affixes, and some derivational affixes, separately from the phonological words, i.e., the major lexical items, on the basis of independent linguistic criteria. Kean's account of the agrammatism in Broca's aphasia presumed that patients omitted phonological clitics, not syntactic elements *per se*. If Kean's notion holds true, both the HELPSS and matrix training procedures afford the agrammatic-apractic patient the opportunity to improve phonological aspects of speech production.

Methods which promote facilitation of articulatory precision

Numerous clinical management suggestions have been found in the literature regarding the facilitation of speech production in apractic speakers. Most are reviewed briefly in Chapter 6. Discussion in this section of the chapter will focus on three general treatment protocols for facilitating articulatory precision in apractic speakers which are not discussed in Chapter 6.

Eight-step task continuum

One of the earliest treatment protocols for facilitating phonologic form in apractic speakers was the eight-step task continuum described by Rosenbek *et al.* (1973). This continuum was based on the notions that treatment for apractic speech should:

1 Focus on articulation and be different from language therapies appropriate for the aphasias
2 Emphasize regaining adequate articulatory gestures and the sequencing of those gestures
3 Facilitate movement of the patient from limited, automatic-reactive speech production to more volitional, propositional speech production.

These investigators provided case examples for three patients who generally required progressively fewer repetitions to reach criterion through the continuum as they learned five unique responses each. A subsequent replication and revision in the use of the continuum by Deal and Florance (1978) also demonstrated efficacy of the approach. Rosenbek *et al.* (1973) cautioned, however, that the continuum should not be considered suitable for all apractic speakers, presumably because of individual differences among patients.

This task continuum may actually represent a methodology for improving repetition abilities rather than motor speech programming, *per se*. Because subtle cognitive deficits such as memory disorders, reduced attention, and diminished sensorimotor integration may be associated with left-hemisphere damage, the task continuum may draw patients' attention to salient features of stimuli. In turn, this enhanced attention may actually only facilitate repetition, a behavior impaired in Broca's aphasic patients. Nonetheless, it has been a successful strategy for improving production in aphasic–apractic speakers.

Speech sound sequencing

Dabul and Bollier (1976) presented a treatment protocol for improving articulatory accuracy in apractic speakers, which was based on the premise that sequencing of speech sounds was the apractic speaker's most characteristic problem. Unlike the Rosenbek and colleagues' continuum which manipulates stimulus conditions, Dabul and Bollier's protocol manipulates the stimuli themselves.

The speech sound sequencing intervention strategy consists of four techniques: mastery of individual phones, rapid repetition of consonant + /a/, build-up of sounds into syllables, and word attack by phone and syllable. Dabul and Bollier (1976) reported that two chronic apractic speakers improved their articulatory precision following one year of relatively intensive treatment, i.e., two to three hours per week.

Their treatment protocol, however, has been criticized on several fronts. First, it is assumed that typical apractic errors are those of anticipation, transposition, and addition, a statement which is controversial relative to the apraxia of speech literature (Rosenbek, Kent and LaPointe, 1984). The use of nonsense syllables in the protocol has also been a source of criticism, although the intent of their use was to concentrate solely on phone sequencing; use of familiar meaningful words was thought to preclude establishment of voluntary control. Finally, linguistic variables which influence articulatory accuracy in apractic speech are ignored (Shewan, 1980). However, despite these limitations the speech sound sequencing protocol may provide clinicians with yet another tactic for improving accuracy of speech sound sequencing and transitionalization among some apractic–aphasic patients.

Content network for verbal dyspraxia treatment program

Shewan (1980) developed an innovative treatment protocol geared toward maximizing the apractic speaker's articulatory precision. Central to this therapy content network were the ideas that:

1 Apractic speakers had difficulty recalling and/or coordinating their articulatory gestures necessary for speech production
2 These articulatory gestures could be imprinted and remembered through the use of tactile, proprioceptive, visual, or other imagery
3 Repetition and drill are essential for the establishment of correct articulatory gestures.

Shewan's therapy content network is presented in Table 5.1. The treatment protocol consists of five areas: stimulation presentation method, stimuli, responses, facilitating response variables, and response criteria. According to Shewan, the goal of treatment using this protocol is to establish, on a volitional basis, the appropriate articulatory gestures for phones, to sequence them into words, and to incorporate them in propositional speech. Training begins at a level at which the patient experiences some success, and difficulty is systematically increased by altering one variable both within and across areas in the content network as each step is mastered.

Stimulus presentation methods include auditory, visual, or tactile modes, used separately or in combination. As much stimulus support as necessary is used to initiate the program, and as the patient becomes

Table 5.1. Shewan's (1980) Content Network for Treatment of Apractic Speech. (Reprinted with permission from Human Communication.)

Stimulus Presentation Method	Stimuli (Easy to Difficult)	Responses	Facilitating Response Variables	Criterion Response
A. *Auditory* Auditory model Phonetic placement	A. *Vowels, Diphthongs*	A. *Clinician-Initiated* *Number* Single responses Multiple responses	A. *Slow Speech Rate* B. *Altered Prosody*	A. *Qualitative* Correct Intelligible
B. *Visual* Watch clinician Mirror use Provide visual feedback to client	B. *Single Consonants* Nasals m,n Glides l,r Plosives p,t,k Fricatives h,s,z,f Dentals th, v	*Time* Unison Immediate repetition Delayed repetition	C. *Compensatory Movements* Approximations D. *Associated Responses* Body Movement Tapping Rhythmical Activity	B. *Quantitative* 80% correct over 20 trails C. *Cumulative* 80% correct
Graphic presentation Written words Anatomical charts	C. *CV,VC Combinations* C + Different V Different C + V Vary C & V	*Propositionality* Automatic drill context		
C. *Tactile* Motokinesthetic method	D. *CVC Monosyllabic Words* Functional words High frequency Concrete words	*Responsive* Responsive to question Sentence completion		
D. *Multimodal* Auditory-Visual Auditory-Tactile Visual-Tactile Auditory-Visual-Tactile	E. *Single Words With C Clusters*	*Spontaneous*		
	F. *Bisyllabic Words.* Two word combinations both syllables or words with primary stress	B. *Client-Initiated* Spontaneous Simple/Short Phonologically Syntactically		
	G. *Syntactic Units* Short			

able to function with less stimulus support, it is diminished. Auditory methods include providing an auditory model or auditory instructions to the patient regarding phonetic placement. Visual methods may involve the patient watching the clinician's placement cues or self-monitoring placement in a mirror, or may take the form of written words, or as a target for the model on anatomical charts which demonstrate placement. Tactile presentation may involve physical manipulation of the patient's articulators into the appropriate position.

Stimuli in the content network are arranged hierarchically from easy to difficult, progressing from vowels and diphthongs to production of phones in the context of syntactically simple sentences. Shewan suggested that since apractic speakers may demonstrate individual variations, this hierarchy should be structured relative to the behavior of each patient. Responses in the content network are of two types: clinician-initiated and client-initiated. Clinician-initiated responses involve a direct model or facilitating context for the client's response. Client-initiated responses are more difficult since they occur without a model and are highly propositional.

Facilitating response variables include speech alterations such as reduced rate and responses used in conjunction with speech such as finger-tapping to facilitate speech production. In addition, phoneme sequences may be altered, such as introducing a schwa within difficult consonant clusters. Prosody may be altered with reduced rate, or with tactics such as equalizing stress, and Shewan advocated that it is often necessary to sacrifice prosody for maintained intelligibility. Qualitative criterion responses refer to the clinician's definition of what constitutes an acceptable response, and quantitative criterion responses reflect the clinician's judgment about what performance should be attained prior to advancing to the next level in the treatment plan.

Shewan cautioned that normal speech production may not be a realistic goal for apractic speakers. Her treatment protocol is devised to move the aphasic-apractic speaker to his own maximum level of functioning. The content network provides a useful schema for clinicians, and is based on principles gleaned from the apraxia of speech literature. While the major goal of Shewan's treatment protocol is to shape phonologic form in apractic speakers, syntactic considerations are introduced. It appears doubtful, however, that patients would derive direct benefits relative to syntax from the content network approach. However, consideration and simplification of syntactic demands reduce the communicative formulation demands for aphasic-apractic speakers thereby facilitating both speech praxis and linguistic expression.

Methods which address both articulatory precision and syntactic form

Several treatment strategies for remediating articulatory and syntactic output deficits associated with Broca's aphasia have been addressed in the treatment literature. One treatment tactic which has been inferred is the manipulation of emphatic stress which serves to facilitate production of articulatory gestures as well as the production of grammatical functors (Goodglass, Fodor and Schulhoff, 1967; Tonkovich and Marquardt, 1977). It is interesting to note that despite Kean's (1977) contention that agrammatism in Broca's aphasia results largely from a phonologic deficit manifested by phonologic simplification of sentences, few speech-language pathologists have attempted to test this notion clinically. Horner's (1983) use of minor hemisphere mediation strategies for treating Broca's aphasia, discussed in this section, represents, in part, some of Kean's influence. Also addressed in this section is the use of singing and melodic intonation therapy for agrammatic-apractic patients.

Minor hemisphere mediation strategies

Horner (1983) provided treatment guidelines which relied heavily on minor hemisphere mediation strategies, i.e., visual-spatial-holistic processing, for moderately and severely impaired Broca's aphasic individuals. The treatment protocol is unique in several ways. First, it addresses the communicative needs of the individual with Broca's aphasia in a 'whole person' way — the phonologic-prosodic, syntactic, and pragmatic aspects of language are integrated in an attempt to maximize the patient's communicative effectiveness and efficiency. Second, capitalized upon are the strengths from a presumably intact minor hemisphere for facilitation and compensation of lost communicative functions within the dominate hemisphere. Horner's emphasis on integrating prosodic contour with syntactic manipulations and phonologic constraints provides a clinical application for Kean's (1977) model of agrammatism, and this is unique as well.

The patient first learns to control linguistic stress patterns in syllables and, then, in words and phrases. This is accomplished via systematic drill, as primary stress is manipulated in the initial, medial, and final positions. In addition, to capitalize on other minor hemisphere contributions, actions are paired with vocalizations. For example, facial expressions may be trained in conjunction with emotionally toned verbalizations to establish basic intonation patterns such as surprise, anger, and negation. Gross body movements may be paired with changes in syllable duration and pauses to help the patient overcome initiation difficulties and to aid in re-establishing prosodic control. This might take the form of moving the patient's arm in a vertical plane to signal stress changes and in the horizontal plane to signal changes in syllable duration and pause.

In training phonological form, Horner advocated first establishing a functional set of single-word utterances, including contentives and expletives initially and gradually adding select functors such as 'wh' words, nominal pronouns, and negatives. Training then centers around gradually increasing utterance length (typically to a ceiling of six to eight syllables) and phonetic complexity. Minor hemisphere strategies are employed in conjunction with the phonological retraining and might include training representational gestures to indicate spatial relationships such as up/down and here/there; training ideographic symbolic gestures; and pairing speech with printed words depicting highly imageable nouns, verbs, and adjectives, thereby encouraging a 'whole word' reading strategy. For the patient with limitations resulting from concomitant dyslexia or limb apraxia, novel pictorial symbols utilized in conjunction with the single-word utterances are advocated to facilitate linguistic retrieval skills.

When training of syntactic form is initiated, a transitional step which serves to establish phonologic-prosodic execution at the phrase level is often useful. This step involves training frequently used phrases such as 'How are you? and 'Time to go', which may be rote memorized in order to stabilize previously learned skills regarding stress, pause, tone, and duration. In the remediation of syntactic form, Horner cautioned that phonological-prosodic gains should not be sacrificed for syntactic normalcy. She stressed the importance of beginning with basic sentence types such as declaratives and imperatives, and of treating nouns, verbs, and adjectives equally to minimize the patient's tendency to rely on nominal forms. Also, redundant morphosyntactic forms should be avoided in early stages of training, since patients with Broca's aphasia tend to omit unstressed inflections and functors which are not informative, especially when the information is sufficiently conveyed by word order and stress. In addition, Horner advocated teaching concatenation, beginning with the conjunction 'and' (e.g., N + V + O *and* N + V + O; NP + is + ADJ *and* NP + VP) as opposed to trying to get the patient to apply the interphrasal syntactic rules associated with more complex syntactic forms such as embedding of relative clauses and conditional constructions.

Specific minor-hemisphere mediating strategies employed at this syntactic level of training may involve pairing speech with symbolic gestures, printed words (using whole word reading) or other ideographic stimuli such as novel pictures. The use of additional visual-enhancement techniques which might include dictionary pronunciation symbols to elucidate phonetic and stress aspects, punctuation marks to signal intonational changes, and grammatical tree diagrams to promote awareness of word order and syntactic constraints was also advocated.

Two features of Horner's approach which presumably aid aphasic-apractic patients in speech production are those which deal with intersystemic reorganization and those with intrasystemic reorganization. Aspects of training such as arm swinging, finger tapping and representational facial and limb gesturing in conjunction with speech production constitute attempts at intersystemic reorganization. The focus on emphatic stress and emotional prosody contours represents an attempt to facilitate intrasystemic organization. Using Horner's approach, patients may improve their syntactic and general communication abilities, while deriving the additional benefit of facilitated motor speech.

Singing and melodic intonation therapy

The use of singing as a speech and language facilitator for aphasic patients with apractic speech has been mentioned in the literature. Gerstman (1964) reported a case study of a mute aphasic patient, presumably of the Broca's variety with apraxia of speech, who first imitated simple song patterns at three months post onset and later learned to respond propositionally in song to simple questions. As treatment progressed, the patient became able to use verbal responses spontaneously and with acceptable affect. Another case, reported by Keith and Aronson (1975), was a Broca's aphasic patient who could sing verbal material such as 'I want coffee', 'Goodbye' and 'See you tomorrow', but was unable to say these words or phrases without the melody pattern. At one month post onset, the patient was involved in a singing therapy which required her to finish open-ended sentence frames sung by the clinician. While intervention was applied during a time when spontaneous recovery may be occurring, the singing seemed to facilitate the patient's production of words and phrases. While it was acknowledged that improvement to a similar extent might have been achieved in conventional therapy or possibly with no intervention, the patient was able to function better communicatively in the singing mode.

The exact relationship between singing and speech-language recovery in aphasic individuals has not been isolated, identified, or discussed to any extent in the literature. Still, clinicians seem to be fascinated by this mysterious relationship when they discover a patient who is able to sing the words to a jingle, but who is otherwise mute. This fascination with singing was perhaps the impetus for the development of Melodic Intonation Therapy (MIT).

MIT is a clinical methodology which aids patients with Broca's aphasia in the re-establishment of both phonologic/phonetic and syntactic aspects of language. The original intention for developing MIT for severely nonfluent aphasic patients, presumably those with both aphasia and apraxia of speech, according to Sparks and Deck (1986), was at least basic recovery of the ability to use language in a meaningful way. However, clinicians have used the technique as one which facilitates speech praxis and/or phonological accessing.

While many consider melodic intonation to be a form of singing, it differs in several ways. Songs have distinct melodies, whereas melodic intonation is based on the prosodic contour of verbal utterances. Unlike songs, melodic intonation typically employs a limited vocal range. Underlying melodic intonation are the prosodic features of melodic line in the spoken phrase or sentence, tempo and rhythm of the utterance, and points of emphatic stress. When utterances are intoned, there is an intensification of spoken prosodic factors associated with an utterance: the tempo is lengthened, the variable pitch of speech is reduced and stylized into a melodic pattern involving the constant pitch of several whole notes; and the rhythm and degree of stress are exaggerated.

The neurophysiological mechanisms underlying MIT are not well understood. Sparks, Helm and Albert (1974) speculated that with increased use of the right hemispheric dominance for the melodic aspects of speech, MIT might promote the role of that hemisphere in interhemispheric control of language, possibly reducing the language dominance of the damaged left hemisphere. Perhaps a more plausible explanation offered by Berlin (1976) was the possibility that good candidates for MIT might have intact pre-Rolandic motor areas without input from a damaged Broca's area on the left. MIT may, therefore, serve to activate the intact right Broca's homologue, which, in turn, may exert transcallosal influences to the intact left motor strip.

Some have hypothesized how MIT might serve to influence the speech production in apractic speakers. Duffy and Gawle (1984) speculated that MIT, which serves to exaggerate vowel duration, might 'normalize' vowel duration to the extent of contributing to the accuracy of surrounding consonants. Tonkovich and Marquardt (1977) posited that the rhythmic hand-tapping in MIT might serve to facilitate the timing of motor speech in apractic speakers and may effect regularity in the central mechanism involved in articulatory programming. Another possibility suggested was that the rhythmic hand-tapping might serve as a distractor, removing some of the volitional aspects of the motor speech act in apractic speakers.

Sparks and Deck (1986) predicted that approximately 75 per cent of carefully selected aphasic candidates will realize the expected degree of recovery associated with MIT. It seems difficult to predict *a priori*, however, which prognostic factors might enable a patient to complete MIT through its final steps of Level Four. Thus, while singing or melodic intonation therapy strategies may not bring agrammatic-apractic patients to a state of voluntary speech fluency, they may shape the outcome of future treatment tactics. MIT may provide patients with imitation skills which are a springboard to other intervention techniques.

When these methods fail

It is not realistic to expect that all agrammatic-apractic patients will be able to function in a communicatively successful manner in the oral mode. Indeed many patients lack the potential for using speech as the primary mode of expression, much to the chagrin of the patients, their family members, and clinicians, as well. While the use of nonvocal communication options for patients with severe apraxia of speech will be discussed in detail by Yorkston and Waugh in Chapter 11 of this volume, some brief, general guidelines will be offered here.

It is imperative that patients with severely limited verbal output have at least some rudimentary form of expression from the outset of intervention procedures. The options may include writing, drawing, gesturing, pointing to pictures or words on a communication board, training the patient to signal 'yes', 'no' and 'I don't know' consistently, or using an electronic device. These tactics may be employed individually or in combination with one another. As the patient's facility with propositional speech increases, the adjunct communication systems may be gradually withdrawn. For those patients who do not demonstrate proficiency in the speech mode after exhaustive attempts with the available methodologies for speech facilitation, treatment should focus on expanding and refining the nonvocal communication system to maximize communicative independence.

What to treat

Thus far in our discussion we have reviewed some aspects of the neuropsychological and neurolinguistic underpinnings of apraxia of speech and treatment strategies developed for improving speech-language production in apractic patients with coexisting aphasia. In order to make rational clinical decisions about whether to focus our intervention efforts on the speech apraxia, the concomitant aphasia, or both, it is necessary to take all of these factors into consideration. So how do we make such decisions? There is no magical formula and much of what we do in the clinical setting is established largely by determining what the patient can and cannot do, recalling our past clinical experiences, reviewing the literature, and possessing knowledgeable intuitiveness.

The following general principles may be helpful to clinicians in making decisions about how to proceed in treatment with apractic patients who are also aphasic:

1 Train basic comprehension skills prior to production and continue to train higher level comprehension skills concurrently with production skills
2 Determine the relative contribution of each disorder (apraxia vs aphasia) with respect to the patient's overall communicative impairment
3 Be realistic about the patient's probable maximal recovery status
4 Encourage self-evaluation and self-cueing (see Chapter 7) as early as possible
5 Use the patient's behavior to determine individual hierarchies for training.

A brief discussion of each of these principles follows.

While much of our treatment discussion centered around managing the apraxia of speech and coexisting syntactic deficits associated with Broca's aphasia, pronounced comprehension difficulties occur in a number of apractic-aphasic patients, particularly in mixed anterior and/or global aphasic patients. In order for these patients to derive maximum benefits from speech-language intervention, training in auditory comprehension (and possibly reading ability as well) takes precedence over work on verbal production. Comprehension training is encouraged until patients have sufficient ability to understand clinical instructions for production tasks. Comprehension training should continue during production training with specific emphasis on self-monitoring. While it is not implausible that such patients might make gains on production tasks in spite of poor comprehension, it has been our clinical experience that this is typically the exception rather than the rule.

The determination of the relative contributions of each symptom to the patient's overall communicative impairment is crucial. Behaviors which should be observed include: the patient's ability to access syntactic operations; the frequency of word initiation difficulties; the degree of muteness; the variety of words and phrases that can be utilized propositionally; and the proportion of utterances which are intelligible. If both apraxia of speech and aphasia appear to contribute equivocally to the patient's inability to communicate (which they often do), a 'safe' but probably efficacious treatment route would be one which focused on both symptoms. For the patient who is totally mute or who has few if any propositional words in the oral mode, initially focusing on the apraxia of speech to establish some sort of core vocabulary would be logical. This would be followed by more language-oriented aphasia interventions. For the patient who produces intelligible speech much of the time, but cannot combine words efficiently, treatment methods focusing on syntactic retraining only would appear to be the clinical decision of choice initially, saving the motor speech 'clean up' for later. When one or the other of these symptoms is disproportionately larger in severity, the clinical decision about what to treat is simple. More often it is the case that we are uncertain about whether the apractic speech or the aphasia interferes more with verbal communication in our patients.

It is highly likely that most apractic-aphasic patients will continue to experience some residual difficulties even after extensive speech-language rehabilitation efforts. These patients may continue to have difficulty executing articulatory movements and/or may persist in being unable to use complex syntactic operations effectively. For this reason, clinicians should maintain a realistic outlook about what each patient's speaking behavior will be at the end of speech-language treatment. When a patient becomes a functional communicator and is essentially satisfied with his/her communicative status, consideration for discharge from treatment is in order. If a patient reaches a plateau in terms of achieving articulatory targets for instance, clinicians should stop treating the apractic speech and move on to other intervention goals. In other words, it is important not only to know *what* disorder to treat, but *when* to stop treating it as well.

By habit, and probably instinct, speech-language pathologists are generally prone to provide feedback to their patients relative to the accuracy of their responses. Since apractic speakers often have so much difficulty with sound initiation and phasing, it is important to develop self-evaluation as early in the course of intervention as possible. In addition to encouraging patients to self-evaluate, clinicians should attempt to look for and implement ways in which patients might self-cue (see Chapter 7).

Finally, the clinician should use the patient's own behavior to shape the course of intervention, despite what the literature says about the 'typical' aphasic-apractic patient. Too often in the literature, individual differences are obscured by group measures of central tendency. That is not to underplay the relevance of the literature in our treatment decisions. Quite the contrary is true. While the literature should shape the course of our treatment decisions in a general way, the patient's behavior should ultimately dictate how we proceed specifically.

Acknowledgments

Drs Tonkovich and Peach wish to Acknowledge *Human Communication* (Canada) for permission to Reprint Table 5.1.

References

ATEN, J.L., JOHNS, D.F. and DARLEY, F.L. (1971) 'Auditory perception of sequenced words in apraxia of speech', *Journal of Speech and Hearing Research*, **14**, pp. 131–43.

BERLIN, C.I. (1976) 'On: Melodic intonation therapy for aphasia by SPARKS, R.W. & HOLLAND, A.L.', *Journal of Speech and Hearing Disorders*, **41**, pp. 298–300.

BRODAL, A. (1981) *Neurological Anatomy in Relation to Clinical Medicine*, New York, Oxford University.

BUCKINGHAM, H.W., Jr. (1979) 'Explanation in apraxia with consequences for the concept of apraxia of speech', *Brain and Language*, **9**, pp. 202–26.

BURNS, M.S. and CANTER, G.J. (1977) 'Phonemic behavior of aphasic patients with posterior cerebral lesions', *Brain and Language*, **4**, 492–507.

CANTER, G.J. (1969) 'The influence of primary and secondary verbal apraxia on output disturbances in aphasic syndromes', Paper presented at the convention of the America Speech and Hearing Association, Chicago.

CANTER, G.J. (1973) 'Dysarthria, apraxia of speech, and literal paraphasia: Three distinct varieties of articulatory behavior in the adult with brain damage', Paper presented at the convention of the American Speech and Hearing Association, San Francisco.

CANTER, G.J., TROST, J.E. and BURNS, M.S. (1985) 'Contrasting speech patterns in apraxia of speech and phonemic paraphasia', *Brain and Language*, **24**, pp. 204–22.

CRYSTAL, D., FLETCHER, P. and GARMAN, M. (1978) *The Grammatical Analysis of Language Disability*, New York, Elsevier.

DABUL, B. and BOLLIER, B. (1976) 'Therapeutic approaches to apraxia', *Journal of Speech and Hearing Disorders*, **41**, pp. 268–76.

DARLEY, F.L. (1967) 'Lacunae and research approaches to them: IV', in MILLIKAN, C.H. and DARLEY, F.L. (Eds.), *Brain Mechanisms Underlying Speech and Language*, New York, Grune and Stratton, pp. 236–40.

DARLEY, F.L. (1968) 'Apraxia of speech: 107 years of terminological confusion', Paper presented at the convention of the American Speech and Hearing Association, Denver.

DARLEY, F.L., ARONSON, A.E. and BROWN, J.R. (1975) *Motor Speech Disorders*, Philadelphia, W.B. Saunders.

DEAL, J.L. (1974) 'Consistency and adaptation in apraxia of speech', *Journal of Communication Disorders*, **7**, pp. 135–40.

DEAL, J.L. and DARLEY, F.L. (1972) 'The influence of linguistic and situational variables on phonemic accuracy in apraxia of speech', *Journal of Speech and Hearing Research*, **15**, pp. 639–53.

DEAL, J. and FLORANCE, C.L. (1974) 'Modification of the eight-step continuum for treatment of apraxia of speech in adults', *Journal of Speech and Hearing Disorders*, **43**, pp. 89–95.

DEUTSCH, S.E. (1984) 'Prediction of site of lesion from speech apraxia error patterns', in ROSENBEK, J.C. *et al.* (Eds.) *Apraxia of Speech: Physiology, Acoustics, Linguistics, Management*, San Diego, College-Hill Press, pp. 113–34.

DUFFY, J.R. and GAWLE, C.A. (1984) 'Apraxic speakers' vowel duration in consonant-vowel-consonant syllables', in ROSENBEK, J.C. *et al.* (Eds.) *Apraxia of Speech: Physiology, Acoustics, Linguistics, Management*, San Diego, College-Hill Press, pp. 167–96.

DUNLOP, J.M. and MARQUARDT, T.P. (1977) 'Linguistic and articulatory aspects of single word production in apraxia of speech', *Cortex*, **13**, pp. 17–29.

ESPER, E.A. (1925) 'A technique for the experimental investigation of associative interference in artificial linguistic material', *Language Monographs*, **1**.

FLECHSIG, P. (1901) 'Developmental (mylogenetic) localization of the cerebral cortex in the human subject', *Lancet*, **2**, pp. 1027–9.

GERSTMAN, H.L. (1964) 'A case of aphasia' *Journal of Speech and Hearing Disorders*, **29**, pp. 89–91.

GESCHWIND, N. (1965a) 'Disconnexion syndromes in animals and man: I', *Brain*, **88**, pp. 237–94.

GESCHWIND, N. (1965b) 'Disconnexion syndromes in animals and man: II', *Brain*, **88**, pp. 585–644.

GILROY, J. and MEYER, J.S. (1975) *Medical Neurology*, New York, Macmillan.

GLEASON, J.B., GOODGLASS, H., GREEN, E., ACKERMAN, N.L. and HYDE, M.E. (1975) 'The retrieval of syntax in Broca's aphasia', *Brain and Language*, **24**, pp. 451–71.

GOLDFARB, R. (1981) 'Operant conditioning and programmed instruction in aphasia rehabilitation', in CHAPEY, R. (Ed.), *Language Intervention Strategies in Adult Aphasia*, Baltimore, Williams & Wilkins, pp. 249–63.

GOODGLASS, H. and KAPLAN, E. (1972) *The Assessment of Aphasia and Related Disorders*, Philadelphia, Lea and Febiger.

GOODGLASS, H., FODOR, I.G. and SCHULHOFF, C.L. (1967) 'Prosodic factors in grammar: Evidence from aphasia', *Journal of Speech and Hearing Research*, **10**, pp. 5–10.

HARDISON, D., MARQUARDT, T.P. and PETERSON, H.A. (1977) 'Effects of selected linguistic variables on apraxia of speech', *Journal of Speech and Hearing Research*, **20**, pp. 334–43.

HELM-ESTABROOKS, N. (1981), *Helm Elicited Language Program for Syntax Stimulation*, Austin, Exceptional Resources.

HOIT-DALGAARD, J., MURRY, T. and KOPP, H. (1983) 'Voice onset time production and perception in apraxic subjects', *Brain and Language,*'**20**, pp. 329–39.

HORNER, J. (1983) 'Treatment of Broca's aphasia,' in PERKINS, W.H. (Ed.) *Language Handicaps in Adults*, New York, Thieme-Stratton.

JOHNS, D.F. and DARLEY, F.L. (1970) 'Phonemic variability in apraxia of speech', *Journal of Speech and Hearing Research*, **13**, pp. 556–83.

JOHNS, D.F. and LAPOINTE, L.L. (1976) 'Neurogenic disorders of output processing: Apraxia of speech,' in WHITAKER, H. and WHITAKER, H.A. (Eds.) *Studies in Neurolinguistics*, **1**, New York, Academic Press, pp. 161–99.

KEAN, M.L. (1977) 'The linguistic interpretation of aphasic syndromes: Agrammatism in Broca's aphasia, an example', *Cognition,* **5**, pp. 9–46.

KEAN, M.L. (1980) 'Grammatical representations and the descriptions of language processes', in CAPLAN, D. (Ed.) *Biological Studies of Mental Processes*, Cambridge, MIT Press, pp. 239–68.

KEITH, R. and ARONSON, A. (1975) 'Singing as therapy for apraxia of speech and aphasia: Report of a case, *Brain and Language*, **2**, pp. 483–8.

KENT, R.D. and ROSENBEK, J.C. (1983) 'Acoustic patterns of apraxia of speech', *Journal of Speech and Hearing Research*, **26**, pp. 231–49.

KERTESZ, A. (1984) 'Subcortical lesions and verbal apraxia', in ROSENBEK, J.C. et al. (Eds.) *Apraxia of Speech: Physiology, Acoustics, Linguistics, Management*, San Diego, College-Hill Press, pp. 73–90.

KURTZKE, J.F. and KURLAND, L.T. (1983) 'The epidemiology of neurologic disease', in BAKER, A.B. and BAKER, L.H. (Eds.) *Clinical Neurology*, Philadelphia, Harper and Row.

LAPOINTE, L.L. and JOHNS, D.F. (1975) 'Some phonemic characteristics in apraxia of speech', *Journal of Communication Disorders*, **8**, pp. 259–69.

MARTIN, A.D. (1974) 'Some objections to the term apraxia of speech', *Journal of Speech and Hearing Disorders*, **39**, pp. 53–64.

MARTIN, A.D. and RIGRODSKY, S. (1974) 'An investigation of phonological impairment in aphasia, Part 1', *Cortex*, **10**, pp. 317–28.

MERRITT, H.H. (1979) *A Textbook of Neurology*, Philadelphia, Lea and Febiger.

MLCOCH, A.G. and NOLL, J.D. (1980) 'Speech production models as related to the concept of apraxia of speech', in LASS, N.J. (Ed.) *Speech and Language: Advances in Basic Research and Practice*, New York, Academic Press, pp. 201–38.

MOHR, J.P. (1976) 'Broca's area and Broca's aphasia', in WHITAKER, H. and WHITAKER, H.A. (Eds.) *Studies in Neurolinguistics*, **1**, New York, Academic Press, pp. 201–35.

MOHR, J.P. PESSIN, M.S., FINKELSTEIN, S., FUNKENSTEIN, H.H., DUNCAN, G.W. and DAVIS, K.R. (1978) Broca aphasia: Pathologic and clinical, *Neurology*, **28**, pp. 311–24.

PEACH, R.K. and TONKOVICH, J.D. (1983) 'Subcortical aphasia: A report of three cases', in BROOKSHIRE, R.H. (Ed.), *Clinical Aphasiology Conference Proceedings*, Minneapolis, BRK Publishers, pp. 244–51.

PEACH, R.K. and TONKOVICH, J.D. (1984) 'Coexisting apraxia of speech and aphasia resulting from subcortical infarction', Paper presented at the convention of the American Speech-Language-Hearing Association, San Francisco.

ROSENBEK, J.C., KENT, R.D. and LAPOINTE, L.L. (1984) 'Apraxia of speech: An overview and some perspectives', in ROSENBEK, J.C. *et al.* (Eds.) *Apraxia of Speech: Physiology, Acoustics, Linguistics, Management*, San Diego, College-Hill Press, pp. 1–72.

ROSENBEK, J.C., WERTZ, R.T. and DARLEY, F.L. (1973) 'Oral sensation and perception in apraxia of speech and aphasia', *Journal of Speech and Hearing Research*, **16**, pp. 22–36.

ROSENBEK, J.C., LEMME, M.L., AHERN, M.B., HARRIS, E.H. and WERTZ, R.T. (1973) 'A treatment for apraxia of speech in adults', *Journal of Speech and Hearing Disorders*, **38**, pp. 462–72.

SCHIFF, H.B., ALEXANDER, M.P., NAESER, M.A. and GALABURDA, A.M. (1983). 'Aphemia: Clinical-anatomic correlations', *Archives of Neurology*, **40**, pp. 720–7.

SHEWAN, C.M. (1980) 'Verbal dyspraxia and its treatment', *Human Communication*, **5**, pp. 3–12.

SPARKS, R.W. and DECK, J.W. (1986) 'Melodic intonation therapy', in CHAPEY, R. (Ed.) *Language Intervention Strategies in Adult Aphasia*, Baltimore, Williams & Wilkins, pp. 320–32.

SPARKS, R., HELM, N. and ALBERT, M. (1974) 'Aphasia rehabilitation resulting from melodic intonation therapy', *Cortex*, **10**, pp. 303–16.

SQUARE, P.A. and MLCOCH, A.G. (1983) 'The syndrome of subcortical apraxia of speech: An acoustic analysis (Abstract)', in BROOKSHIRE, R.H. (Ed.) *Clinical Aphasiology Conference Proceedings*, Minneapolis, BRK Publishers, pp. 239–43.

SQUARE-STORER, P., DARLEY, F.L. and SOMMERS, R.K. (1988) 'Nonspeech and speech processing skills in patients with aphasia and apraxia of speech, *Brain and Language*, **33**, pp. 65–85.

THOMPSON, C.K., MCREYNOLDS, L.V. and VANCE, C.E. (1982) 'Generative use of locatives in multiword utterances in agrammatism: A matrix-training approach', in BROOKSHIRE, R.H. (Ed.) *Clinical Aphasiology Conference Proceedings*, Minneapolis, BRK Publishers, pp. 289–97.

TONKOVICH, J.D. and LOVERSO, F. (1982) 'A training matrix approach for gestural acquisition by the agrammatic patient', in BROOKSHIRE, R.H. (Ed.) *Clinical Aphasiology Conference Proceedings*, Minneapolis, BRK Publishers, pp. 283–8.

TONKOVICH, J.D. and MARQUARDT, T.P. (1977) 'The effects of stress and melodic intonation on apraxia of speech', in BROOKSHIRE, R.H. (Ed.) *Clinical Aphasiology Conference Proceedings*, Minneapolis, BRK Publishers, pp. 97–102.

TROST, J.E. and CANTER, G.J. (1974) 'Apraxia of speech in patients with Broca's aphasia: A study of phonemic production accuracy and error patterns', *Brain and Language*, **1**, pp. 63–79.

WERTZ, R.T., LAPOINTE, L.L. and ROSENBEK, J.C. (1984) *Apraxia of Speech: The Disorder and its Treatment*, New York, Grune and Stratton.

WERTZ, R.T., ROSENBEK, J.C. and DEAL, J.L. (1970) 'A review of 228 cases of apraxia of speech: Classification, etiology, and localization', Paper presented at the convention of the American Speech and Hearing Association, New York.

Chapter 6

Traditional Therapies for Apraxia of Speech — Reviewed and Rationalized

Paula Square-Storer

The traditional definition of apraxia of speech (AOS) as put forth by Darley (1968) highlighted two aspects of the impairment — difficulty in positioning the speech musculature accurately and impaired ability to sequence multiple speech movements. It is the purpose of this chapter to review the traditional therapy techniques used for the treatment of apraxia of speech and to discuss them within the framework of Darley's definition, i.e., those which facilitate spatial targeting and, most probably the 'phasing' or temporal activation of speech muscles groups at the segmental and/or syllabic levels, and those which facilitate temporal integration and 'phasing' of multiple speech movements in longer utterances. These latter approaches probably influence the sequencing of phonemes as well. In addition, constructs for the efficacious selection of traditional treatment methods and techniques for AOS will be put forth; this information is generally obtained from results of assessment of apraxia of speech as discussed by Collins in Chapter 4 and/or diagnostic therapy. The final sections of the chapter are directed towards discussions of methods for reducing motor speech perseveration, those methods for bringing speech under volitional control, and the use of linguistic/symbolic facilitators to enhance motor speech programming.

Methods which Enhance Spatial Targeting and 'Phasing' at the Segmental and Syllable Levels

Those methods of therapy which appear to be more directed towards facilitating the positioning of the speech musculature, and/or the coordinated phasing of speech subsystems and muscles or muscle groups to signal manner, voicing, and place of articulation at the segmental and syllabic levels include, among others, phonetic derivation, progressive approximation, phonetic placement, and the key-word technique. These techniques are not always mutually exclusive; some aspects of the methods overlap. Further, several of these methods may be used simultaneously. They, most probably, are appropriately applied for the remediation of errors of initiation and spatial targeting as discussed in Chapter 2 by Square-Storer and Roy. Each was proposed in the early works of Van Riper (1939, 1963) for the treatment of articulation disorders and was further refined by Rosenbek (1978, 1985) and Wertz, LaPointe and Rosenbek (1984) for the treatment of apraxia of speech. Imitation of phonetic contrasts, a method highlighted in the writings of Van Riper (1939, 1963) and Fairbanks (1940), may also achieve the above stated goals; it, too, has been refined for use with verbally apractic patients (Rosenbek, 1978, 1985; Wertz, LaPointe and Rosenbek, 1984).

Phonetic derivation

Phonetic derivation, or the shaping of speech sounds from nonspeech sounds, orofacial postures, and postures combined with other speech actions such as nasal/oral resonance, speech respiration, and phonation, has been reported to be a potential approach for deriving speech segment production, i.e., phoneme production. However, the patients for whom such a method is used should not have significant impairment of oral nonverbal praxis. As reviewed in Chapter 2, the coexistence of oral apraxia with verbal apraxia or, at least, 'phonetic/phonemic' disturbances in aphasia, is quite high. Thus, patients with verbal apraxia for whom phonetic derivation techniques are considered, should be screened thoroughly for the presence and severity of oral apraxia. The following questions should be answered from a thorough examination of oral praxis function.

Is the patient able to produce consistently and effortlessly nonspeech sounds? This is particularly relevant when attempting to shape segment production from nonspeech sounds such as deriving /p/ from a popping sound, /b/ from a bubble sound, /k/ from a coughing sound, or /t/ from tongue clicking.

Is the patient able to produce consistently and accurately oral postures? An answer to this question is relevant when attempting to derive vocalics from oral-facial postures such as /a/ from the 'open wide' posture or /i/ from the 'smile' posture.

Finally, *is the patient able to produce consistently and accurately complex oral actions by successively adding oral tract actions to orofacial postures?* For instance, is the patient able to first bite his lower lip and then add a blowing action to achieve an approximated /f/, or close his lips, achieve velar closure in order to puff out his cheeks, and, then, release the imploded air abruptly by releasing lip closure to achieve a /p/?

Progressive approximation

Progressive approximation refers to the process of gradually shaping speech segments from other speech segments. Before applying this method, the clinician should have thoroughly assessed both speech and oral apraxia (see Chapter 4 for a discussion). With regard to speech praxis, the following question is most important — *Is the patient able to produce consistently and effortlessly several phonemes in isolation?* An answer to this question may be obtained from the results of the 'repetition of individual phonemes' subsection of verbal apraxia batteries as described elsewhere by Wertz, LaPointe and Rosenbek (1984) and in this volume by Collins in Chapter 4. However, when contemplating the use of progressive approximation, knowledge of the consistency of accurate production of facilitative target phonemes is vital, particularly since 'inconsistency' of production is a primary symptom of apraxia of speech (see Chapter 2). Thus, it is recommended that the 'repetition of phonemes' subsection of any apraxia screening battery be administered several times for the purpose of establishing consistency of phoneme production. Also, of interest here would be the issue of differential performance as a result of input modality. For some patients, consistent and effortless production of phonemes may be better derived from graphemic input than auditory-verbal input as required in repetition (Wertz, LaPointe and Rosenbek, 1984). Also, in the repetition mode, the astute clinician will assess the effects of auditory-verbal input versus auditory-verbal input plus visual input (facial mime) (see, for instance, Johns and Darley, 1970; LaPointe and Horner, 1976).

A thorough assessment of oral apraxia is indeed needed to determine the answer to the following vital question — *May the phoneme(s) that is/are produced effortlessly and consistently, be modified by making appropriate and usually small oral adjustments?* i.e., can the patient produce from /s/, /ʃ/ by slowly drawing his tongue body posteriorly or /Θ/ by slowly easing the tongue anteriorly and interdentally? times, such adjustments can be better achieved with kinesthe' than with verbal instructions. Thus, clinicians should also a effect of kinesthetic input such as drawing the index finge' buccal region posteriorly to achieve a more appropriate positioning of the tongue body. Such input may maximize speech accuracy for some patients with apraxia of speech.

Phonetic placement

Phonetic placement techniques may also be used to maximize the positioning of the speech musculature and the coordinated activation of speech subsystems. Techniques include providing the patient with descriptions of how speech sounds are made; using graphs, models and drawings of the vocal tract to facilitate descriptions; manipulating the oral structures; and/or developing onomatopoetic associations such as humming for /m/ or hissing for /s/. For effective use of the first two techniques, *there should be evidence that the patient possesses an accurate spatial representation or 'spatial coordinate system' of the vocal tract* (MacNeilage, 1970; Hardy, 1970; Scott and Ringel, 1971). Previous studies have indicated that many verbally apractic patients, indeed, have orosensory perceptual deficits (Rosenbek, Wertz and Darley, 1973; Teixeira, Defran and Nichols, 1974; Square, 1976). Such deficits, however, probably coexist with the disorder rather than being an integral part of the disorder (see Chapter 5). Traditionally, orosensory perception has been tested using the following:

1 Oral stereognosis tests in which a patient must recognize what shape he is manipulating lingually or discriminate between two geometric oral forms introduced orally in succession
2 Two-point discrimination in which a caliper is used to determine the distance between two points required for the patient to perceive that two points are being stimulated rather than one
3 Quadrant localization in which the patient must identify the lingual quadrant being stimulated by point pressure
4 Mandibular kinesthesia in which the patient bites on a caliper and determines whether two successively presented items are the same with regard to degree of jaw opening or whether the second is of a greater or lesser distance than the first (see Mlcoch and Square, 1984 for a discussion).

Impairments on these types of crude tests *may* be indicative that a patient may not be able to profit from descriptions of segment production and/or the use of graphs, models, and drawings. If, however, such orosensory deficits exist, manipulation of the oral structures and the larynx *may* be beneficial in that such techniques *enhance* kinesthetic feedback. Finally, the use of onomatopoetic sounds may tap a completely different level of speech formulation, i.e., intrasystemic reorganization (Rosenbek, 1978), in that the production of these sounds may be of a more automatic nature than the application of speech production rules to linguistic tokens such as phonemes or words. Informal testing of a patient's ability to produce such 'noises' consistently and with ease may provide the clinician with a starting point in therapy for severely impaired patients.

Key word technique

This technique capitalizes upon the patient's ability to emit consistently *some* words, usually monosyllabic ones, accurately. Typical examples are names of spouses or children. The patient is then encouraged to practise the words under less and less automatic conditions. Once such control is established, attention is drawn to the 'feel' of the words, i.e., the kinesthetic feedback that results from their production. Finally, practise is extended from the key word to other words which are comprised of the same phoneme(s). An example of the process follows. If a patient emits consistently and correctly his wife's name, 'Sue', production of that word is encouraged under less automatic conditions such as in response to questions. Once the name is emitted consistently and correctly under these less automatic conditions, it is practised repeatedly with instructions to the patient to think how the 's' feels. Words which are initiated by /s/ are then presented for training. These may include such items as 'soap', 'sit', and 'sun'. Two major questions must be answered concerning a patient's behavior before applying this method:

1 *Is the patient able to utilize kinesthetic and proprioceptive information from the vocal tract?*
2 *Does this patient lack a propensity towards perseveration?*

Imitation of phonetic contrasts

This method is directed towards the facilitation of producti particular phoneme target as it occurs in varying phonetic cont instance, /t/ may be a target which is easily produced w

environments such as, 'tea', 'toe', 'tie, 'two', etc. Once having established a patient's ability to produce such individual items consistently
and effortlessly, contrastive phonetic pairs are practised in order to
achieve consistent control of a phoneme which differs 'minimally', such
as /s/. For example, contrastive pairs might include 'tea-sea', 'toe-sew',
'tie-sigh', and 'two-Sue'. The patient's attention is again drawn to the
'feel' of the words. Task demands are gradually increased in that the
predictability of the pair to be imitated is reduced. That is, in some
pairs, /t/-initiated words might occur first and, in others, /s/-initiated
words. Bisyllabic words, such as 'sitter', 'city', 'tootsie', etc., are
eventually used as targets for practice.

The key question here is: *is the patient able to imitate verbal tokens and
under what conditions is imitation best facilitated?* Some indication of a
patient's ability to imitate may be derived from the subtests of the
apraxia of speech examination which assess repetition of individual
phonemes and monosyllabic words (see Chapter 4). In the Neuropraxis
Research Laboratory in Toronto codirected by Dr Roy and myself, we
have expanded the monosyllabic repetition subtest to sixty-nine items
in which most consonants occur three times in the initiating and three
times in the terminating positions of CVCs. While we have retained the
traditional symmetrical CVC items such as 'sis', 'judge', and 'church',
the majority of the monosyllabic words are not symmetrical. All,
however, are highly familiar and frequently occurring words. This
expanded version provides us with a greater sampling of items from
which to assess a patient's repetition abilities within various phonetic
contexts.

Aside from general ability to repeat, we must also determine *the
conditions under which the patient repeats best.* Controversy exists in the
literature regarding the best modality(ies) of input. For some patients,
integral stimulation (Rosenbek, 1978, 1985), in which the patient is
instructed, 'Watch me, listen to me, do what I do', appears to facilitate
better repetition (Johns and Darley, 1970; Dabul and Bollier, 1976).
However, some patients may benefit most from auditory input alone
(LaPointe and Horner, 1976). Also, some patients, when instructed
how to use it, may benefit from visual monitoring using a mirror
(Darley, Aronson and Brown, 1975; Deal and Darley, 1972). Finally,
repetition of stimuli may not be the most facilitative; reading or naming
may enhance motor speech production to a greater degree (LaPointe
and Horner, 1976).

When selecting stimuli for treatment, *phonetic complexity* must also
be considered (Deal and Darley, 1972; Johns and Darley, 1970;
Shankweiler and Harris, 1968; Trost and Canter, 1974). For instance, if

the target is /s/ in the initial position of CVCs, we will probably avoid words ending in affricates, other fricatives, or clusters, e.g., 'such', 'soothe', etc. And, finally, because most of our patients are aphasic as well as verbally apractic, *linguistic variables* such as word class and abstractness (Deal and Darley, 1972), and word familiarity and frequency (Schuell and Jenkins, 1961) warrant our attention. There are indications in the literature that, with Broca's aphasic patients, even verbs may be too difficult to process (Miceli *et al.*, 1984); thus, nominal stimuli may be the clinician's best choice for the treatment of AOS. For a comprehensive discussion of issues regarding the treatment of aphasic-apractic patients, the reader is referred to Chapter 5 in this volume by Tonkovich and Peach.

Stimulus-response variables constitute the final area of concern when using repetition methods. Those areas of concern include the *number of models* provided for the patient, *immediate responses versus delayed ones*, and the *number of responses or reattempts* allotted the patient (Johns and Darley, 1970; Deal and Darley, 1972; LaPointe and Horner, 1976). Bugbee and Nichols (1980) tested ten verbally apractic patients with regard to their abilities to repeat thirty concrete nouns under five conditions:

1 A clinician-controlled delay of three seconds
2 Clinician-controlled number of rehearsals which was always four
3 Patient-controlled delay
4 Patient-controlled number of rehearsals
5 Immediate repetition.

Results indicated that patients were able to imitate nouns with significantly greater accuracy under the self-determined number of spoken rehearsals than in the immediate response condition, the clinician-controlled-number-of-rehearsals condition, or the clinician-imposed-delay-of-three-seconds condition. With regard to the self-determined-number-of-rehearsals condition, it was reported that subjects rarely chose more than three rehearsals, stopped rehearsing after a correct production, did not go beyond their best response to a less accurate one, could and did evaluate their own speech accuracy, and improved their responses when they controlled their own number of repetitions. It was suggested that the overt rehearsals of patients might be shaped into covert rehearsals by instructing patients to wait to respond until they felt they could produce the target correctly. Such a method m' ᵇᵉ thought of as a self-cueing technique. This and other self-/ techniques are discussed in Chapter 7 of this volume by R Golper.

Facilitating the Temporal Schemata of Speech and the Sequencing of Segments in Longer Utterances

Several methods of treatment appear to have as their major focus, the enhancement of the coordinated interaction of multiple speech movements by different muscles or muscle groups and, to a lesser degree, the sequencing of speech segments, i.e., phonemes. Each method uses, as one facilitative component, rhythm. The rationale is that rhythm underlies the control of *all* motor behavior (Shaffer, 1982), speech not withstanding (Kent, 1976; Lenneberg, 1967). Along a similar line but from a slightly different standpoint, Öhman (1965) proposed that consonantal production is superimposed upon a *melodic* vocalic line.

Four methods will be discussed in this section — Melodic Intonation Therapy, vibrotacticle stimulation, facilitators including intersystemic timing gestures and intrasystemic suprasegmental facilitators, and PROMPTs. It is hypothesized that these methods enhance motor speech programming (see Chapter 9) in that, as one of each of their components, they provide a temporal schemata for the organization of multiple speech movements.

Melodic Intonation Therapy

As discussed in Chapter 5 by Tonkovich and Peach and in Chapter 7 by Rau and Golper, Melodic Intonation Therapy (Sparks, Helm and Albert, 1974; Sparks and Holland, 1976; Sparks, 1981; Naeser and Helm-Estabrooks, 1985) was originally developed for the treatment of aphasia in order to encourage verbal expression at the phrase and sentence level. It has since been reported to be quite useful for facilitating verbal expression among patients with apraxia of speech and coexisting aphasia. The method is hierarchically graded into four major levels which encourage the patient's volitional control of speech output. The method capitalizes upon 'intoning' output and facilitating that output, at lower levels of difficulty, with hand tapping. The hand tapping provides an even more definite basis for rhythm than the use of intoning alone, probably because it encourages intersystemic reorganization (Luria, 1970; Rosenbek, 1978, 1985), i.e., the pairing of a more intact motor system with one which is impaired. Intrasystemic reorganization is also stressed within this method in that speech, itself, is brought to a different level of output, a modified singing level or 'sprechgesang'. Since melody is processed by the nondominant or usually right hemisphere, it has been hypothesized by Sparks (1981) that the intact hemisphere may be facilitating the output of that which has been linguistically formulated in the dominant hemisphere. We, like others, have observed this method to be an efficacious one, even for patients who are grossly disorganized and demonstrate unintelligible speech due to initiation, and spatial and temporal speech difficulties (see Chapter 2). It is especially *useful for patients who have great difficulty repeating*, even when integral stimulation methods such as those developed by Rosenbek *et al.* (1973) are used. Recently a program called Melodic Apraxia Training: Stop Consonants (Smith and Engle, 1984) has been published which uses principles of Melodic Intonation Therapy but focuses on the segmental level of production. Results of application of this program are lacking but may add further to our knowledge of the use of rhythm and/or melodic lines as facilitators of speech organization. Readers must be cautioned, how-ever, with regard to using rhythm as the sole basis of therapy. Wertz, LaPointe and Rosenbek (1984) pointed out that methods which capitalize solely or primarily on rhythm for the treatment of AOS have been found, in their experience, to be less efficient than other methods.

Vibrotactile stimulation

Another therapy technique which capitalizes on intersystemic reor-ganization is vibrotactile stimulation (Rubow, Rosenbek and Collins, 1982). In this method tactile stimulation is applied to the finger simultaneously with speech production. Specifically, Rubow and col-leagues applied a 50 Hz vibration to the volar surface of a patient's right index finger. The clinician controlled the intensity, timing, and duration of the vibrotactile stimulation, applying a greater intensity and duration to stressed syllables of polysyllabic words. Thus, in this method, rhythm was paired with stress similarly as they are in contrastive stress drills (Wertz, LaPointe and Rosenbek, 1984). However unlike contras-tive stress drill therapy which is thought to reorganize speech intra-systemically, vibrotactile stimulation hypothetically capitalizes upon intersystemic reorganization.

A single patient with moderate apraxia of speech and mild to moderate aphasia was reported by Rubow, Rosenbek and Collins (1982). Two lists of polysyllabic words, one loaded with plosives, and the other with fricatives were used as stimuli. Although initial perform-ance on the two lists of words, as measured from repetition, was similar as indicated by multidimensional scoring system (see Chapter 4 for a description of such scoring methods), application of vibrotactile stimulation improved performance dramatically for the fricative-loaded list while imitative performance on the plosive-loaded list improved marginally. It was suggested by the experimenters that afference from the vibrotactile stimulation induced intersystemic reorganization and, hence, the reorganization of central motor programs.

Other intra- and intersystemic facilitators

In his writings on the treatment of apraxia of speech in adults, Rosenbek (1978, 1985) spoke of using suprasegmental facilitators' to enhance speech production. Among those mentioned were rate, segment duration, pause time, and loudness–pitch variations. It may be that the use of each of these suprasegmental variations provides for patients an enhanced temporal schemata which underlies the regulation of the timing of speech events. As mentioned previously, the use of contrastive stress drills as outlined by Rosenbek (1978, 1985) and Wertz, LaPointe and Rosenbek (1984) provides another example of intrasystemic reorganization techniques which pair rhythm and stress and which have been reported to be highly successful clinically although empirical data is not available.

Intersystemic timing gestures have been used extensively in the treatment of apraxia of speech among children (Yoss and Darley, 1974) but to a lesser extent with adults. Such techniques may include squeezing one's fist rhythmically, tapping the thigh or foot, finger tapping, and using baton accents. These methods may have great value in the treatment of apraxia of speech in adults as well in that they encourage intersystemic reorganization and possibly an enhanced internal temporal–spatial schemata. The efficacious use of finger tapping for the treatment of apraxia of speech was, in fact, demonstrated by Simmons (1978). One subject who had enjoyed good success in therapy for nine months, henceforth demonstrated a five-month plateau in performance. The patient was trained to tap his index finger and thumb together in accompaniment to the production of each word in 'Pronoun + Verb + Preposition + Article + Noun' utterances. The patient's speech efficiency greatly improved in therapy and there was generalization in that his PICA verbal subtest scores improved a remarkable twenty-one percentile points.

There is some evidence that the 'intersystemic reorganization', or the pairing of a more or less intact motor system with another less intact one, is responsible for the improvement of speech production for each of the previously mentioned methods: that is, the mere application of an external source of rhythm does not appear responsible for improvement. This was demonstrated by Shane and Darley (1978) who applied an external source of rhythm, a metronome, and paired it with speech production while apractic patients read. The metronome was set for normal speaking rate as well as a slower rate and a faster one. There were no significant differences in articulatory accuracy among the three conditions. Further, and most important to our hypothesis, is the fact that the intersystemic incorporation of rhythm with other parameters such as stress enhance an internal temporal schemata which accounts for improved speech performance. In fact, the external source of rhythm applied by Shane and Darley (1978) actually had a deleterious effect on speech. Overall, patients were more accurate in their speech production with no metronome.

PROMPTs

PROMPTs or Prompts for Restructuring Oral Muscular Phonetic Targets was developed by Chumpelik (1984) as a method of treating apraxia of speech among children. The method was applied with successful results to adult patients with apraxia of speech and Broca's aphasia by Square, Chumpelik and Adams (1985) and Square *et al.* (1986). The method is best described as a dynamic phonetic placement/action technique which provides, simultaneously, intersystemic reorganization for spatial and temporal aspects of speech production. This method is the topic of Chapter 8 and is described fully there.

Methods for Treating Motor Speech Perseveration

The nature of and the mechanism(s) responsible for perseverations among left-hemisphere-damaged (LHD) patients continues to be debated in the literature. That is, *does the presence of perseveration indicate, in some cases, a severe disorder of praxis?* Lebrun, in Chapter 1, thinks not. Square-Storer and Roy, in Chapter 2, provide evidence that perseverative behavior, in some cases, relates to or, at least, coexists with disorders of praxis for the limb and nonverbal oral motor systems and, most probably, the speech system. And, Santo-Pietro and Rigrodsky (1986) have indicated that among LHD patients, some perseverations are motorically based while others are linguistically based.

Although the underlying bases of oral–verbal perseverative behavior among LHD patients remains debatable and is a fruitful area for further research, two methods of treatment have been reported to decrease such behaviors. The first, Voluntary Control of Involuntary Utterances, was originally proposed by Helm-Estabrooks (1983) and appears to be directed towards the remediation of perseverations at the linguistic level. Multiple Phoneme Input Therapy, originally presented by Stevens and Glasser (1983), is elaborated upon by Stevens in Chapter 9 of this volume. The rationale for this method hinges on the tenet that verbal perseverations have a motoric basis and a goal is to bring under voluntary control the inhibition of this type of pathological behavior. Novel utterances are then shaped from some elements of the motoric actions contained in the patient's stereotypy(ies).

Encouraging Volitional Control of Speech in Verbal Apraxia

It is generally believed that automatic-reactive speech is better produced than purposeful, volitional speech and that imitative speech is produced with greater accuracy than spontaneous speech among verbally apractic speakers (Darley, 1968; Johns and Darley, 1970). There have been exceptions to the imitative-spontaneous tenet, however. Trost and Canter (1974) found that phoneme accuracy was not greater in the former than in the latter condition among Broca's aphasic patients with AOS. And, Lebrun, in Chapter 1 of this volume, has proposed conversely that, in patients with 'anarthria' not complicated by aphasia, a similar phenomenon exists. Contrarily, in the North American literature, it has been generally reported that imitation is an easier mode of motor speech production than is spontaneous speech for patients with AOS (and usually coexisting aphasia) (Wertz, LaPointe and Rosenbek, 1984). Bearing this in mind, Rosenbek and colleagues (1973) set forth an eight-step hierarchy for assisting the apractic speaker to bring under volitional control increased speech efficiency from the imitative mode (Steps 1 through 4), to the written mode (Steps 5 and 6), and finally to the self-formulation of speech (Steps 7 and 8). Throughout this hierarchy, supportive cues are gradually decreased in order to aid the patient to become more self-reliant for controlling speech accuracy. Other methods which encourage patient independence for controlling speech accuracy are presented by Rau and Golper in Chapter 7 of this volume.

Intersystemic Symbolic/Linguistic Facilitators

Discussion of symbolic gestures as facilitators of motor speech production has been reserved for this latter section of the review because we do not understand *how* the use of such communicatively significant gestures facilitates speech production. That is, because most of our patients with verbal apraxia are aphasic as well, when the pairing of a symbolic gesture with speech attempts improves the speech emitted, it is difficult to say whether *the use of gesture has facilitated language retrieval at the lexical and/or phonological levels, or motor speech programming, per se.* This question is of great theoretical and neuropsychological interest and deserves further attention. Nonetheless, when a patient has lost his/her ability to communicate functionally and the use of this technique is facilitative and efficacious, the answers to the preceding questions become moot issues. When choosing a methods of symbolic gestural facilitators, whether emblems or gestures which can replace the meaning of words, or a modified sign language such as Amer-Ind (Skelly, 1979; Skelly *et al.*, 1974), several key issues must be addressed about the neuropsychological status of the patient. First, *does the patient demonstrate limb praxis skills commensurate for learning pantomimes and/or limb posturings,* or, *has the patient retained a set of symbolic gestures which he uses spontaneously in environmental contexts and which can be paired with speech output?* Latter types of gestures may include, for example, waving goodbye or shrugging the shoulders. If affirmative answers to either of the above two questions do not exist then the pairing of symbolic gestures with speech output for the purpose of improving speech accuracy will probably not be an efficient therapeutic technique. The purpose of such techniques is to facilitate intersystemic reorganization. Thus, if both 'systems' are impaired, intersystemic reorganization should, logically, be compromised or, at least, be less efficient.

There are, to our knowledge, no empirical reports of the efficacious use of gestural language as an intersystemic reorganizer for enhancement of *motor speech programming* (see Chapter 8), although clinical reports are numerous. However, there are several published reports of the successful training of other means of communication among verbally apractic patients. Amer-Ind was taught successfully to one apractic patient as an alternate means of communication (Dowden, Marshall and Thompkins, 1981) and successful use of instruments such as the Handi-Voice have appeared in the literature (Rabidoux, Florence and McCauslin, 1980). Yorkston and Waugh, in Chapter 11 of this book, address the use of other forms of augmentative and alternative communication for verbally apractic patients.

Summary

It has been the purpose of this chapter to review the current approaches used most frequently for the treatment of apraxia of speech and to provide a conceptual model which sets out principles for selection of these methods. Specific procedures for each were not presented; readers are urged to refer to the original reports. Also, little empirical data have been provided regarding the efficacy of many of these methods although numerous clinical reports have indicated most to be effective for at least some patients. Further research, particularly using single case study designs (McReynolds and Kearns, 1982), is needed to isolate those features which account for the effectiveness of each treatment approach and/or technique and to delineate specifically the behavioral profiles of patients for whom each is most effective. Descriptions of speech symptomatology alone and/or severity of verbal apraxia may not be the best means of selection of appropriate treatment approaches. However, severity of AOS has been the method of choice advocated by Wertz, LaPointe and Rosenbek (1984). We propose, instead, the investigation of each patient's speech dynamics in combination with neuropsychological and linguistic profiles. These holistic behavioral profiles, most probably, deserve greater consideration when selecting the most efficacious treatment approaches for aphasic–verbally apractic individuals.

Acknowledgments

Dr Square-Storer acknowledges the assistance of the Graduate Department of Speech Pathology and Department of Rehabilitation Medicine for their assistance in the preparation of this chapter and the Faculty of Medicine, University of Toronto for continued support in her research endeavors.

References

BUGBEE, J. and NICHOLS, A. (1980) 'Rehearsal as a self-correction strategy for patients with apraxia of speech', in BROOKSHIRE, R. (Ed.), *Clinical Aphasiology Conference Proceedings*, Minneapolis, BRK Publishers, pp. 279–84.

CHUMPELIK, D. (1984) 'The Prompt system of therapy', in ARAM, D. (Ed.), *Seminars in Speech and Language*, **5**, pp. 139–56.

DABUL, B. and BOLLIER, B. (1976) 'Therapeutic approaches to apraxia', *Journal of Speech and Hearing Disorders*, **41**, pp. 372–6.

DARLEY, F.L. (1968) 'Apraxia of speech: 107 years of terminological confusion', Paper presented to the American Speech and Hearing Association, Chicago.

DARLEY, F.L., ARONSON, A.E. and BROWN, J.R. (1975) *Motor Speech Disorder*, Philadelphia, W.B. Saunders.

DEAL, J.L. and DARLEY, F.L. (1972) 'The influence of linguistic and situational variables on phonemic accuracy in apraxia of speech', **15**, pp. 639–53.

DOWDEN, P.A., MARSHALL, R.C. and TOMPKINS, C.A. (1981) 'Amer-Ind sign as a communicative facilitator for aphasic and apractic patients', in BROOKSHIRE, R. (Ed.), *Clinical Aphasiology Conference Proceedings*, Minneapolis, BRK Publishers, pp. 133–40.

FAIRBANKS, G. (1940) *Voice and Articulation Drillbook*, New York, Harper and Row.

HARDY, J.C. (1970) 'Development of neuromuscular systems underlying speech production', *ASHA Reports, No. 5*, Rockville, Maryland, American Speech Language and Hearing Association, pp. 49–68.

HELM-ESTABROOKS, N. (1983) 'Treatment of subcortical aphasia', in PERKINS, W. (Ed.), *Language Handicaps in Adults*, New York, Thieme and Stratton, pp. 97–103.

JOHNS, D.F. and DARLEY, F.L. (1970) 'Phonemic variability in apraxia of speech', *Journal of Speech and Hearing Research*, **13**, pp. 556–83.

KELSO, J.A.S. and TULLER, B. (1981) 'Toward a theory of apractic syndromes', *Brian and Language*, 12, pp. 224–45.

KENT, R. (1976) 'Models of speech production', in LASS, N. (Ed.), *Contemporary Issues in Experimental Phonetics*, New York, Academic Press, pp. 79–104.

LaPOINTE, L.L. and HORNER, J. (1976) 'Repeated trials of words by patients with neurogenic phonological selection-sequencing impairments (apraxia of speech)', in BROOKSHIRE, R. (Ed.), *Clinical Aphasiology Conference Proceedings*, Minneapolis, BRK Publishers, pp. 261–77.

LENNEBERG, E.H. (1967) *Biological Foundations of Language*, New York, Wiley.

LURIA, A.R. (1970) *Traumatic Aphasia: its Syndromes, Psychology and Treatment*, The Hague, Mouton.

MACNEILAGE, P.F. (1970) 'Motor control of the serial ordering of speech', *Psychological Review*, **77**, pp. 182–96.

MCREYNOLDS, L. and KEARNS, K. (1983) *Single Subject Experimental Designs in Communicative Disorders*, Baltimore, University Park Press.

MICELI, G., SIVERI, M., VILLA, G. and CARAMAZA, A. (1984) 'On the basis for agrammatics' difficulty in producing main verbs', *Cortex*, **20**, pp. 207–20.

MLCOCH, A.B. and SQUARE, P.A. (1984) 'Apraxia of speech: Articulatory and perceptual factors', in LASS, N. (Ed.) *Speech and Language: Advances in Basic Research and Practice*, **10**, Orlando, Academic Press, pp. 1–58.

NAESER, M.A. and HELM-ESTABROOKS, N. (1985) 'CT localization and response to MIT in nonfluent aphasia', *Cortex*, **21**, pp. 203–22.

ÖHMAN, S.E.G. (1965) 'Coarticulation in VCV utterances: spectrographic measurements', *Journal of the Acoustical Society of America,* **39**, pp. 151–68.

RABIDOUX, P.C., FLORENCE, C.L. and MCCAUSLIN, L.S. (1980) 'The use of the handivoice in the treatment of a severely apractic patient' in BROOKSHIRE, R. (Ed.), *Clinical Aphasiology Conference Proceedings*, Minneapolis, BRK Publishers, pp. 294–302.

ROSENBEK, J.C. (1978, 1985) 'Treating apraxia of speech', in JOHNS, D.F. (Ed.), *Clinical Management of Neurogenic Communicative Disorders*, Boston, Little Brown, pp. 191–241 and 267–312.

ROSENBEK, J.C., WERTZ, R.T. and DARLEY, F.L. (1973) 'Oral sensation and perception in apraxia of speech and aphasia', *Journal of Speech and Hearing Research*, **16**, pp. 22–36.

ROSENBEK, J., LEMME, M., AHERN, M., HARRIS, E. and WERTZ, R. (1973) 'A treatment for apraxia of speech in adults', *Journal of Speech and Hearing Disorders*, **38**, 462–72.

RUBOW, R.T., ROSENBEK, J.C. and COLLINS, M.J. (1982) 'Vibrotactile stimulation for intersystemic reorganization in apraxia of speech', *Archives of Physical Medicine and Rehabilitation*, **63**, pp. 150–3.

SANTO PIETRO, M.J. and RIGRODSKY, S. (1986) 'Patterns of oral-verbal perseveration in adult aphasics', *Brian and Language*, **29**, pp. 1–17.

SCHUELL, H. and JENKINS, J.J. (1961) 'Reduction of vocabulary in aphasia', *Brain*, **84**, pp. 243–61.

SCOTT, C.M. and RINGEL, R.L. (1971) 'Articulation without oral sensory control', *Journal of Speech and Hearing Research*, **14**, pp. 804–18.

SHAFFER, L.H. (1982) 'Rhythm and timing in skill', *Psychological Review*, **89**, 109–22.

SHANE, H. and DARLEY, F.L. (1978) 'The effect of auditory rhythmic stimulation on articulatory accuracy in apraxia of speech', *Cortex*, **14**, pp. 444–50.

SHANKWEILER, D. and HARRIS, K.S. (1966) 'An experimental approach to the problem of articulation in aphasia', *Cortex*, **2**, pp. 277–97.

SIMMONS, N. (1978) 'Finger counting as an intersystemic reorganizer in apraxia of speech', in BROOKSHIRE, R. (Ed.), *Clinical Aphasiology Conference Proceedings*, Minneapolis, BRK Publishers, pp. 174–9.

SKELLY, M. (1979) *Amerind Gestural Code Based on Universal American Hand Talk*, New York, Elsevier.

SKELLY, M., SCHINSKY, L., SMITH, R.W. and FUST, R.S. (1974) 'American Indian Sign (Amerind) as a facilitator of verbalization for the oral verbal apraxic', *Journal of Speech and Hearing Disorders*, **39**, pp. 445–56.

SMITH, P.K. and ENGEL, B.J. (1984) Melodic apraxia training: Stop consonants', Tuscon, Communication Skill Builders Inc.

SPARKS, R. (1981) 'Melodic intonation therapy', in CHAPEY, R. (Ed.), *Language Intervention Strategies in Adult Aphasia*, Baltimore, Williams and Wilkins, pp. 265–82.

SPARKS, R. and HOLLAND, A. (1976) 'Method: Melodic intonation therapy', *Journal of Speech and Hearing Disorders*, **41**, pp. 287–97.

SPARKS, R., HELM, N. and ALBERT, M. (1974) 'Aphasia rehabilitation resulting from melodic intonation therapy, *Cortex*, **10**, pp. 303–16.

SQUARE, P.A. (1976) 'Oral sensory perception in adults demonstrating apraxia of speech', Unpublished Master's Thesis, Kent State University.

SQUARE, P., CHUMPELIK, D. and ADAMS, S. (1985) 'Efficacy of the PROMPT system of therapy for the treatment of acquired apraxia of speech', in

BROOKSHIRE, R. (Ed.), *Clinical Aphasiology Conference Proceedings*, Minneapolis, BRK Publishers, pp. 319–20.

SQUARE, P., CHUMPELIK, D., MORNINGSTAR, D. and ADAMS, S. (1986) 'Efficacy of the PROMPT system of therapy for the treatment of apraxia of speech: A follow-up investigation', in BROOKSHIRE, R. (Ed.) *Clinical Aphasiology Conference Proceedings*, Minneapolis, BRK Publishers, pp. 221–6.

STEVENS, E. and GLASSER, L. (1983) 'Multiple input phoneme therapy: an approach to severe apraxia and expressive aphasia', in BROOKSHIRE, R., *Clinical Aphasiology Conference Proceedings*, Minneapolis, BRK Publishers, pp. 148–55.

TEIXEIRA, L.A., DEFRAN, R.H. and NICHOLS, A.C. (1974) 'Oral stereognostic differences between apraxics, dysarthrics, aphasics, and normals', *Journal of Communication Disorders*, **7**, pp. 213–25.

TROST, J.E. and CANTER, G.J. (1974) 'Apraxia of speech in patients with Broca's aphasia: A study of phoneme production accuracy and error patterns, *Brain and Language*, **1**, pp. 63–79.

VAN RIPER, C. (1939, 1963) *Speech Correction: Principles and Methods*, Englewood Cliffs, New Jersey, Prentice Hall.

WERTZ, R.T., LAPOINTE, L.L. and ROSENBEK, J.C. (1984) *Apraxia of Speech in Adults: The Disorder and Its Management*, Orlando, Florida, Grune and Stratton.

YOSS, K.A. and DARLEY, F.L. (1974) 'Therapy in developmental apraxia of speech', *Language Speech and Hearing Services in the Schools*, **5**, pp. 23–31.

PART THREE
Efficacy of Intervention

Chapter 7

Cueing Strategies

Marie T. Rau and Lee Ann C. Golper

A Tradition of Cueing

The use of cues to assist communicatively impaired patients to produce a desired response or to retrieve an elusive word is a venerable notion in our treatment literature. Clinicians have observed that providing a priming stimulus in the form of a description of function, a written word, an open-ended sentence, an associated word, or a phonetic cue can result in the accurate production of a verbal target. Various authors describe a variety of cueing techniques and systematic cueing hierarchies (LaPointe, 1985; Rosenbek, 1985; Chapey, 1986; Darley, 1982; Wertz, LaPointe, and Rosenbek, 1984). Tests for aphasia and apraxia of speech contain standardized prompts, such as those used with the Porch Index of Communicative Ability (Porch, 1981) and even whole subtests which incorporate cueing techniques (for example, Kertesz, 1982; Porch, 1981; Schuell, 1972). Likewise, cueing formats are common in the many therapy manuals and workbooks available for use with aphasic and apractic adults. This widespread acceptance of the value of cueing strategies appears to be independent of the theoretical orientation of the clinician–researcher and of the treatment approach employed. Stimulation approaches (Duffy, 1986; Linebaugh and Lehner, 1977) and programmed approaches (Bollinger and Stout, 1976) examine the relative power of particular cues to elicit accurate verbal responses. Pragmatically based, natural conversation approaches (Davis and Wilcox, 1985; Davis, 1986) encourage the patient to maximize both the communicative content of messages sent to the listener and comprehension of messages received by utilizing available cues. Most of what clinicians do can be viewed as cueing in one form or another.

Broad and Focused Research Questions

Researchers have examined cueing techniques and behaviors from a variety of perspectives, and with different questions in mind. Some have employed group designs, asking such questions as: are some types of cues more effective than others across groups of patients; or is there a hierarchy of effective cueing techniques that can be generalized to large numbers of apractic or aphasic patients (Love and Webb, 1977; Pease and Goodglass, 1978)? Other investigators have utilized individual case study approaches or single-subject research designs to determine the effectiveness of a particular cueing strategy (Rao and Horner, 1978; Simmons, 1978), or the relative effectiveness of two or more types of cues in eliciting target verbal responses (Golper and Rau, 1983; Simmons, 1980). These researchers have asked such questions as: for this apractic patient, is an auditory–visual cue more or less effective than an auditory–visual plus a tactile cue (Rubow *et al.*, 1982; Simmons, 1980)? If this patient uses an association cue, or a verbal description prompt, does it result in a more intelligible target response than a graphic cue, or an attempt to sound out the word (Golper and Rau, 1983)? Do gestural cues result in improved verbal performance or more effective overall communication for this aphasic–apractic patient (Kearns, Simmons, and Sisterhen, 1982; Rao and Horner, 1978)? Is rhythmic cueing effective, or relatively more effective than other types of cues for improving verbal fluency in this moderately apractic patient (Golper and Rau, 1983; Simmons, 1978)?

Some authors have described the types of facilitators that aphasic and apractic speakers use spontaneously. They have asked such questions as: what types of self-generated cues do communicatively impaired adults utilize in word retrieval efforts? What is the relative frequency of use of different types of cues (Marshall, 1976)? What types of patient-generated cues are most effective for eliciting an intended response (Berman and Peelle, 1967; Marshall, 1976; Tompkins and Marshall, 1982)? What have these researchers learned about cueing techniques and strategies?

Group Studies of Cueing Effectiveness

With regard to investigations using group designs, there is little data available concerning the types of cueing strategies which help apractic patients. Most of what we know about facilitating the verbal performance of apractic patients relates to characteristics of the stimuli themselves, such as word frequency, word length, characteristics of individual phonemes (relative difficulty, frequency, visibility, position in the word, etc.), and other features such as the number of repetitions of the stimulus by clinician or patient, and the effects of imposing delay (see Wertz, LaPointe and Rosenbek, 1984, for an excellent and complete review of this literature). Group studies specifically focused on cueing strategies have been most often conducted with aphasic subjects, although many probably have included patients with apraxia of speech as well as aphasia. A brief review of the results of some representative studies follows.

Love and Webb (1977), in looking at four types of clinician generated cues, found some evidence for a systematic hierarchy of cueing effectiveness. In a word retrieval task, they found imitation of the target word the most potent facilitator, followed by initial syllable stimulation. Sentence completion and printed word cues were equally facilitative. Of particular interest to us, however, were Love and Webb's findings of the differential effects of cueing as it related to overall severity of impairment. Results indicated a systematic hierarchy of cueing potency for severely impaired subjects, while mildly impaired subjects exhibited an idiosyncratic, unsystematic pattern of response to the various cues.

Pease and Goodglass (1978) also found phonemic cueing to be a potent cue in facilitating verbal responses. They examined patterns of response to cues on a naming task in relationship to type of aphasia, severity of naming impairment, and auditory comprehension level. Initial syllable cues were found to be significantly more effective than all other types of cues, regardless of severity of naming impairment or type of aphasia. Pease and Goodglass also found that completion cues were more facilitative than superordinate, function, or location cues. In general, the same pattern of responsiveness to different facilitators occurred across aphasic types but not across levels of severity of naming impairment. The only type of cue that most of the severely impaired subjects found facilitative was the initial syllable cue, while moderately and mildly impaired subjects were able to utilize all types of cues.

In contrast to the results reported above, Podraza and Darley (1977) found no particular hierarchy of cueing facilitation when they looked at the relative effectiveness of five cueing conditions (auditory prestimulation) on picture naming ability. Naming performance was about equally facilitated by prestimulation with the initial phoneme plus schwa, an open-ended sentence, and the target word together with unrelated foils. Interestingly, prestimulation with the target word and two semantically related foils worsened, rather than improved naming performance.

We have cited only three representative group studies of the effects of a variety of types of cues on the verbal performance of communicatively impaired adults. Darley (1982) reviews more completely the large number of group investigations which have looked at variables which influence verbal performance in this population. What can we generalize from these studies? First, severity of verbal impairment is inversely related to the number and types of cues to which the patient is responsive. Second, there is conflicting evidence that a cueing hierarchy which can be applied to all patients exists. Pease and Goodglass (1978) found evidence for a pattern of cueing potency while Love and Webb (1977) found one only for their most severely impaired subjects. Podraza and Darley (1977), on the other hand, found no evidence for a systematic cueing hierarchy that could be generalized to large numbers of patients.

Group Studies of Apractic Speakers

There have been some group studies which have looked specifically at aspects of response to cueing in apractic speakers. The two most important ones were reviewed by Square-Storer in Chapter 6. Shane and Darley (1978) examined the effects of an external timing cue, rhythmic auditory stimulation provided by an electronic metronome, on the articulatory accuracy of a group of apractic speakers with minimal aphasic language involvement. No significant effects of auditory rhythmic stimulation upon articulatory accuracy were found. In fact, articulatory performance tended to deteriorate with this form of externally imposed cueing. Shane and Darley speculated that externally imposed rhythmic cues may be different from reportedly successful rhythmic cues such as finger or hand tapping (Simmons, 1978; Sparks and Deck, 1986), or rhythmic hand gestures which the patient may internalize (Golper and Rau, 1983) or from which he or she may receive *combined* cues including visual and tactile–kinesthetic feedback.

Bugbee and Nichols (1980) studied the articulatory accuracy of a group of apractic adults under four experimental conditions. These were reviewed in Chapter 6. As a group, the apractic subjects were significantly more accurate when they controlled the number of rehearsals than when they repeated immediately, attempted the target word after a clinician-imposed number of four rehearsals, or repeated following a clinician-imposed delay of three seconds. Though not statistically significant, there was also a trend toward improved articulatory performance when subjects controlled delay intervals. The potency of allowing apractic patients to control response time is suggested by this study.

Studies of Patients' Self-Generated Cueing Behaviors

The relative effectiveness of self-cueing behaviors commonly demonstrated by apractic and aphasic speakers is another potential source of information for treatment planning. Investigators have identified several types of such behaviors used by patients in conversation including delay, semantic association, description, and generalization or the use of empty or general words (Marshall, 1976). They have also examined the relative effectiveness of different self-cueing strategies in communicating an intended target utterance to a listener when the actual stimulus was not known (Tompkins and Marshall, 1982). These studies have provided some useful information about patient self-cueing behaviors:

1 Verbal associations and descriptions were found to be the most frequently used self-cueing behaviors, followed by delay and generalization (Marshall, 1976).
2 Delay was found to be the most successful self-cueing behavior, although associations and verbal descriptions were moderately successful (Marshall, 1976).
3 Severity of communication impairment influenced both the type and amount of self-cueing used. The least impaired speakers were the only ones who used delay strategies, and they were more successful in the overall use of self-cues. Generalization, a rarely successful self-cue, was used only by the most severely impaired speakers (Marshall, 1976).
4 The most successful types of self-generated cues in helping listeners to guess or predict an intended message were functional description, gestural cues, and combined cues (Tompkins and Marshall, 1982).
5 Patient-generated cueing behaviors should be viewed as ways of transferring information to listeners regardless of whether the specific verbal target is produced. When correct listener 'guesses' are combined with successful patient word retrieval efforts significant improvement in the number of successfully communicated targets may be achieved (Tompkins and Marshall, 1982).

Clinician–Determined Cueing Hierarchies

Much of the treatment literature related to cueing strategies has described hierarchies which serve as the basis for more or less complete therapy programs designed to improve verbal performance. These programs have generally been based on logical assumptions about the relative potency of different types of cues. Some have utilized data from the verbal apraxia literature related to characteristics of stimuli and kinds of tasks which are easiest to most difficult for the majority of aphasic–apractic speakers. Although each approach has been described previously in this volume in Chapters 5 and 6, they will be briefly reviewed here with special reference to cueing. Table 7.1 summarizes and compares several of these treatment programs.

Rosenbek *et al.* (1973) described one of the earliest systematic task hierarchies specifically designed for the treatment of acquired apraxia of

Table 7.1: Summary of Cueing Strategies Described in Representative Treatment Programs

Type of cue	Program				
	Dabul and Bollier (1976)	Florance and Deal (1977)	Linebaugh and Lehner (1977)	Rosenbek et al. (1973)	Sparks and Deck (1986)
Auditory					
Repetition	X	X	X	X	X
Phoneme			X		X
Syllable			X		
Unison	X	X		X	X
Intonational				X	X
Rhythmic					X
Plus visual		X		X	X
Plus gestural					X
Visual	X	X	X		X
Phonetic placement	X			X	
Gestural					
Limb			X		X
Rhythmic					X
Graphic	X	X		X	
Linguistic					
Associative			X		
Question		X	X	X	X
Verbal description	X		X		
Pseudoconversation/ conver.		X		X	
Situational					
Delay				X	X
Multiple repetitions	X	X		X	

speech. Their eight-step task continuum was clinician-controlled and incorporated many types of cueing techniques (see Chapter 5). In addition, Rosenbek and his co-workers advocated the use of a variety of 'facilitators' which could also be considered cues, such as the use of slowed rate and exaggerated stress. The Rosenbek hierarchy is ordered from maximum cueing, i.e., auditory and visual stimulation with the model followed by simultaneous production by clinician and patient, to minimal cueing, i.e., use of target responses in role-playing situations.

Dabul and Bollier (1976) described a systematic cueing hierarchy in which the focus was on the process of sequencing speech sounds, and ordering of stimuli, rather than on the product or the specific stimulus conditions. It is a drill-like approach, beginning with individual phonemes and proceeding through consonant–vowel (CV), consonant–vowel–consonant (CVC) and CVCV combinations, with criteria specified for each level. Nonsense syllables, rather than real words, comprise the stimuli. An important aspect of the Dabul–Bollier program is multiple rapid repetitions at all levels beyond the isolated phoneme production level. This approach employs several types of clinician-generated cues as listed in Table 7.1.

Florance and Deal (1977) advocated a clinician-determined, clinician-controlled cueing hierarchy in a three-step program with several sublevels in each. The program was described as appropriate for 'nonverbal' stroke patients. The aim of the Florance–Deal program was to train groups of target sentences to generalization and to stimulate novel utterances. While there is no mention of self-cueing in this program, target sentences are selected on the basis of potential usefulness to the patient, and patient preference. Thus, some external or environmental cueing might be presumed.

Some highly structured programs have been shown to be useful with apractic patients, although not perhaps originally intended for this clinical group. The most widely used is Melodic Intonation Therapy (MIT) (Sparks and Deck, 1986). As described in Chapters 5 and 6, this program utilizes intoned stimuli (phrases or sentences) and incorporates strong rhythmic tapping cues as well as auditory cues of words and melody. Cues are gradually faded, and delays incorporated at each of the four levels, with the final product being responses to questions produced with natural conversational prosody. All cues in the MIT program, as in other programs described in this section, are clinician-generated and controlled, although phrases and sentences are selected on the basis of functional value and patient success.

A general cueing hierarchy for developing and improving word retrieval abilities in aphasic and apractic patients has been described by Linebaugh and Lehner (1977). This hierarchy proceeds in the direction of minimum cue ('What's this called?') to maximum cue ('Say -----'), with the patient being provided cues of appropriate potency to facilitate the desired response. Although this approach uses a clinician-specified hierarchy, determination of individual patient hierarchies and incorporation of patient-generated cues into the program are encouraged.

Another general program of cueing hierarchies applicable to a broad range of communicative impairments including apraxia of speech is that of Bollinger and Stout (1976). They emphasized the concept of cue potency, i.e., the likelihood that a particular type of cue will elicit a desired target response. Small-step increments in task difficulty contingent on high rates of patient success were also advocated.

Others have incorporated communicative systems such as gesture in apraxia treatment programs based on cueing hierarchies (Rosenbek, Collins, and Wertz, 1976; Skelly *et al.*, 1974). Improvement in the verbal skills of some apractic patients has been reported with use of gestural stimulation cues, although others have questioned whether it was gestural facilitation *per se* that was responsible for the verbal improvement (Kearns, Simmons and Sisterhen, 1982).

Thus a variety of different cueing techniques, including auditory, visual, graphic, semantic associational, gestural, intonational, and rhythmic cues have been incorporated into these hierarchically structured treatment regimens. Some general observations can be made about these programs. First, while success has been reported for each of the treatment approaches, and objective patient improvement data have been included, no published, controlled group studies of the relative efficacy of such treatment programs exist. Second, there appear to be certain kinds of patients for whom these highly structured treatment programs are most appropriate. They are probably most applicable, for example, to patients who have very severe verbal impairment and for whom other, more traditional stimulation approaches have been ineffective for improving motor speech programming. Furthermore, these approaches do not appear to be suitable for treating the globally aphasic patient with severe auditory comprehension and other linguistic deficits. Finally, most reports of the use of these programs caution against rigid application of the described cueing hierarchy without regard for individual patient needs, strengths, and ability to move through the program. In fact, successful modification of existing treatment protocols based on individual patient response to the program have been reported (Deal and Florance, 1978; Marshall and Holtzapple, 1976).

Individual Case Studies and Single-Case Experimental Designs

It has become increasingly common for clinician–researchers to employ well conceived and well controlled single subject experimental designs (McReynolds and Kearns, 1983) to answer questions about the efficacy of specific cueing techniques. Nevertheless, some earlier reports utilizing a more traditional case study approach and including both objective and descriptive data about patients' verbal improvement have made valuable contributions.

One of the first papers to give systematic attention to patient self-cueing was published by Berman and Peelle in 1967. These authors outlined a series of steps which they had used for individualized treatment programs with several verbally apractic and aphasic adults. Their program was based on cueing strategies leading to patient-generated cues. First, on an individual patient basis, the types of cues which were successful in eliciting desired responses were determined. Next, cueing strategies were systematically taught to the patient or skills were strengthened to encourage self-initiation. Third, the patient was assisted in recognizing that specific cues could lead to successful communication. The final step was to condition the patient to use self-produced associations to cue desired responses. Descriptive summaries of individual patient progress provided support for Berman and Peelle's approach.

Further evidence that particular cueing approaches can be effective with individual patients has been provided by a number of researchers using case study approaches. Rao and Horner (1978) explored the relative efficacy of gestural cueing and gestural training as facilitators of functional communication. Simmons (1978) demonstrated that training in the use of pacing provided by finger counting as the words in a sentence were spoken resulted in substantial improvement in verbal fluency in a moderately apractic speaker. Dowden, Marshall and Tompkins (1981), with two severely aphasic–apractic patients, found that while both speakers were able to learn a series of gestural signs based on Amer-Ind (Skelly *et al.*, 1974) and communicate them intelligibly, only one of the two patients showed generalization to untrained signs. Furthermore, there was no evidence that Amer-Ind facilitated improvement in verbal scores on subsequent PICA testing. Thus, Dowden and her co-workers, as well as Kearns, Simmons and Sisterhen (1982) obtained results which conflicted with earlier claims that gestural cueing training *per se* was responsible for noted improvements in verbal expressive scores.

Recently, carefully designed single-case experimental studies have added to our knowledge base regarding the efficacy of specific cueing approaches. Investigations by Hoodin and Thompson (1983), Kearns, Simmons and Sisterhen (1982), Rubow *et al.* (1982), and Simmons (1980) have demonstrated that combined cueing approaches have been more effective than the use of single modality cues for individual patients. Because different types of cueing strategies were employed in each of these studies, and because several different patients were involved, the effectiveness of combined cueing approaches may be emerging as a general principle. Results of these studies have been compatible with those obtained by Weidner and Jinks (1983) using a group design. Other examples of efficacious treatment for verbal apraxia using single-case experimental design approaches have been reported by Collins *et al.* (1980), Golper and Rau (1983), and LaPointe (1984).

In summary, case reports and single-case design studies have contributed to our knowledge of the effectiveness of cueing approaches by focusing on areas that had previously received little attention, e.g., the importance of developing patients' abilities to self-cue, and by providing specific answers to specific questions about types and combinations of cues.

Summary of the Literature

From the literature on cueing techniques and strategies, the following generalizations can be made:

1 There is not much evidence for the existence of a systematic potency hierarchy of cues that can be applied generally to all patients. Less severely impaired patients, especially, show great variability of response to different types of cues, and tend to be more idiosyncratic in the types of self-cues they employ.
2 There is conflicting evidence regarding the effectiveness of specific types of cues, e.g., verbal descriptions, depending upon whether the cue is generated by the clinician or the patient and whether the measured outcome is elicitation of a target response or simply successful communication.
3 It appears that most apractic patients benefit from multimodality cues and multiple simultaneous cues rather than cues that stimulate only one input modality or utilize only one output modality.

4 Reports of programmed treatment approaches caution against rigid application and urge individualizing the program based upon individual hierarchies of responsiveness.

5 Clinicians have been creative about adapting existing treatment hierarchies, such as MIT, to suit individual patient needs, and about testing the application of less traditional cueing techniques.

6 Apractic speakers do generate effective self-cues and can learn to generalize the use of these cues to real communicative situations.

7 More carefully designed and controlled studies exploring different types and combinations of cueing strategies with individual patients are needed before generalizations regarding efficacy can be made.

The Rationale for Using Cueing Strategies

Cueing techniques as facilitators and reorganizers

Cueing, as we have used the term in this chapter, refers to external events, either initiated by the listener/clinician (Can you tell me what this is? You use it to cut wood with. It has sharp teeth...) or by the patient himself or herself (It's a k-e-y. I use it in the door... it's a key) which appear to stimulate associations or initiate recall of speech sequences within the impaired speaker's brain. The use of facilitating techniques presumes that an external stimulus can serve to stimulate internal processes.

Cues are facilitative and may serve a 'deblocking' function, especially in the early stages of recovery and therapy (Weigl, 1974; Weigl and Bierwisch, 1977). The term 'deblocking' refers to the use of intact or relatively intact modes of responding and processing information to facilitate the use of modalities that are functioning at less optimum levels (Weigl and Bierwisch, 1977). In apraxia and aphasia therapy, 'deblocking' involves maximizing residual skills by stimulating the channel that is most functional for the patient. For example, presenting a written or printed word to an apractic patient may aid the sequential aspects of motor speech programming.

If deblocking is a *function* which cueing serves, the *process* within which the function operates may be, in some instances 'transcoding'. Transcoding is the interaction of two language systems or codes, for example writing to dictation or reading aloud (Weigl, 1974). If one functional part of the communication system is impaired by brain damage, but the ability to switch from one functional system to another is intact, then the more intact mode (which, for many apractic speakers might be writing) can serve to stimulate responding in more impaired modalities. Many cueing strategies, such as the use of graphic or reading cues, would appear to use transcoding processes to deblock impaired response channels. Especially in mildly impaired speakers, and those in whom rapid recovery occurs, cueing techniques likely serve a deblocking or disinhibiting function.

In the case of severe, chronic apraxia and aphasia, some researchers have suggested that Luria's (1970) concept of intra- and intersystemic reorganization may underlie the successful use of cueing approaches. Intrasystemic reorganization refers to shifting a specific function *down* to a more primitive, automatic level or *up* to a higher cortical level of control (Luria, (1970). Cueing techniques employing singing or intonation, or building upon a patient's automatic, involuntary utterances (see Helm and Barresi, 1980) would appear to be accomplishing intrasystemic functional reorganization. Intersystemic reorganization, on the other hand, accomplishes reorganization by incorporating an entirely different functional system in the re-establishment of the impaired function. Rosenbek, Collins and Wertz (1976), Rao and Horner (1978), and others have suggested that intersystemic reorganization is the underlying rationale for the use of gestural cueing strategies in apraxia therapy (see also Chapter 6). Rosenbek (1985) and his colleagues (Rosenbek, Collins and Wertz, 1976) have speculated that MIT works with some patients through the mechanisms of both intra- and intersystemic reorganization.

Cueing strategies, then, may be both facilitative–disinhibitory in that they serve a deblocking function, and reorganizing in that the function of restructuring a response mode is served. Many of the treatment hierarchies for apraxia of speech, e.g., the Rosenbek *et al.* eight-step continuum and MIT, may serve the severely apractic speaker to reorganize motor speech initiation and programming.

Some Basic Principles in the Use of Cueing Therapies

Our overriding treatment goal for apraxia of speech is the selection of therapy tasks and materials which will make the most significant functional improvement in the patient's verbal communication ability in the shortest amount of time. To this end, it is important to establish effective compensatory strategies *with* the patient, which then can be employed away from the clinic and the clinician. With these goals in mind, some basic principles in the use of cueing approaches can be formulated:

1 From the earliest stages of therapy, any productive self-cueing techniques which the patient employs should be brought to a conscious level of control, reinforced, and utilized in speaking tasks of gradually increasing difficulty and complexity. If, as Rosenbek (1978) maintains, the goal of therapy with apractic patients from the first day of therapy is to point them toward the door (and we agree with this principle), emphasis on self-cueing therapies for those patients who demonstrate such potential is crucial.

2 Systematic, well-planned cueing hierarchies should be developed on an individual patient basis with the guiding principle being to provide the minimum amount of cueing necessary to ensure consistently successful responses and to reduce struggle behavior.

3 Therapy materials and cueing techniques should incorporate principles regarding the relative difficulty of phonetic and linguistic stimuli for apractic speakers. Even when patient-generated cues are the focus of therapy, stimuli (words, phrases, sentences, pictures) need to be selected to optimize successful patient responses.

4 From the initiation of therapy, the apractic speaker must understand the value and purpose of successful cues and self-cues. Thus, strategies for developing patients' awareness of their self-cueing abilities must be part of treatment.

Treatment Steps: Preliminaries to Using Self-Cues

Initially, an individual patient may be so severely apractic that he or she is not able to generate self-cues. Extremely limited verbal output may be confined to a few stereotyped utterances or overlearned automatic verbalizations. Verbal associations or descriptions are not within the patient's behavioral repertoire. Gestural ability may be limited or defective and not facilitative of verbal production. Graphic abilities may also be nonfacilitative. Such individuals have severe verbal apraxia and probably moderately severe aphasia. They initially have minimal abilities to respond to clinician-generated cues and it may be most facilitative to begin treatment with highly structured, clinician-controlled programs such as MIT (Sparks and Deck, 1986), Voluntary

Control of Involuntary Utterances (VICU) (Helm and Barresi, 1980), a gestural facilitation program (Skelly *et al.*, 1974; Rosenbek, Collins and Wertz, 1976), or one of the highly structured therapy hierarchies for apraxia of speech (see Table 7.1). Concurrent with the application of a structured program, the clinician should accumulate detailed data on the patient's progress, be continually alert for any evidence of emerging self-cueing behaviors, and note the patient's responsiveness to different types of cues.

Some patients who may not be able to initiate self-cues early on may, nevertheless, be responsive to clinician-generated cues, as determined from initial assessments and early therapy sessions. For example, an individual may be totally unable to name any of the items of the PICA on subtest IV, yet will be able to produce the desired target word when a carrier phrase is provided; or, while unable to generate a written self-cue, he or she will be able to produce the verbal target when the clinician writes or prints the referent word. It may also be observed that, while the patient is unable to self-cue verbal responses, he or she can imitate clinician-modeled phonemes, words, or phrases.

In these situations, the clinician needs to determine:

1 Which cues or combinations of cues are most successful in facilitating production of target responses
2 What the most efficient cueing hierarchy is, i.e., a hierarchy that will permit the maximum number of successful patient responses while permitting the fading of cues as rapidly as possible (Linebaugh and Lehner, 1977)
3 Which successful cues the patient may be likely to generate for himself or herself
4 What steps are necessary to shape successful self-cueing from successful clinician-facilitated responses.

In the preliminary stages of treatment, novel steps in the program may be needed to promote self-cueing. For example, error recognition strategies may be implemented. While many patients with motor speech programming disorders are acutely aware of their off-target responses, some apractic–aphasic individuals are not. As Tonkovich and Berman (1981) point out, inherent in the encouragement of self-generated cues is the assumption that the patient is able to recognize his or her own errors and unsuccessful communicative attempts. Knowledge of a cueing strategy alone will not aid communication. The patient must also know *when* to use the strategy. Tonkovich and Berman suggested that error recognition can be shaped using a variety of methods. A hierarchy that begins with clinician judgment and expression of the adequacy of a patient response proceeds to clinician-assisted client judgment, and finally to independent client judgment is the most facilitating. The clinician must carefully determine for each patient whether treatment aimed at heightening error awareness is necessary. The patient who is already sufficiently aware of errors demonstrates consistent attempts at self-correction and self-cueing.

Whitney (1975) outlined four basic steps in conditioning the apractic–aphasic patient to incorporate self-produced cues:

1 Identify and isolate effective cues
2 Determine the skills necessary for development of the volitional use of cues, e.g., the patient may need to strengthen or relearn associations between phonemes and their graphic representations before employing an initial letter cue as a facilitator
3 Heighten the patient's awareness of the utility of the chosen cue
4 Teach the patient to use self-produced cues.

This conditioning process may involve direct instruction, indirect prompting, and/or reinforcement of the appropriate use of cues.

In the following sections, we summarize the rationale for employing patient-generated cues in therapy, provide a description of the process for determining the presence and relative effectiveness of self-cueing behaviors, and provide illustrative case examples in which the steps involved in successful self-cueing were accomplished utilizing single case experimental design approaches. These techniques can be effectively employed for those patients who are relatively mildly impaired, i.e. patients who are capable of initiating some successful self-cueing behaviors.

Summary of the Rationale: Self-Cueing Therapy

Treatment which focuses on the patient's self-cueing behavior rests on three basic assumptions. First, chronically apractic–aphasic individuals who can use and apply self-cueing strategies should have greater *independence and flexibility* in their communicative interactions. Patients who demonstrate self-cueing and self-correction behaviors appear to have a good prognosis for positive changes in their communicative abilities (Wepman, 1958). Furthermore, the cues and revisions they use have an inherent value in communicating the intended message, thus providing an advantage to the listener (Tompkins and Marshall, 1982). Second, the progression of treatment for patients who display self-cueing should be *hierarchical*, beginning with a highly controlled context in which the patient is encouraged to use his or her most productive self-cues and culminating in an application of those strategies at the most independent level of communication. Finally, the *uniqueness* of each individual should be recognized when selecting the treatment approach and structuring a method for evaluating outcome. Thus, the variety and types of self-cues used and their relative success must be analyzed individually. This analysis will guide the selection of a treatment approach, the stimuli and materials used in treatment, and the emphasis of treatment. It may also help to predict the potential for generalizing the treatment.

Stages of Analysis

Preliminary analysis of self-cueing abilities

The analysis stages in verbal self-cueing therapy begin with broad observations of the patient in a variety of expressive tasks. The clinician focuses on the *processes* and *strategies* the patient uses, i.e., the clinician looks for tangible evidence of an intangible process. What does the patient do to come up with a word or phrase? Under what circumstances is fluency enhanced? If the patient communicates part of the message, how does he or she do it? The clinician begins by identifying every facilitative behavior displayed by the patient as indicative of residual strengths that can be tapped to improve communicative efficiency.

Four standard conditions under which these observations can be made include:

1 Object naming
2 Object description
3 Story picture description
4 Conversation requiring the communication of content.

It is helpful to use more than one observer and to videotape the samples for purposes of evaluation and for comparison with subsequent evaluations which repeat the initial sampling procedures. Further, McReynolds and Kearns (1983) recommend taking multiple samples during the pretreatment condition to determine whether the pretreatment baseline is relatively stable, or whether changes are developing in a positive direction such that treatment effects are not independent of the trend.

By way of illustration, sample analyses are provided in Figures 7.1

SELF-CUEING ANALYSIS FORM

PATNT _____ *J. H.* _____ DATE ___ *9-31* ___

CLINICIAN (S): _____ *L. A.* _____

METHOD OF RECORDING: (CIRCLE) (VTR) AUDIOTAPE LIVE OBSERVATION

CONDITION	TYPES OF SELF-CUES	FACILITATIVE-*
Obj. Naming	*Revisions*	
	mid-word	✻
	pauses	
Obj. Description	*mid-word / Sentence*	
	pauses	✻
	Hand gestures	✻
	Subvocalizations	✻
Picture Descrip.	*Hand gestures*	✻
	Pauses	✻
	Subvocalizations	✻
	Revisions	✻
Conversation	*Revisions*	
	Hand gestures	✻
	Pauses	✻
	Subvocalizations	✻

SUMMARY OF FINDINGS *Fluent utterances usually preceded by gestures and pauses.*

PLAN *Alternating tx. design: evaluate pauses, pauses with subvocal rehearsal, syllable tapping.*

Figure 7.1   *Self-cueing behaviors of patient JH*

and 7.2. The eliciting conditions, stimuli, and behavioral observations are recorded. A composite list of self-cueing strategies, their frequencies of occurrence, and rate of success across sampling conditions is derived. Figure 7.1 describes the self-cueing behaviors of patient JH, a man with relatively mild aphasia and a moderate degree of verbal apraxia. Analysis revealed three types of self-cues occurring before or during his more fluent productions of multisyllabic words and short phrases. In each of the four sampling conditions the patient was noted to pause as though he were mentally rehearsing or subvocalizing. In the object description, story telling, and conversation conditions, he used a hand waving or pointing gesture as he paced his production of the utterance.

Figure 7.2 depicts the performance of a more severely impaired patient. JS could accurately express only a few single words or short phrases on the sampling tasks, but employed several types of self-cues. He gestured, wrote part of the word, expressed the initial phoneme of a word, or said a related word, even though the accuracy of his responses was poor. In conversation, he occasionally could circumlocute to give the listener a vague notion of the intended message. These preliminary

SELF-CUEING ANALYSIS FORM

PATIENT _J. S._ DATE _8-11_

CLINICIAN (S): _L. G._

METHOD OF RECORDING: (CIRCLE) VTR AUDIOTAPE (LIVE OBSERVATION)

CONDITION	TYPES OF SELF-CUES	FACILITATIVE-*
Obj. Naming	Initial sound / syll.	
	Pointing gesture	✶
	Related word	✶
	Delays	✶
Conversation	Pointing	✶
	Descriptive gesture	✶
	Initial sound	
	Write - first letter	
	Related word	✶

SUMMARY OF FINDINGS *Can't move on after he starts a word; gives up; comes up with name when gesturing or with circumlocutions.*

PLAN *Systematic analysis: relative effectiveness of patient's self-cues.*

Figure 7.2 Self-cueing behaviors of patient JS

analyses gave the clinician some direction for the second analysis stage, a systematic look at the efficacy of the patient's self-cues.

Multiple baseline analyses of self-cues

After preliminary observations are made, the efficacy of various self-cues is analyzed by taking repeated samples using similar tasks. Figure 7.3 illustrates the application of an alternating treatments design (McReynolds and Kearns, 1983) for analyzing the first patient's most predominant types of self-cues. The sampling task involved having the patient read ten short sentences containing multisyllabic words. The sentences were read under three imposed conditions:

1 With pauses at phrase intervals, but with no subvocal rehearsal of the next phrase
2 With pauses during which the patient was instructed to sub-vocally rehearse the next phrase prior to saying it
3 With the patient tapping each syllable as he read the entire sentence.

Order of presentation was varied for each sampling session. Tape recorded samples were randomized for review and scored using an adaptation of Porch's (1981) multidimensional scoring system. When the scores were plotted across six sessions, the syllable-by-syllable tapping condition emerged as the strongest type of self-cue in eliciting

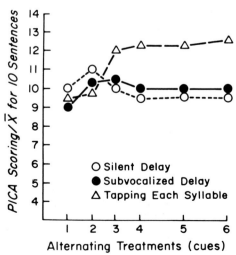

Figure 7.3   Application of alternating treatment design to compare cueing conditions

fluent and more accurately articulated speech utterances. Following this analysis, treatment focused on the patient's use of pacing cues. Treatment moved through the following steps:

1 Using syllable-by-syllable pacing in reading
2 Pacing in sentence completions
3 Pacing in short answers
4 Pacing in conversational interactions.

Figures 7.4 and 7.5 illustrate how frequency and success scores for the second patient, with moderately severe aphasia and apraxia of speech, were analyzed. While the patient was engaged in PACE therapy interactions (Davis and Wilcox, 1985; Davis, 1986), the frequency and success percentages of different self-cues were tabulated. The most frequently occurring self-cue was the use of the initial phoneme(s) of the target word; however, less frequently occurring cues were much more likely to elicit a correct or nearly correct response. Thus, multiple baseline comparisons of frequency and success percentages supported a

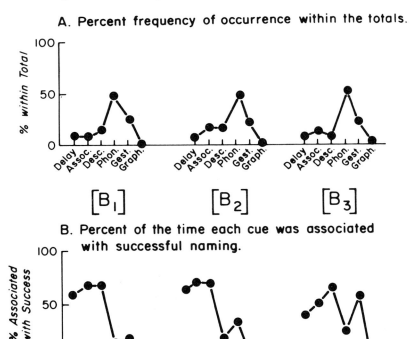

Figure 7.4   Baseline comparisons of different types of cues (Assoc = Association; Desc. = Description; Phon. = Initial Phoneme; Gest. = Gestural; Graph = Graphic)

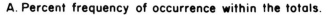

A. Percent frequency of occurrence within the totals.

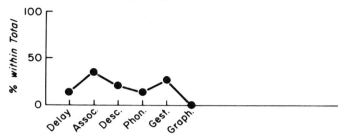

B. Percent of the time each cue was associated with successful naming.

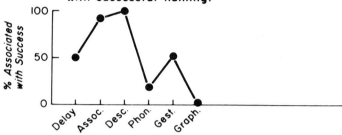

Figure 7.5   Final treatment probe of comparisons of different types of cues (Assoc = Association;   Desc. = Description;   Phon. = Initial   Phoneme;   Gest. = Gestural; Graph = Graphic)

treatment approach focused on encouraging the patient to increase his use of delay, gesture, association, and description. PACE therapy was interrupted briefly to devote explicit attention to the patient's self-cueing behavior. Treatment hierarchies were developed by taking the most frequently occurring successful cues (gestures), and pairing those with verbal descriptions and verbal associations using tasks and stimuli that required progressively more complex verbal utterances and pro-gressively less reliance on the clinician. Throughout this stage of treatment the patient was discouraged from merely trying to say the name of an object, since his apractic repetitions of the initial phoneme or syllable seldom led to successful naming and were misleading cues for the listener, creating frustration on both sides. By selectively focusing interim treatment on what appeared to be his more successful self-cues, this patient gradually began to use more gestures and verbal associa-tions and fewer initial phoneme cues. When PACE therapy was resumed, he continued to apply this approach and his response scores demonstrated considerably less reliance on the clinician to communicate a message.

Conclusion: Patient and Clinician Participation in Treatment

In these two examples, both the patient and the clinician were active participants in the treatment. Tests and assessments of aphasic–apractic patients are a means for finding out what the patient is or is not capable of doing when given certain communicative tasks, but tests and assessments more often than not are aimed at measuring 'rights' and 'wrongs' rather than *how* the response occurred. Identifying and analyzing the patient's self-cues require an examination of what the patient is contributing in both effective and ineffective ways towards the generation of messages. Self-cueing tells the clinician something about the patient's communicative patterns, patterns that are likely to be used by the patient in interactions outside of the clinic and remain with the patient after discharge from treatment.

The processes leading towards successful communication of a message will differ among patients. We can surmise differences in their internal schemata, but must rely on the patient's behavior as the best evidence of these mental processes. The patient provides the evidence for strategies he or she will naturally use, and the clinician provides a therapy to lead the patient towards applying those strategies as often and as effectively as possible. Self-cueing therapy is tangible, in the sense that the clinician says to the patient, 'These are the things I see you doing; this seems to be working pretty well but that doesn't seem to help at all, and we're going to work together so you'll start doing more of this and less of that'. The patient is not passive and there is no mystery to the intent of therapy. At the end of therapy patients should come to know what their self-cueing strategies are and how to use those strategies as effectively as they can. As chronically aphasic–apractic speakers they should leave treatment not with the feeling that they have been 'left to their own devices', but that they are left *with* their own devices.

References

BERMAN, M. and PEELLE, L.M. (1967) 'Self-generated cues: A method of aiding aphasic and apractic patients', *Journal of Speech and Hearing Disorders,* **32**, pp. 372–6.

BOLLINGER, R.L. and STOUT, C.E. (1976) 'Response-contingent small-step treatment: Performance-based communication intervention', *Journal of Speech and Hearing Disorders,* **41**, pp. 40–9.

BUGBEE, J.K. and NICHOLS, A.C. (1980) 'Rehearsal as a self-correction strategy for patients with apraxia of speech', in BROOKSHIRE, R.H. (Ed.) *Clinical Aphasiology Conference Proceedings 1980*, Minneapolis, BRK Publishers, pp. 279–84.

CHAPEY, R. (Ed.) (1986) *Language Intervention Strategies in Adult Aphasia*, 2nd ed., Baltimore, Williams and Wilkins.

COLLINS, M.J., CARISKI, D., LONGSTRETH, D. and ROSENBEK, J.C. (1980) 'Patterns of articulatory behavior in selected motor speech programming disorders', in BROOKSHIRE, R.H. (Ed.) *Clinical Aphasiology Conference Proceedings 1980*, Minneapolis, BRK Publishers, pp. 196–208.

DABUL, B. and BOLLIER, B. (1976) 'Therapeutic approaches to apraxia', *Journal of Speech and Hearing Disorders,* **41**, pp. 269–76.

DARLEY, F.L. (1982) *Aphasia*, Philadelphia, W.B. Saunders.

DAVIS, G.A. (1986) 'Pragmatics and treatment', in CHAPEY, R. (Ed.) *Language Intervention Strategies in Adult Aphasia*, 2nd ed., Baltimore, Williams and Wilkins, pp. 251–65.

DAVIS, G.A. and WILCOX, M.J. (1985) *Adult Aphasia Rehabilitation*, San Diego, College-Hill Press.

DEAL, J. and FLORANCE, C.L. (1978) 'Modification of the eight-step continuum for treatment of apraxia of speech in adults', *Journal of Speech and Hearing Disorders,* **43**, pp. 89–95.

DOWDEN, P.A., MARSHALL, R.C. and TOMPKINS, C.A. (1981) 'Amerind sign as a communicative facilitator for aphasic and apractic patients', in BROOKSHIRE, R.H. (Ed.) *Clinical Aphasiology Conference Proceedings 1981*, Minneapolis, BRK Publishers, pp. 133–40.

DUFFY, J.R. (1986) 'Schuell's stimulation rehabilitation', in CHAPEY, R. (Ed.) *Language Intervention Strategies in Adult Aphasia*, 2nd ed., Baltimore, Williams and Wilkins, pp. 187–214.

FLORANCE, C.L. and DEAL, J.L. (1977) 'A treatment protocol for non-verbal stroke patients', in BROOKSHIRE, R.H. (Ed.) *Clinical Aphasiology Conference Proceedings 1977*, Minneapolis, BRK Publishers, pp. 59–67.

GOLPER, L.C. and RAU, M.T. (1983) 'Systematic analysis of cueing strategies in aphasia: Taking your "cue" from the patient', in BROOKSHIRE, R.H. (Ed.) *Clinical Aphasiology Conference Proceedings 1983*, Minneapolis, BRK Publishers, pp. 52–61.

HELM, N. and BARRESI, B. (1980) 'Voluntary control of involuntary utterances: A treatment approach for aphasia', in BROOKSHIRE, R.H. (Ed.) *Clinical Aphasiology Conference Proceedings 1980*, Minneapolis, BRK Publishers, pp. 308–15.

HOODIN, R. and THOMPSON, C. (1983) 'Facilitation of verbal labeling in adult aphasia by gestural, verbal, or verbal plus gestural training' (abstract), in BROOKSHIRE, R.H. (Ed.) *Clinical Aphasiology Conference Proceedings 1983*, Minneapolis, BRK Publishers, pp. 62–4.

KEARNS, K.P., SIMMONS, N.N. and SISTERHEN, C. (1982) 'Gestural sign (Amer-Ind) as a facilitator of verbalization in patients with aphasia', in BROOKSHIRE, R.H. (Ed.) *Clinical Aphasiology Conference Proceedings 1982*, Minneapolis, BRK Publishers, pp. 183–91.

KERTESZ, A. (1982) *Western Aphasia Battery*, New York, Grune and Stratton.

LAPOINTE, L.L. (1984) 'Sequential treatment of split lists: a case report', in

ROSENBEK, J.C. *et al.* (Eds.) *Apraxia of Speech: Physiology, Acoustics, Linguistics, Management*, San Diego, College-Hill Press, pp. 278–86.

LAPOINTE, L.L. (1985) 'Aphasia therapy: Some principles and strategies for treatment', in JOHNS, D.F. (Ed.) *Clinical Management of Neurogenic Communicative Disorders*, 2nd ed., Boston, Little-Brown, pp. 179–241.

LINEBAUGH, C. and LEHNER, L. (1977) 'Cueing hierarchies and word retrieval: A therapy program', in BROOKSHIRE, R.H. (Ed.) *Clinical Aphasiology Conference Proceedings 1977*, Minneapolis, BRK Publishers, pp. 19–31.

LOVE, R. and WEBB, W.G. (1977) 'The efficacy of cueing techniques in Broca's aphasia', *Journal of Speech and Hearing Disorders*, **42**, pp. 170–8.

LURIA, A.R. (1970) *Traumatic Aphasia*, The Hague, Mouton.

MCREYNOLDS, L.V. and KEARNS, K.P. (1983) *Single-Subject Experimental Designs in Communicative Disorders*, Baltimore, University Park Press.

MARSHALL, N. and HOLTZAPPLE, P. (1976) 'Melodic intonation therapy: variations on a theme', in BROOKSHIRE, R.H. (Ed.) *Clinical Aphasiology Conference Proceedings 1976*, Minneapolis, BRK Publishers, pp. 115–41.

MARSHALL, R.C. (1976) 'Word retrieval behavior of aphasic adults', *Journal of Speech and Hearing Disorders*, **41**, pp. 444–51.

PEASE, D.H. and GOODGLASS, H. (1978) 'The effects of cueing on picture naming in aphasia', *Cortex*, **14**, pp. 178–89.

PODRAZA, B. and DARLEY, F.L. (1977) 'Effect of auditory prestimulation on naming in aphasia', *Journal of Speech and Hearing Research*, **20**, pp. 669–83.

PORCH, B.E. (1981) *Porch Index of Communicative Ability*, **II**, 3rd ed., Palo Alto, Consulting Psychologists Press.

RAO, P.R. and HORNER, J. (1978) 'Gesture as a deblocking modality in a severely aphasic patient', in BROOKSHIRE, R.H. (Ed.) *Clinical Aphasiology Conference Proceedings 1978*, Minneapolis, BRK Publishers, pp. 180–7.

ROSENBEK, J.C. (1978) 'Treating apraxia of speech', in JOHNS, D.F. (Ed.) *Clinical Management of Neurogenic Communicative Disorders*, Boston, Little-Brown, pp. 191–241.

ROSENBEK, J.C. (1985) 'Treating apraxia of speech', in JOHNS, D.F. (Ed.) *Clinical Management of Neurogenic Communicative Disorders*, 2nd ed., Boston, Little-Brown, pp. 267–312.

ROSENBEK, J.C., COLLINS, M.J. and WERTZ, R.T. (1976) 'Intersystemic reorganization for apraxia of speech', in BROOKSHIRE, R.H. (Ed.) *Clinical Aphasiology Conference Proceedings 1976*, Minneapolis, BRK Publishers, pp. 255–60.

ROSENBEK, J.C., LEMME, M.L., AHERN, M.B., HARRIS, E. and WERTZ, R.T. (1973) 'Treatment of apraxia of speech in adults', *Journal of Speech and Hearing Disorders*, **38**, pp. 462–72.

RUBOW, R.T., ROSENBEK, J.C., COLLINS, M.J. and LONGSTRETH, D. (1982) 'Vibrotactile stimulation for intersystemic reorganization in the treatment of apraxia of speech', *Arhives of Physical Medicine and Rehabilitation*, **63**, pp. 150–3.

SCHUELL, H. (1972) *The Minnesota Test for Differential Diagnosis of Aphasia*, Revised Edition, Minneapolis, University of Minnesota Press.

SHANE, H. and DARLEY, F.L. (1978) 'The effect of auditory rhythmic stimulation on articulatory accuracy in apraxia of speech', *Cortex,* **14**, pp. 444–50.

SIMMONS, N.N. (1978) 'Finger counting as an intersystemic reorganizer in apraxia of speech', in BROOKSHIRE, R.H. (Ed.) *Clinical Aphasiology Conference Proceedings 1978*, Minneapolis, BRK Publishers, pp. 174–9.

SIMMONS, N.N. (1980) 'Choice of stimulus modes in treating apraxia of speech: A case study', in BROOKSHIRE, R.H. (Ed.) *Clinical Aphasiology Conference Proceedings 1980*, Minneapolis, BRK Publishers, pp. 302–7.

SKELLY, M., SCHINSKY, L., SMITH, R.W. and FUST, R.S. (1974) 'American Indian sign (Amerind) as a facilitator of verbalization for the oral verbal apraxic', *Journal of Speech and Hearing Disorders,* **39**, pp. 445–56.

SPARKS, R.W. and DECK, J.W. (1986) 'Melodic intonation therapy', in CHAPEY, R. (Ed.) *Language Intervention Strategies in Adult Aphasia*, 2nd ed., Baltimore, Williams and Wilkins, pp. 320–32.

TOMPKINS, C.A. and MARSHALL, R.C. (1982) 'Communicative value of self-cues in aphasia', in BROOKSHIRE, R.H. (Ed.) *Clinical Aphasiology Conference Proceedings 1982*, Minneapolis, BRK Publishers, pp. 75–82.

TONKOVICH, J.D. and BERMAN, M.S. (1981) 'Use of the two-alternative forced-choice paradigm in training aphasic error recognition', in BROOKSHIRE, R.H. (Ed.) *Clinical Aphasiology Conference Proceedings 1981*, Minneapolis, BRK Publishers, pp. 128–32.

WEIDNER, W.E. and JINKS, A.F.G. (1983) 'The effects of single versus combined cue presentations on picture naming by aphasic adults', *Journal of Communication Disorders,* **16**, pp. 111–21.

WEIGL, E. (1974) 'Neuropsychological experiments on transcoding between spoken and written language structures', *Brain and Language,* **1**, pp. 227–40.

WEIGL, E. and BIERWISCH, M. (1970) 'Neuropsychology and linguistics: Topics of common research', *Foundations of Language,* **6**, pp. 1–18.

WEPMAN, J. (1958) 'The relationship between self-correction and recovery from aphasia', *Journal of Speech and Hearing Disorders,* **23**, pp. 302–5.

WERTZ, R.T., LAPOINTE, L.L. and ROSENBEK, J.C. (1984) *Apraxia of Speech in Adults*, New York, Grune and Stratton.

WHITNEY, J.L. (1975) 'Developing aphasics' use of compensatory strategies'. Paper presented at the annual meeting of the American Speech and Hearing Association, Washington, D.C. (unpublished).

Chapter 8

PROMPT Treatment

Paula Square-Storer and Deborah (Chumpelik) Hayden

The PROMPT System (Prompts for Restructuring Oral Muscular Phonetic Targets), is a dynamic tactile method of treatment for motor speech disorders which capitalizes upon touch pressure, kinesthetic, and proprioceptive cues. The method was developed by Chumpelik (Hayden) (1984) originally for the treatment of verbally apractic children. Subsequently, however, it was reported to facilitate verbal expression among adults with apraxia of speech and Broca's aphasia (Square, Chumpelik (Hayden), and Adams, 1985; Square *et al.*, 1986). Depending on the nature of the speech disorder or needs of the patient, PROMPTs provide the clinician with almost total motor control of the peripheral and some proximal articulators through manipulation. In turn, this manipulation provides for the patient, a framework for spatial and temporal motor speech programming. Prompts are applied to the mylohyoid muscle, facial musculature, and through manipulation of the mandible. Depending on the nature and degree of severity of the motor speech disorder, PROMPTs may provide input for some or all of the following parameters: spatial targeting for place and sometimes manner of production; degree of mandibular excursion; protrusion or retraction of facial muscles; the number of speech muscles required to contract; and relative segment and syllable durations. The purpose of this chapter is to describe the rationale and components of the PROMPT System, and to demonstrate the efficacy of the method by providing preliminary results of single-case research.

Rationale

Recent theories of initiation and control of movement specify three processes — *planning, programming,* and *execution* (Allen and Tsukahara, 1974; Brooks, 1979). Marsden (1982) described the motor *plan* as

190

conceiving the 'strategy for action', specification of 'where..., when..., and how to act', and putting 'together the package of motor actions...' (pp. 521–2). *Programming*, on the other hand, was described as including the 'assembly of simple single sequences specifying the activity of agonists, antagonists, synergists and postural fixators' plus 'assembly of subroutines and complex sequences of the program' (p. 522). Motor *execution* was said to entail 'initiating or beginning the movement sequence, running necessary programs, ... controlling the course of movement, and terminating or ceasing action' (p. 552). To our way of thinking, motor *planning* is roughly analogous to the generation of the phonological matrix which, according to the motor theory of speech production (Liberman *et al.*, 1967), is an *abstract* representation of patterns of neural activity for sets of distinctive features; for example, stridency may have one representation of neural activity while retroflexion, another. As such, this level of control of speech may be thought of as the generation of higher order linguistic phonological rules or the planning of phonemic templates. It is at this level that disruptions result in phonemic paraphasias marked by phoneme substitutions and/or phoneme sequencing disorders. Remediating such impairments may entail using transcoding between phonemes and graphemes (Wiegl and Bierwisch, 1970), since each represents linguistic units.

Programming is thought to be the disrupted control mechanism in the apraxias. It is at this level of motor control that 'motor pretuning' (Kelso and Tuller, 1981), and 'phasing' (Kent and Rosenbek, 1983) of the neuromotor commands are disrupted resulting in temporospatial disorganization of movements (see Chapter 2). Finally, it is usually the level of motor *execution* that is disrupted in the dysarthrias in that neural activation of the muscles of the speech system is disrupted; this precludes the efficient running of programs and control of the course of movement.

Although the exact neurophysiologic mechanisms cannot be fully specified, it is known that somatosensory information from muscles, joints, and skin not only influences execution via direct routes to the intermediate cerebellum and motor cortex, but also the *programming* of motor events via input to the association cortex. According to Brooks (1979) the basal ganglia and cerebellar hemisphere communicate with the association cortex in programming volitional movements. Marsden (1982) stated '... the pars intermedia (of the cerebellum) updates the intended movement, based upon the motor command originally issued and somatosensory description of ... position and velocity on which the movement is to be superimposed' (p. 522); and, 'to execute a motor plan, one has to move from point to point of a sequence, the signal of arrival at each point being the trigger to delivery of the motor program required to shift to the next point in a sequence (Marsden, 1982, p. 535).

It is upon this model that we predicate the efficacy of PROMPT treatment. The skilled and experienced PROMPT clinician provides for the patient an enhanced and, initially, clinician-controlled somatosensory description of the postural fixators or articulatory end-points, velocities, and trajectories of movements, and the 'phasing' or temporal assembly of motor subroutines. The clinician acts as an 'external programmer' and, once having mapped in the program, ensures that the patient remains motorically but not sensorily passive. Immediately after, the patient is allowed motoric control while the clinician continues to provide somatosensory support for the constraints and patterns of movement. Eventually, the patient appears to internalize the program for each target and, especially among children, begins to generate related programs (Chumpelik (Hayden), 1984) in that principles of motor equivalence (Hebb, 1949) seem to be learned.

Method

In this section the components of the PROMPTs used for treatment will be discussed. Our readers must be aware that PROMPT treatment is multifaceted treatment and that many principles beyond those reported here comprise the method. Further, because the PROMPT System is a dynamic method, extensive training and practice are required in order to competently and efficiently administer this form of treatment. Attempts to learn the PROMPT System from the skeletal information presented here will be impossible.

When initiating a PROMPT treatment session, the clinician engages the patient by first establishing a sitting position that allows for maintenance of head control. For example, the clinician stabilizes the patient using one hand behind his/her head, while using the other hand to control and provide cues to the oral apparatus. The patient is then instructed to allow the clinician complete control through the instruction, 'let me do it'. The clinician, thus, has full liberty to program in the target phoneme, word, or phrase. Integral stimulation, that is, the instruction, 'watch me, listen to me', (Rosenbek, 1978) are also used for multimodality input. For some patients, attention to all modalities, i.e., auditory, visual, tactile, and kinesthetic may prove to be overstimulating. In those cases, the patient is encouraged not to watch the clinician but rather to 'feel the movement'. The patient's attention if further directed to the 'sequenced' aspects of the production. That is, cues for the temporal aspects of speech movements are stressed.

The PROMPT System cannot elicit speech where there is an extremely severe neuroinnervation impairment (dysarthria). The patient must have, minimally, breath support, phonation ability for an open vowel, some ability to cooperate, and minimal/basic comprehension skills. The System can guide the articulators to specific postures and actions sequentially, and, thus, stimulate motor speech programming. If the clinician is skilled, the PROMPT System can help the patient to approximate phonemes successfully and independently produce programmed words/phrases, i.e., depending upon the patient's preserved abilities and extent of disability with regard to language and motor speech processes, spontaneous generalization is more or less probable but seems to occur to a much lesser degree, in aphasic–apractic adults than among verbally apractic children.

Given the above considerations, PROMPTs work to establish the patterning of several different speech parameters. They are: place of contact; extent of mandibular excursion; resonance and phonation; number of muscles in the contracted state; duration of segments relative to one another; manner of production; and coarticulation. Each will be discussed below.

Place of contact

Place of contact is traditionally seen as the end point of a target 'movement' (Lindblom, 1963; Stevens and House, 1963). Traditional treatment identifies areas of orofacial structures, i.e., upper/lower lips, alveolar ridge, hard palate, and soft palate, as 'places' where various structures articulate. For example, in the production of /t/ the tongue tip touches the alveolar ridge. In the PROMPT System, four places of contact are prompted. These are designated as A, B, C, and D in Figure 8.1. They traverse the mylohyoid muscle from just behind the mandible (point A), to just above and behind the larynx (point D). Through digital manipulation of these placements the tongue may be prompted to articulate with the palate at the most anterior lingua–alveolar position to the most posterior linguavelar place. For example, an A position is used for all tongue tip/blade productions (/t/, /d/, /n/, /s/, /z/), and D for velar productions (/k/, /g/, /ŋ/). Points B and C are used for midpalatal productions, (/I/, /ɛ/, /ʃ/, /ɜˆ/, etc.). The clinician uses either one, two, or three fingers to stimulate the approximate *area* of the lingual surface (width) needed to produce the target phoneme. Through cues related to

PLACE OF CONTACT FOR TARGET POSITIONS
MYLOHYOID PLACEMENTS

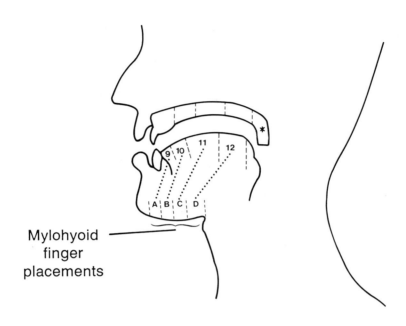

Mylohyoid
finger
placements

9. tongue tip

10. apex

11. blade front

12. dorsum

Figure 8.1   Place of contact for target positions and mylohyoid placements. (Adapted by permission from Chumpelik, D.: Seminars in Speech and Language, Vol. 5, No. 2, Thieme Medical Publishers, New York, 1982)

lingual width, the placement of production and amount of lingual excursion in the superior/inferior plane (depth of movement as signaled by amount of pressure), the clinician can:

1 Partially manipulate the structures into the placement position
2 Approximate the neuromuscular pattern needed for production
3 Stimulate kinesthetically the lingual musculature required for moving to the correct target position.

Place of contact is also signaled on the facial muscles. These prompted positions are most often bilateral using two digits, usually the thumb and index finger to provide information to the facial muscles for the labial postures of spreading and rounding, or for degree of mandibular excursion. On the face, all prompts are worked from midline or bilaterally to stimulate symmetrical action, an important goal of such training. This is especially desirable for those patients with various degrees of neuromuscular innervation dysfunction or unilateral facial paresis. As with the mylohyoid prompts, pressure is provided as a cue that deeper muscles or muscle groups which cannot be directly stimulated, are to be activated. Duration cues are also added to represent timing of activity.

In Figure 8.2, placements 1 and 2 are used to stimulate labial rounding as for /o/ or /u/, or retraction as for /s/; placements 3 and 4, the upper for /i/ and the lower for /Θ/; placement 5 for /f/ or /v/ (labial manipulation only); placement 6 and 7 for /ʃ/ and one component of /tʃ/ (contraction); placement 8 for indicating velar lowering to signal nasality (cue only); placement 9 indicating phonation for voicing (cue only); and placement 10 for jaw excursion. The latter three 'place' cues indicate major speech 'actions' while the former seven indicate movements towards spatial targets.

Mandibular excursion

Mandibular excursion relates to the amount of jaw opening needed for each target position. The proper balance of tongue–jaw action 'phased' with the coordinated contraction of facial muscles to achieve actions such as labial rounding, or spreading, are also critical for coarticulation. Correct extent of mandibular excursion is a crucial component of normal speech production although, in the management of some dysarthrias, mandibular stabilization may be desirable (Rosenbek and LaPointe, 1978). For some patients with AOS, mandibular kinesthesia impairments may complicate the primary motor speech programming impairment (Rosenbek, Wertz and Darley, 1973). Thus, place of contact may be correct, but segmental production may be distorted due to exaggerated or restricted mandibular action. The PROMPT System provides kinesthetic manipulation for the degree of opening required for each target, segment, or syllable as well as mandibular changes required during transitions between segments.

The four positions shown in Figure 8.3 are used by the clinician to signal different degrees of mandibular excursion. Depending on the

FACIAL PROMPTS

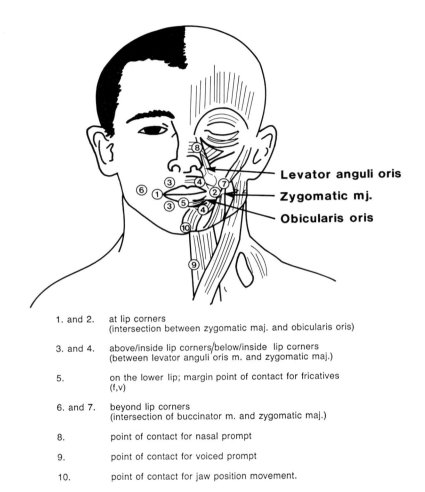

Levator anguli oris

Zygomatic mj.

Obicularis oris

1. and 2. at lip corners
(intersection between zygomatic maj. and obicularis oris)

3. and 4. above/inside lip corners/below/inside lip corners
(between levator anguli oris m. and zygomatic maj.)

5. on the lower lip; margin point of contact for fricatives
(f,v)

6. and 7. beyond lip corners
(intersection of buccinator m. and zygomatic maj.)

8. point of contact for nasal prompt

9. point of contact for voiced prompt

10. point of contact for jaw position movement.

Figure 8.2   Facial PROMPTS. (Adapted by permission from Chumpelik, D.: Seminars in Speech and Language, *Vol. 5, No. 2, Thieme Medical Publishers, New York, 1982)*

patient's jaw length, facial, dental, or palatal structures, there will be differences in the maximal degree of opening, i.e., the distance between the extreme positions, 1 and 4, as well as between each of the four positions. Thus, the clinician must take all structural aspects into account when determining the maximum jaw opening position.

Although vowel segments are primarily influenced by jaw excursion, consonants also need varying jaw heights to achieve place of contact or to enable the tongue to move semi-independently of the jaw.

JAW POSITIONS FOR VOWEL PRODUCTION

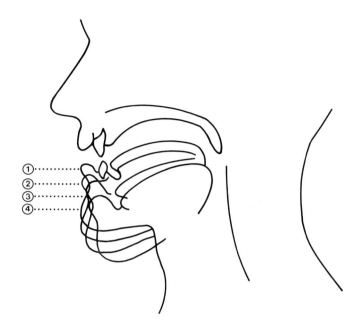

Jaw Positions for Vowel Production

		FRONT	CENTRAL	BACK
HIGH	1.	[i] heed	[ə] above	[u] who'd [ʊ] hood
	2.	[e] hate	[ʌ] hut	[o] hoe
	3	[ɛ] head		
	4	[æ] had		[a] hot

Figure 8.3   Jaw positions for vowel production. (Adapted by permission from Chumpelik, D.. Seminars in Speech and Language, Vol. 5, No. 2, Thieme Medical Publishers, New York, 1982)

Segments produced at jaw position 1 include the /i/, /u/, /p/, /f/; at 2, /o/, /n/, /ʃ/, and /Θ/; at 3, /dʒ/, /ɜˆ/, and /ɛ/; and at 4, /k/, /g/, /æ/, and /a/. For syllabic coarticulation within phrases, jaw position is never extended beyond the 2 or 3 position. When specifically training the phonemes, /k/ and /g/, in isolation or the neutral environment of /ʌ/, the jaw may be extended to a 4 position to encourage the movement of the dorsum of the tongue to articulate with the soft palate (place of contact). Although the patient may receive slightly exaggerated tactile and kinesthetic cues for some positions, the prompting will facilitate the integration of this information for coarticulation, and especially when rate of speaking becomes faster.

Orality/nasality and voicing/devoicing actions

The patient learns that resonatory and phonatory control is required for production of all speech segments. Nasality is signaled by facial prompt 8 shown in Figure 8.2. The thumb provides tactile stimulation to the side of the nose and this prompt is incorporated with a mylohyoid finger prompt for place of production of /n/ or /ŋ/, or lip closure for /m/. The nasality cue is always provided for the client to ensure consistency of production. As stated above, the degree of mandibular excursion is also provided as needed, e.g., position 4 for /ŋ/.

In adult apractic patients, devoicing/voicing and nasality/orality confusions often occur (Itoh and Sasanuma, 1984). With the PROMPT System, the clinician can cue the patient for nasality, and/or voicing. A devoiced airstream may also be cued along with manipulation of other structures to achieve targets. This latter type of cueing utilizes principles of phonetic derivation (see Chapter 6). For example, /f/ may be obtained by first eliciting an airstream as for /h/ and, then, manipulating the jaw to the 1 position while using facial prompt 5 to move the lower lip into the correct labiodental position.

Once patients are clearly in control of actions for signaling voicing/devoicing and orality/nasality and are observed to associate the cued actions for achieving these end-point targets with the intended perceptual features, the clinician will usually need only to touch the area to remind the client of the added or omitted articulatory feature.

Tension

Cues for tension relate specifically to the number of muscles or muscle group(s) which should be activated in the facial or lingual systems and the relative length of time they should be activated (Shriberg and Kent, 1982). The degree of pressure applied by the clinician signals these two parameters. Also the deeper the muscles to the periphery, the higher the prompted degree of tension. For specific phonemes, lingual and facial tensions vary. Thus, increased pressure is applied for tense vowels such as /i/ and /u/, and reduced pressure for lax vowels such as /ʋ/. Further, prompts delivered to the mylohyoid are greater in pressure than those delivered to the face, as there are more layers of tissue to work through before cues for contraction of the varying lingual muscles become salient to the patient. For example, different degrees of tension and thus prompted pressure, exist for /a/, /ɛ/ and /ɜˆ/. For /a/, when trained in isolation, the jaw is at a full open 4 position and there is little or no specific pressure applied to the tongue via the mylohyoid. For /ɛ/, the jaw is at an open 3 position and there is tension in the blade area of the tongue, at the mylohyoid C position. Adjunctively, two fingers are used and quick, firm pressure is applied. This pressure provided in such a quick manner signals the lingual muscles which should contract, as well as the duration of muscle contraction. For /ɜˆ/, the jaw is loosely opened at a 1 position and consistent, firm pressure is placed on the mylohyoid at position C using three fingers. This firm consistent pressure signals the activation of deep lingual muscles of the blade and dorsum. Facial prompts at the 1 and 2 position also increase the overall tactile impression.

Relative duration of segments

Prompts for the *relative* timing of segments is essential for normal speech production. As noted above in 'tension', the prompt may be quick or held longer to indicate duration of a phoneme. When there is a high amount of tension, duration will not normally signal features which require that few muscle groups be contracted. For example, little tension and a longer relative duration may signal features such as nasality. Relative duration over segments will influence the relative timing of segments at the syllable level as well as the timing of transitions between segments, i.e., coarticulation. Since coarticulation in AOS has been found to be deviant (Ziegler and von Cramon, 1985, 1986), these prompts may be of utmost importance. Further, vowel durations among apractic speakers are often deviant (see Square-Storer, 1987 for a review) and, thus, in need of timing control. The PROMPT System provides coordinated input for the programming of coordinated output.

Manner

Manner, or airstream management, is handled by combining the critical prompts for place (facial or mylohyoid), degree of mandibular excursion (of jaw opening), orality/nasality, duration, and pressure cues. That is, airstream management in this treatment approach is always depend-ent on the adequate prompting of other articulatory actions. For example, if a patient is producing a stop consonant, /t/, for the fricative, /s/, duration is a critical factor as well as the facial prompts for placements 1 and 2. For each manner class, different prompts may be emphasized. For example, for bilabial stop plosion, the lips need to be occludea lightly and quickly released after appropriate imploding of the airstream. Thus, PROMPTs for position, pressure, and timing are critical. For production of frication, the tongue or the cutting edge of the incisors is involved. Depending on the effectors required for each phoneme, different PROMPT parameters will be emphasized. For /f/, the lower lip would be manipulated. Contrarily, for /ʃ/, the width and placement of tongue involvement (three fingers at a C position) as well as facial prompts 6 and 7, for labial protrusion anteriorly and buccal contraction bilaterally, are important. Airstream management (manner) is always a dynamic process and depending on the phoneme, or coarticulatory influences on phonemes, differing amounts of input by the clinician will be needed. Inherent to all of the above, is imparting to the patient the knowledge of what muscle groups must contract under specific constraints in order to achieve the appropriate action. Equally important is cueing for the coarticulation of muscle groups in a tightly 'phased' manner. That is, temporal prompting for the integration of all the articulatory subfeatures of phonemes and parameters of coarticula-tion between the articulatory features is necessary.

Coarticulation

One of the most unique functions of the PROMPT System is that it is a *dynamic* treatment approach. Thus, once segments can be elicited using PROMPTs, treatment immediately focuses on transitionalization between them and, to a lesser extent, sequencing of the units (phonemes) themselves. For the clinician, this may mean working predominantly at the phrase level with occasional steps back to the phoneme or syllable level to improve phoneme precision. At this level the clinician uses 'surface' prompts to cue key elements of the motor pattern. When prompting at the 'surface level', the clinician provides place and timing cues. 'Deep prompting' delivers more specific cues for muscle contraction and duration. During segmental production, coar-ticulation influences are significant and variables such as jaw height and labial rounding or retraction are dictated by the constraints of the phonetic environment. Coarticulation influences may be noted in that, consonant features are easily distorted and/or determined by the preceding or following vowel. For example, in 'coat' the lips are rounded while the /k/ and /t/ are produced. When needed, the clinician can provide anticipatory and regressive assimilation cues, i.e., coarticulatory cues, for such influences. The clinician, thus, focuses on these variables in order to achieve coordinated coarticulated muscle activation which results in appropriately perceived speech. If specific target production continues to be in need of prompting, the clinician may isolate the phoneme, prompt it alone and then return to the word or phrase. In adult aphasic–apractic patients, phrases are usually the preferred stimuli for treatment as they can be 'programmed in' as easily as a single word. With phrases, however, the clinician prompts all targets dynamically. This skill demands a complete understanding of the normal dynamics of speech production as well as experience with PROMPT treatment. Excellent clinical results, however, are achieved. In the next section, we present our pilot research regarding PROMPT treatment for adults with acquired apraxia of speech with coexisting aphasia and, possible, coexisting mild dysarthria.

Evidence of the Efficacy of PROMPT Treatment

Subjects

The subjects of this investigation were three patients, two males, PW and RJ, aged 58 and 59, and one female, SS, aged 38. Each demonstrated at least ten symptoms of apraxia of speech as discerned from administration of both the Apraxia of Speech Battery for Adults (Dabul, 1979) and the Mayo Clinic Screening Battery for Apraxia of Speech. The latter is similar to the battery described by Wertz, LaPointe and Rosenbek (1984). The characteristics of apraxia of speech demonstrated by each are summarized in Table 8.1. All subjects were classified as Broca's aphasic subjects on the Western Aphasia Battery (WAB) (Kertesz, 1982). Their aphasia quotients (AQ) were 23.2 (PW), 45.5 (RJ), and 52.8 (SS). Informal testing revealed that one subject, (SS), was severely agrammatic; the other two subjects demonstrated agrammatism to a lesser degree. Each had suffered a single left-hemisphere thromboembolic accident. There was confirmation that PW's lesion was a deep one extending into the internal capsule. It was suspected that SS's lesion was also a deep one, based upon her dense hemiplegia and pervasive yet mild hypernasality. RJ's neuropsychologic profile was

Table 8.1: Characteristics of Apraxia of Speech Demonstrated by Each Patient Undergoing PROMPT Treatment

	S1 (PW)	S2 (RJ)	S3 (SS)
Phonemic anticipatory errors			
Phonemic perseverative errors	X		X
Phonemic transposition errors			
Phonemic voicing errors	X	X	X
Phonemic vowel errors	X	X	X
Visible/audible searching	X	X	X
Numerous/varied off-target attempts	X	X	X
Errors highly inconsistent	X	X	X
Errors increase with length	X	X	X
Fewer errors, in automatic speech	X	X	X
Marked difficulty initiating speech	X	X	X
Intrusive schwas, CCs	N/A*	X	
Abnormal prosody	N/A*	N/A*	X
Awareness of errors/inability to correct	X	X	X

* N/A: due to the severity of their disorders, reliable judgements of these parameters could not be attained.

consistent with those for cortical frontoparietal lesions. Each subject was at least one year post-onset, severely limited with respect to functional verbal expression, and had been discharged from formal speech–language treatment due to lack of evidence of progress.

Procedures

Performances of each subject were baselined over three days on three types of repetition tasks. These included imitation of minimally contrastive phoneme pairs, polysyllabic words, and functional phrases. On each of three consecutive days, twenty-four pairs of minimally contrastive phonemes listed in Table 8.2 were repeated three times in different random orders. Thus, an overall total of 216 productions for each subject were obtained. Production of twenty polysyllabic words, ten laden with plosives and ten with fricatives, was probed. The words are listed in Table 8.3. Each was repeated ten times on each of three baseline days, totaling 600 polysyllabic productions for each subject. Ten functional phrases consisting of three two-syllable imperatives, three three-syllable, and four four-syllable common phrases were probed. The phrases are listed in Table 8.4. Each was repeated ten times on each baseline day, for a total of thirty productions of each or, 300 tokens per subject. Productions of all baseline stimuli were scored as correct or incorrect by two clinicians. A third investigator who had not observed the patients' on-line performances selected, from the scored data,

Table 8.2: Minimal Pairs Tested

		(List one)				(List two)				(List three)	
V	1.	s-z	—	M	1.	s-t	—	V	1.	v-f	—
P	2.	t-k	—	P	2.	p-t	—	P	2.	t-p	—
M	3.	tʃ-t	—	V	3.	dʒ-tʃ	—	M	3.	t-s	—
M	4.	dʒ-d	—	P	4.	g-d	—	M	4.	z-d	—
P	5.	ʃ-s	—	M	5.	t-n	—	P	5.	d-b	—
V	6.	t-d	—	V	6.	f-v	—	V	6.	k-g	—
P	7.	g-d	—	V	7.	b-p	—	P	7.	g-b	—
V	8.	f-v	—	P	8.	b-d	—	V	8.	p-b	—
M	9.	t-n	—	M	9.	d-z	—	M	9.	ʃ-tʃ	—
V	10.	g-k	—	M	10.	dʒ-d	—	V	10.	s-z	—
P	11.	p-t	—	P	11.	ʃ-s	—	P	11.	t-k	—
M	12.	s-t	—	V	12.	t-d	—	M	12.	tʃ-t	—
M	13.	d-z	—	P	13.	b-g	—	M	13.	tʃ-ʃ	—
P	14.	b-d	—	M	14.	tʃ-ʃ	—	P	14.	b-g	—
V	15.	b-p	—	V	15.	g-k	—	V	15.	g-k	—
P	16.	b-g	—	V	16.	s-z	—	P	16.	ʃ-s	—
V	17.	dʒ-tʃ	—	P	17.	t-k	—	V	17.	t-d	—
M	18.	tʃ-ʃ	—	M	18.	tʃ-t	—	M	18.	dʒ-d	—
V	19.	z-s	—	M	19.	ʃ-tʃ	—	V	19.	b-p	—
P	20.	k-t	—	P	20.	g-b	—	P	20.	b-d	—
M	21.	t-tʃ	—	V	21.	p-b	—	M	21.	d-z	—
M	22.	d-dʒ	—	P	22.	d-b	—	M	22.	t-n	—
P	23.	s-ʃ	—	P	23.	z-d	—	P	23.	g-d	—
V	24.	d-t	—	V	24.	k-g	—	V	24.	f-v	—

M: manner difference
P: place difference
V: voice difference

*Table 8.3: Polysyllabic
words tested*

Bisyllables

Plosives	*Fricatives*
cookie	seafood
daddy	scissor
baby	father
puppy	fussy
table	chiffon

Trisyllables

cantelope	sensation
cabinet	fanciful
getaway	faithful
tobacco	vaseline
decorate	fatherly

stimuli for the investigation. For each patient, four pairs of minimally
contrasting phonemes were selected; none had ever been produced
correctly during the baseline sessions. Two pairs were randomly
selected for training using PROMPTs and two pairs acted as controls

Table 8.4: *Functional Phrases Tested*

A. *Two syllables* (score 0–2)
  1 Help me
  2 Stop it
  3 Come here

B. *Three syllables* (score 0–3)
  1 I am fine
  2 I want more
  3 How are you?

C. *Four syllables* (score 0–4)
  1 What do you want?
  2 I want to go
  3 See you later
  4 Give it to me

for probing using imitation. For two subjects (PW and RJ), four polysyllabic words were randomly selected, two for training using PROMPTs and two for probing. For the third subject (SS), six polysyllabic words were selected, three for training and three for probing. For two subjects, functional phrases were trained. For one subject (PW), two phrases were trained and two were probed. For the other subject (RJ), one phrase was trained and a second was not. Training of phrases for the third subject (SS) was not undertaken due to her severe agrammatism. Instead the subject's performances on additional polysyllabic words, as described above, were observed.

It was decided *a priori* to score and analyze the data in two ways. The first was to use a binary system of correct–incorrect. The second scoring system graded each minimal pair production or each polysyllabic word response using a 2, 1, 0 categorical system in which '2' represented a response which was spatially and temporally correct, i.e., totally correct. 'Spatially correct' was defined as a response in which targeting for each phoneme (segment) was correct with regard to place of production and in which there were no gross distortions, additions, nor omissions of segments nor any initial gropes. 'Temporal correctness' denoted several parameters including the perception of correct onset and termination of voicing, correct 'phasing' of all articulatory features, correct relative segment durations, and, in the case of polysyllabic words and phrases, no intersyllabic or word pauses. A slow rate of speech was acceptable. A '1' denoted a response which was marked by a spatial or temporal error, while a '0' was given for a response which was spatially and temporally incorrect or characterized by more than one spatial or temporal error. For phrases only, each word produced correctly both spatially and temporally received one point; that is, the graded scoring system was not used. Point-to-point, inter-rater reliability using the graded scoring system was found to be acceptable in that it ranged from 81.4 per cent to 70.1 per cent. Point-to-point, inter-rater reliability using the correct–incorrect system was found to range from 89.3 per cent to 91.1 per cent. Mean reliability was 91.09 per cent.

The PROMPT training procedure was as follows. First, the patient was presented with an auditory model of a minimal pair, word, or functional phrase. No prompts were given. The patient attempted to repeat the target according to a model and a score of '0', '1' or '2' was given. If a score of '2' was received, the next item was presented for a total of twenty tokens. If, however, a score of '1' or '0' was received, the clinician prompted as follows: the subject was instructed not to respond as the clinician 'mapped in' the correct motor pattern for the sequence of phonemes to be produced using the PROMPT System. The clinician then instructed the subject to attempt the target phoneme, word, or phrase as the clinician simultaneously prompted the motor pattern again. The response was scored as a '0', '1' or '2'. The next token in each train of twenty was then presented auditorily for imitation and the same procedure was followed based upon the subject's ability to imitate the token after the first presentation. Untrained series of items were presented auditorily only and the subject's ability to repeat those items was scored using the same scoring methods.

Results

The results are reported for each patient according to accuracy of production of each type of stimulus item, i.e., minimal pairs, polysyllabic words, and phrases, during the course of treatment.

Minimal pairs

As graphically depicted in Figure 8.4, using the plus–minus scoring system, PW demonstrated accelerated learning curves for the phonemes which were trained using PROMPT. These are observed at the top of the figure and are indicated by the solid line. Results for those phoneme contrasts which were not prompted are shown in the lower part of Figure 8.4. No acquisition of the nontrained pairs occurred when accuracy of production was scored using the correct–incorrect method. Results using the graded 0, 1, 2 scoring system were essentially the same

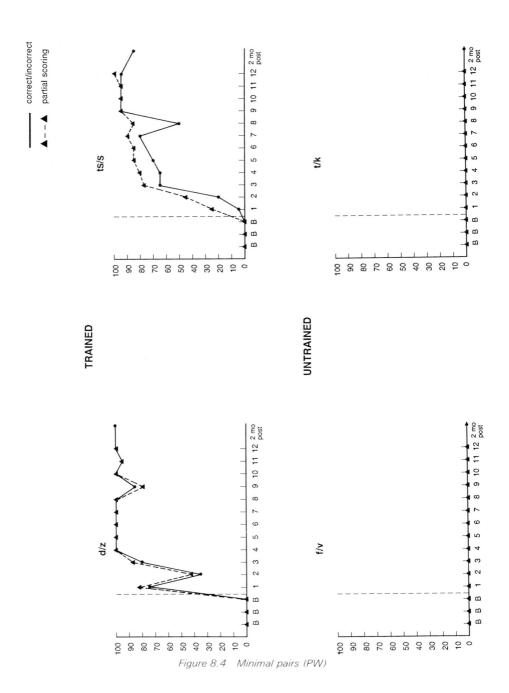

Figure 8.4   Minimal pairs (PW)

as indicated by the dotted lines on all graphs. A slightly improved performance for the trained pair, tʃ/ʃ, was discerned when partial credit was given; no differences were seen for production of the untrained items, i.e., performance remained at 0 per cent correct. We were able to obtain measures of PW's performances on these minimal pairs two months after termination of PROMPT treatment. It is interesting to note that the patient maintained production of the trained contrasts even though treatment had ceased.

As shown in Figure 8.5, RJ performed similarly to PW. Using the correct–incorrect scoring system shown in the solid lines at the top of the figure, he demonstrated accelerated learning curves for the prompted minimal pairs. Further, he demonstrated poor performances on the untrained items, with the exception of one training session in which he produced 50 per cent of d/z contrasts correctly. Use of the partial scoring system reflected by the broken lines, however, demonstrated some learning of the untrained minimal pairs by RJ. Thus, it appeared that use of repetition alone facilitated some minimal and/or variable performances.

Figure 8.6 summarizes the results for SS, with regard to production of minimal pairs. Using the correct–incorrect scoring system (solid line), she demonstrated accelerated and fairly stable learning curves for the trained items as shown in the top portion of the figure. Results of performances on the untrained stimuli were not as convincing in that, for the d/z pair, considerable positive results were demonstrated, but at a slower rate and with greater variability. It may be that learning was demonstrated for this pair because the features of place and voicing were contrasted in the trained pairs. As well, plosion was PROMPT trained as it occurred in /t/. Results of production of minimal pairs by SS, as derived using the partial credit scoring system, revealed even more learning of the untrained pair, d/z: 95 per cent accuracy was achieved by session 12. The learning of that pair, however, was not as accelerated as for the trained pairs. Nonetheless, the partial-credit scoring system, indeed, revealed relatively stable improvement curves. For the minimal pair tʃ/ʃ, some learning, although minimal and variable, was discerned from the use of the partial-credit scoring system.

Polysyllabic words

As demonstrated in Figure 8.7, PW demonstrated rapidly accelerated learning curves for the trained stimuli, 'cabinet' and 'sensation'. Using the partial scoring system (broken lines), performances on the trained stimuli were only slightly enhanced from the results obtained using the

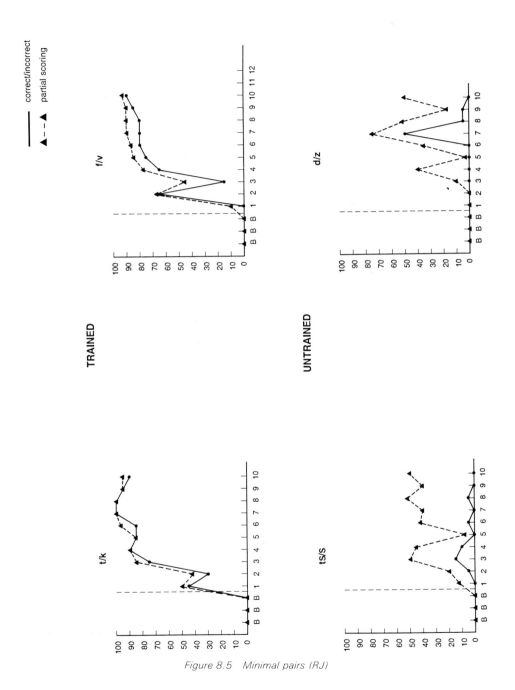

Figure 8.5   Minimal pairs (RJ)

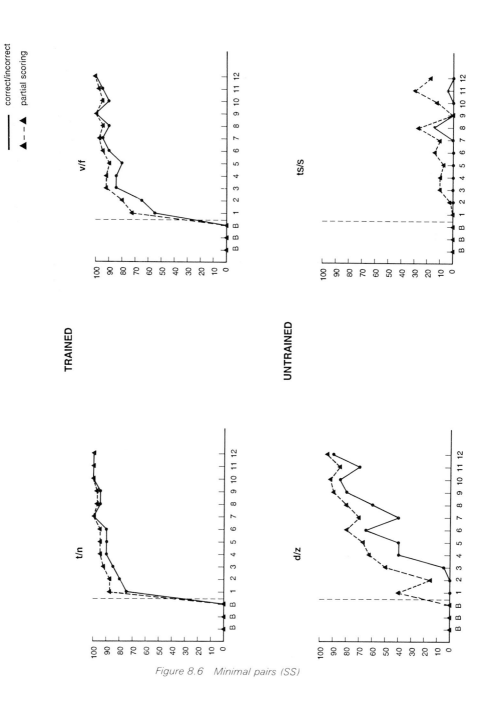

Figure 8.6 Minimal pairs (SS)

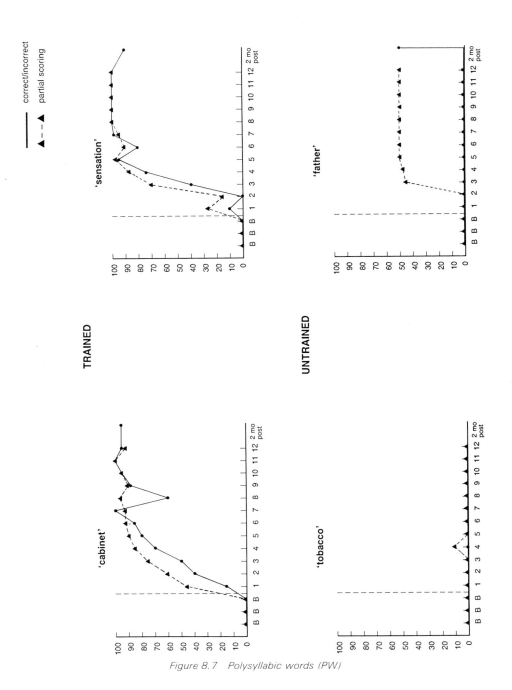

Figure 8.7   Polysyllabic words (PW)

correct–incorrect system. Upon retesting two months after completion of PROMPT therapy, performances for production of these words maintained as they had for the minimal pairs. For the untrained word, 'tobacco', accuracy of performance using the two scoring systems was essentially the same and hovered around 0. However, accuracy of production of the untrained word, 'father', was shown to improve using the graded scoring system. PW, from session two onwards, attained a 48 per cent to 50 per cent accuracy of production for the word using a partial-credit scoring system. A score of '1' was given to most of his repetition productions, since only one phoneme remained erroneous in most productions of that word, $/\partial/$. Thus, again there was some evidence of improvement using repetition only; however, that improvement was not nearly as dramatic as that observed for those items trained using the PROMPT System.

Results of the performances of RJ are shown in Figure 8.8. Rapidly accelerated learning curves were demonstrated using both scoring systems for PROMPT trained items. No progress was demonstrated for the untrained item, 'cantelope', using either scoring system. For the untrained word, 'father', no improvement was discerned using the $+/-$ scoring system; application of the graded error system demonstrated improvement, but not until the seventh session. Again, although the partial-scoring system revealed some learning under the repetition mode of stimulation, improvement occurred later and to a lesser degree than for the PROMPT trained items.

Subject SS demonstrated similar trends of acquisition. As shown in Figure 8.9, application of both scoring systems revealed that the three PROMPT trained words, 'decorate', 'chiffon' and 'fanciful' were produced with at least 85 per cent accuracy by the fifth session. Using the correct–incorrect scoring system, performances on the untrained items, 'cantelope' and 'seafood', demonstrated no improvement and only limited improvement for the untrained word 'sensation'. Application of the partial-credit scoring system also revealed no learning for production of the word, 'cantelope'. For the words, 'seafood' and 'sensation', some improvement occurred over time, but degree of accuracy and consistency of production were inferior to that achieved for the trained items.

Functional phrases

Functional phrases were trained for PW and RJ only. As described previously, only the correct–incorrect scoring method was used and the correctness of each word was evaluated. Thus, in a two–word phrase

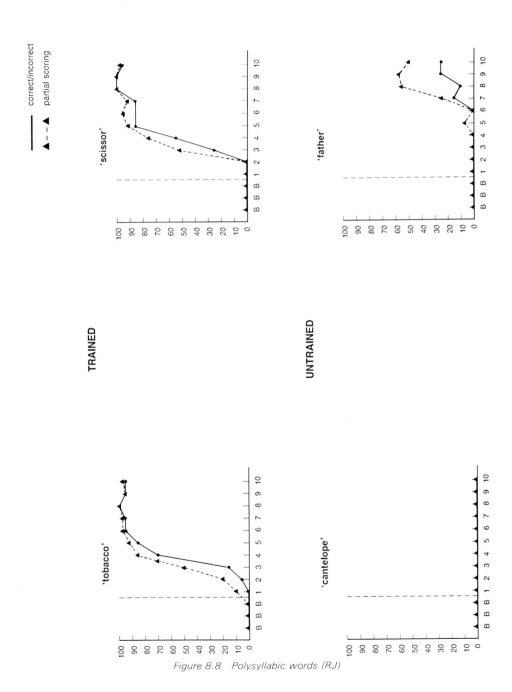

Figure 8.8   Polysyllabic words (RJ)

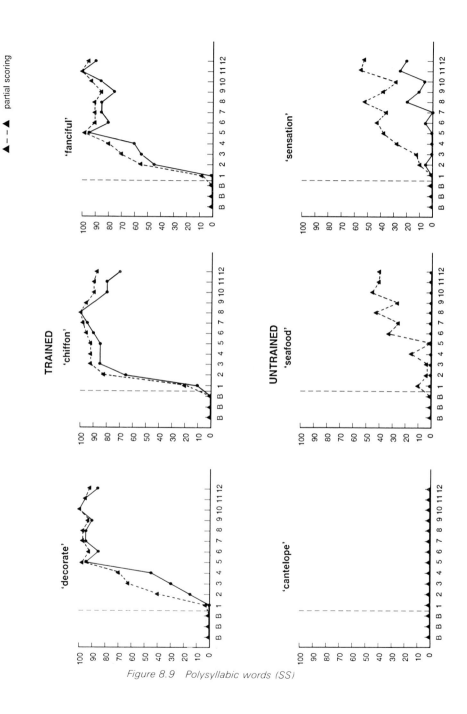

Figure 8.9   Polysyllabic words (SS)

such as, 'Help me', a patient could receive a score of 50 per cent for correct production of only one word.

The data for PW, on the trained and untrained phrases, are presented in Figure 8.10. Again, rapidly accelerated learning curves were demonstrated for the two trained phrases while minimal and variable performances were demonstrated for the untrained items. It should be noted that for both of the untrained phrases, some learning appeared to take place. In the phrase, 'Stop it', partial learning was due to correct yet variable production of the word 'it'. For 'Give it to me', the learning effect reflected was due to the correct yet variable production of the words, 'it' and 'me'.

For RJ, two phrases were used. Prompts were used for the longer phrase. Again, as shown in Figure 8.11, rapidly accelerated learning curves for all words of the trained phrase were demonstrated. For the untrained phrase, only the word, 'it' improved but the patient's performance on that word was variable.

Implications

Administration of PROMPT therapy was found to be highly efficacious for all three subjects involved in this study. For PW, little or no improvement of phoneme contrasts and polysyllabic word stimuli occurred for untrained items using either scoring system. Some minimal yet variable improvement was demonstrated for several words in untrained phrases as reflected through the use of the partial-credit scoring system.

For the other two chronic subjects of this study, PROMPT treatment resulted in rapidly accelerated and stable performance curves for all trained items using both scoring systems. These two patients also benefitted somewhat from repetition as measured by the partial-credit scoring system, but learning was much slower, less dramatic, and performances more variable.

It, thus, appears that PROMPT therapy may be highly efficacious for the training of accurate target verbalizations among chronic apractic–aphasic patients for whom more traditional methods of treatment have failed. For other chronic apractic–aphasic patients, intensive repetition training may, in itself, be appropriate in that some learning occurred which could not be attributed solely to PROMPTs. This was reflected in the application of the partial-credit scoring system used in this pilot study. Commonalities between and differences among patients who derived differential benefits from PROMPT treatment were, thus,

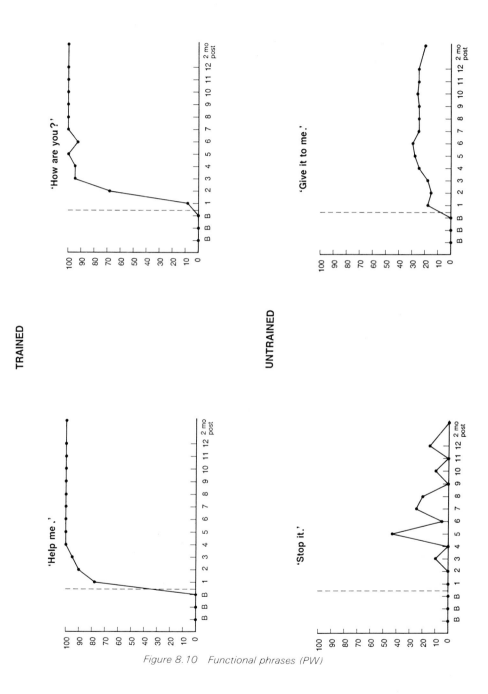

TRAINED

'How are you ?'

'Help me .'

UNTRAINED

'Give it to me.'

'Stop it.'

Figure 8.10   Functional phrases (PW)

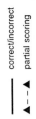

correct/incorrect
partial scoring

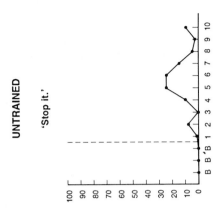

UNTRAINED

'Stop it.'

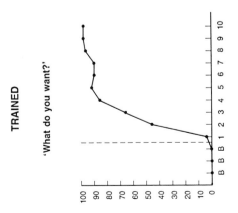

TRAINED

'What do you want?'

Figure 8.11   Functional phrases (RJ)

explored. Subjects of the present study were all participants in the Neuropraxis Research Program, codirected by Dr Paula Square-Storer and Dr Eric Roy. As such, each had undergone an extensive battery of cognitive, aphasia, motor, and sensory testing which included fourteen standardized tests. Those data were scrutinized for each subject in order to determine whether any standardized measures revealed patient differences. Only results of the WAB did. The AQs, (Kertesz, 1982) for the two subjects who demonstrated some learning under the repetition mode alone had higher AQs: 45.5 (RJ) and 52.8 (SS) versus 23.2 (PW). While, the WAB repetition scores did not show consistent differences between the subjects, the spontaneous speech scores did. PW, who appeared not to profit from intensified repetition demonstrated a much lower spontaneous speech score of 2; RJ's was 9, and SS's, 10. From this preliminary and informal analysis, it would appear that those subjects who are most limited in their spontaneous output may be the ones who derive more benefit from PROMPTs. Subjects with better spontaneous output may also derive benefit from repetition, albeit with less consistent and accelerated positive benefits. These tentative impressions are in need of further investigation.

Future Research Directions

Future research regarding PROMPT treatment will address several issues. These will include the application of alternating treatment designs (McReynolds and Kearns, 1982) in which the effects of imitation using integral stimulation (Rosenbek, 1978), rhythmic inter-systemic timing using buccal tapping, phonetic placement (see Chapter 6), and PROMPTs will be investigated. Treatment will be applied only to the learning of functional phrases in chronic apractic–aphasic patients who are severely limited in their verbal output. Environmental probes exploring transfer of training will also be incorporated in future investigations. It is our hope that these areas of investigation will better delineate the efficacy of PROMPTs as well as indicate the 'types' of patients, for whom PROMPT treatment is most appropriate.

Acknowledgments

Dr Square-Storer and Ms Hayden wish to acknowledge their colleagues, Scott Adams and Debra Morningstar for the contribution made towards the efficacy investigations for the PROMPT system.

Portions of these data were reported at the Clinical Aphasiology Conference, 1985 and 1986. Partial funding for this research was derived from three sources: Dean's Fund, Faculty of Medicine, University of Toronto; the Ontario District SPEBSQSA; and Health and Welfare, Canada, for the project entitled 'Disruptions to Limb, Oral and Verbal Praxis: Assessment and Remediation'. Support for the preparation of the graphics within this chapter was provided by Bell Canada in conjunction with their support of the Bell Canada Speech and Language Centre for Children, Speech Foundation of Ontario. Permission was granted from Thieme Medical Publishers for use of Figures 8.1, 8.2, and 8.3. Highly similar figures originally appeared in Chumpelik, D. *Seminars in Speech and Language* Vol. 5, No. 2, 1984.

References

ALLEN, G.I. and TSUKAHARA, N. (1974) 'Cerebrocerebellar communication systems', *Physiology Review,* **54**, pp. 957–1006.

BROOKS, V.B. (1979) 'Motor programs revisited', in TALBOTT, R.E. and HUMPHREYS, D.R. (Ed.) *Posture and Movement*, New York, Raven Press, pp. 13–49.

CHUMPELIK (HAYDEN), D. (1984) 'The Prompt System of therapy', in ARAM, D. (Ed.) *Seminars in Speech and Language,* **5**, pp. 139–56.

DABUL, B. (1979) *Apraxia Battery for Adults*, Tigard, Oregon, C.C. Publications.

HEBB, D.O. (1949) *The Organization of Behavior: A Neuropsychological Theory*. New York, John Wiley and Sons.

ITOH, M. and SASANUMA, S. (1984) 'Articulatory movements in apraxia of speech', in ROSENBEK, J. *et al.* (Eds.) *Apraxia of Speech: Physiology, Acoustics, Linguistics and Management*, San Diego, College Hill Press, pp. 133–65.

KELSO, J.A.S. and TULLER, B. (1981) 'Toward a theory of apractic syndromes', *Brain and Language,* **12**, pp. 224–45.

KENT, J.C. and ROSENBEK, J.C. (1983) 'Acoustic patterns of apraxia of speech', *Journal of Speech and Hearing Research,* **26**, pp. 231–49.

KERTESZ, A. (1982) *The Western Aphasia Battery*, New York, Grune and Stratton.

LIBERMAN, A.M., COOPER, F.S., SHANKWEILER, D.P. and STUDDERT-KENNEDY, M. (1967) 'Perception of the speech code', *Psychological Review,* **74**, pp. 431–61.

LINDBLOM, B.E.F. (1963) 'Spectographic study of vowel reduction', *Journal of Acoustical Society of America,* **35**, pp. 1773–81.

MARSDEN, C.D. (1982) 'The mysterious motor function of the basal ganglia: The Robert Wartenberg Lecture', *Neurology,* **32**, pp. 514–39.

MCREYNOLDS, L. and KEARNS, K. (1982) *Single Subject Experimental Designs in Communicative Disorders*, Baltimore, Maryland, University Park.

ROSENBEK, J.C. (1978) 'Treating apraxia of speech', in JOHNS, D.F. (Ed.) *Clinical Management of Communicative Disorders*, Boston, Little, Brown and Co., pp. 191–241.

ROSENBEK, J.C. and LAPOINTE, L.L. (1978) 'The dysarthrias: Description, diagnosis and treatment', in JOHNS, D.F. (Ed.) *Clinical Management of Communicative Disorders*, Boston, Little, Brown and Co., pp. 251–310.

ROSENBEK, J.C., WERTZ, R.T. and DARLEY, F.L. (1973) 'Oral sensation and perception in apraxia of speech and aphasia', *Journal of Speech and Hearing Research,* **16**, pp. 22–36.

SHRIBERG, L. and KENT, R. (1982) *Clinical Phonetics*, New York, John Wiley.

SQUARE, P., CHUMPELIK (HAYDEN), D. and ADAMS, S. (1985) 'Efficacy of the PROMPT system of therapy for the treatment of acquired apraxia of speech', in BROOKSHIRE, R. (Ed.) *Clinical Aphasiology Conference Proceedings*, Minneapolis, BRK Publishers, pp. 319–320.

SQUARE, P., CHUMPELIK (HAYDEN), D., MORNINGSTAR, D. and ADAMS, S. (1986) 'Efficacy of the PROMPT system of therapy for the treatment of apraxia of speech: A follow-up investigation', in BROOKSHIRE, R. (Ed.) *Clinical Aphasiology Conference Proceedings*, Minneapolis, BRK Publishers, pp. 221–6.

SQUARE-STORER, P. (1987) 'Acquired apraxia of speech', in WINITZ, H. (Ed.) *Human Communication and Its Disorder*, Norwood, New Jersey, pp. 88–166.

STEVENS, K.N. and HOUSE, A.S. (1963) 'Perturbation of vowel articulation by consonantal context: An acoustical study', *Journal of Speech and Hearing Research,* **16**, pp. 22–36.

WERTZ, R.T., LAPOINTE, L. and ROSENBEK, J.C. (1984) *Apraxia of Speech in Adults: The Disorder and Its Management*, Orlando, Florida, Grune and Stratton.

WIEGL, E. and BIERWISCH, M. (1970) 'Neuropsychology and linguistics: Topics of common research', *Foundations of Language,* **6**, pp. 1–18.

ZIEGLER, W. and VON CRAMON, D. (1985) 'Anticipatory coarticulation in a patient with apraxia of speech', *Brain and Language,* **26**, pp. 117–30.

ZIEGLER, W. and VON CRAMON, D. (1986) 'Disturbed coarticulation in apraxia of speech: Acoustic evidence', *Brain and Language,* **29**, pp. 34–47.

Chapter 9

Multiple Input Phoneme Therapy

Elaine R. Stevens

Frequently in clinical practice we are confronted with patients who demonstrate such severe expressive involvement that they either fail in therapy or are considered not to be appropriate candidates for traditional treatment methods. The verbal output of these individuals, whether they are two months or five years post-onset, is limited to repetitive verbal behaviors consisting of stereotypies, automatisms, or recurring utterances as described by Brunner *et al.* (1982). A significant oral apraxia as well as apraxia of speech is usually present, although the latter is difficult to assess due to the complete absence of repetition, even for highly probable words or isolated speech sounds.

Often there is a concomitant impairment in initiating or copying gestures. In addition, standardized diagnostic tests reveal minimal responses on all verbal tasks and in many cases auditory comprehension scores are little better. Although the alert examiner may detect some environmental comprehension, despite inability to perform simple picture pointing tasks, the appropriate diagnosis would appear to be global aphasia combined with limb, verbal, and oral apraxia. However, a specific disorder of language comprehension cannot be proven on the basis of poor performance on motor tasks, as difficulties in maintaining sequences or disturbance in the ability to carry out motor activities on verbal command (apraxia) may be responsible (Benson, 1979).

Despite difficulties in precisely classifying these individuals according to major aphasic syndromes, their clinical behavioral characteristics can be enumerated as described in Table 9.1. Specifically, it should be noted that these individuals display significant language impairment, marked dyspraxia, cannot repeat, and are generally regarded as having a guarded or poor prognosis due to the combination of a severe communication deficit as well as neuromotor and neurobehavioral disabilities. Therefore, the following management questions arise:

Table 9.1: Characteristics of Candidates for MIPT

1 Left hemisphere CVA (cortical–subcortical)
2 Verbal output limited to stereotypies
3 Absence of repetition skills
4 Labeled as 'poor prognosis'
5 Questionable auditory comprehension
6 Poor performance on standardized tests of aphasia
7 Verbal apraxia
8 Marked–moderate oral apraxia
9 Reduced gestural skills
10 Marked–moderate reading impairment
11 Marked–moderate impairment of writing and/or copying
12 Failure with previous aphasia and/or apraxia of speech therapy approaches
13 Range of physical impairment with right hemiparesis

should the patient be treated? If so, what technique(s) should be used? And, what should be treated first, the aphasia or verbal apraxia?

Generally the literature has indicated that the prognosis for severe apractic patients with coexisting aphasia is guarded (Hill, 1978; Wertz, LaPointe and Rosenbek, 1984). Treatment failure of the speechless person is even more predictable when production of isolated phonemes cannot be stimulated. As discussed in this volume by Collins (see Chapter 4) and by Tonkovich and Peach (see Chapter 5), apraxia and aphasia are different disorders and require different treatment techniques. This issue is further addressed in this chapter with specific reference to the functionally nonexpressive chronic apractic–aphasic patient.

Many patients with severe long-term expressive aphasia with verbal output limited to meaningless grunts, stereotyped phonemes, or repetitive words have been successfully treated with Melodic Intonation Therapy when other forms of therapy have failed (Albert, Sparks and Helm, 1973). However, typical patients, as described here, either create their own melodies or substitute their perseverative utterance for the stimulus phrase.

Another therapeutic approach, Voluntary Control of Involuntary Utterances (VCIU), has been advocated for individuals who emit stereotypies (Helm and Barresi, 1980). It was reported that successful control of perseverative utterances could be achieved by presenting patients with printed words or phrases which the patients had been heard to utter, thus bringing at least some aspects of verbalization under voluntary control. Although Multiple Input Phoneme Therapy (MIPT) and VCIU are similar in concept in that both attempt to control involuntarily produced utterances, their methodologies are quite different. Whereas VCIU utilizes a visual–verbal mode, MIPT stimulates an auditory–verbal connection, developing repetition skills prior to stimulating a response to written material. Helm-Estabrooks (1983), in a later report, described the use of VCIU for patients with subcortical damage. It appears that MIPT is also useful for patients with subcortical lesions. Although subjects participating in earlier studies of MIPT were not given CT scans, a number of them demonstrated characteristics which implicated combined subcortical and cortical damage. CT scans have confirmed subcortical damage in two recent MIPT subjects.

Clinicians typically strive to imprint the correct patterns of articulatory movements in individuals with apraxia of speech (see, for example, Shewan, 1980). Inherent to such approaches is the ability to repeat an utterance with an approximated response. However, individuals at a prerepetition level, who cannot even produce utterances simultaneously with the clinician and who fail traditional techniques for apraxia or aphasia would appear to have little hope of developing functional verbal communication.

Numerous authors have emphasized the futility of employing aphasia therapy techniques to address dyspraxic impairment and have stressed the need to devise effective therapy techniques for patients with combined severe apraxia and expressive aphasia. Therefore, an approach to verbal expression at a subrepetition level which controls and alters non-functional stereotypies and subsequently facilitates access to underlying phonemic and linguistic competencies would be appropriate. It is the purpose of this chapter to introduce a newly developed therapeutic approach, Multiple Input Phoneme Therapy (MIPT), which appears to achieve these goals. Theoretical rationale, methodology, clinical observations, and two case studies will be presented.

Theoretical Basis of Multiple Input Phoneme Therapy

It is hypothesized that the severely apractic–aphasic patient who produces stereotypies is locked-in to a verbal motor loop (Stevens and Glaser, 1983). The utterance(s) may originally have been self-generated or environmentally stimulated. However, due to the severity of neurological damage, once the utterance(s) is created and utilized repetitively, the motor loop becomes strengthened such that access to residual phonological, semantic, and syntactic competencies is prevented. Thus, each volitional speech attempt elicits the automatic motor loop. As the patient struggles to self-correct the perseverative utterance or to initiate a new utterance, speech efforts become more volitional and the patient appears to become increasingly locked-in to the motor loop. As described by Shindler, Caplan, and Hier (1984), patients such as these fail to generate appropriate responses to stimuli and fail to inhibit incorrect perseverative stereotyped responses.

Levy, Nebes and Sperry (1971) proposed that a hemisphere intrinsically better equipped to handle particular tasks may also more easily dominate the motor pathways. Taking this a step further, in patients with damage so severe as to result in exclusive use of verbal stereotypies, not only does one hemisphere dominate, but also one motor response dominates. Therefore, a request for verbal output is referred to the damaged left hemisphere and the patient is locked-in to the motor-loop response(s), such as, for example, 'wata, wata'. Also, the left hemisphere may inhibit or suppress the right hemisphere's attempt to process information linguistically through inhibitory influences across the cerebral commissures (Moscovitch, 1973). This may explain why patients, regardless of severely depressed auditory comprehension scores, succeed with MIPT, yet fail techniques which tap right-hemisphere strengths (see Chapter 5). The occurrence of automatisms and recurring utterances in patients with combined cortical and basal ganglia lesions as opposed to aphasic syndromes with only cortical infarctions has been described by Brunner, *et al.* (1982), as well as Kornhuber (1977), and Kornhuber, Brunner and Wallesch (1979). The phenomenon of recurring utterances may be due to inadequately disinhibited motor speech patterns which are unintentionally elicited when defective programming of motor-speech sequences fail to produce a desired verbal response; and, as more CT scans become available, the existence of subcortical damage in MIPT patients may be further documented.

Repetition tasks typically provide only one or two stimulus inputs prior to the required patient response. However, due to weakened transmission pathways as well as the overriding strength of the perseverative motor loop, one or two inputs is not sufficient. Strengthening these pathways via multiple input, utilizing a stimulus which is in the patient's repertoire, and removing all volitional intent of speech through a controlled stimulus–response pattern significantly increases the probability of a correct response. MIPT thus enables the clinician to gain control over the inhibitory influence of the stereotypies in the motor loop, and this control is progressively transferred to the patient as he/she moves through the therapy hierarchy. In viewing the stereo-typies as a motor programming dysfunction, this technique may initially treat the apractic component prior to the aphasia.

It has traditionally been assumed that the process of verbal repetition involves the integrity of Wernicke's and Broca's areas and the arcuate fasciculus of the dominant hemisphere. In fact, recently Selnes *et al.* (1985) have implicated Wernicke's area as being the primary site responsible for repetition disorders. Hypothetically, as depicted in Figure 9.1(A), an utterance may be processed and comprehended in the temporal lobe (1). The auditory image, in turn, evokes kinesthetic memories of the movements associated with the utterance (2). These memories are transmitted to the premotor areas via association fibers (3). In the premotor area the actual motor program is accessed (4) and then transmitted to the motor strip for execution (5).

Figure 9.1(B) represents the hypothesized pathologic condition which may account for a verbal repetition disability as well as the pathological process of perseveration, specifically as it applies to verbal stereotype production. Although verbal utterances may be processed correctly in the temporal lobe and may evoke correspondingly correct kinesthetic patterns in the parietal lobe, the motor program corres-ponding to the sensory inputs from these lobes cannot be accessed in the frontal lobe. Instead only one motor program which is elicited in a loop fashion is activated (2). This results in perseverative stereotypies

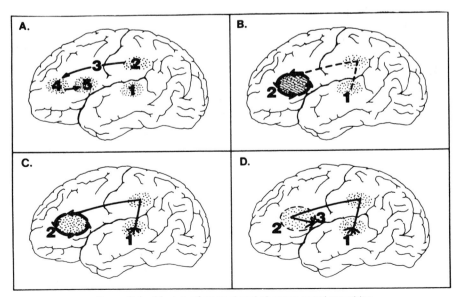

Figure 9.1   Models of normal and aberrant word repetition

which occur each time repetition is attempted. Further, any attempt at a verbalization results in this one motor pattern being evoked.

Throughout the process of MIPT, the clinician endeavours to shape from the stereotypies a variety of utterances which eventually may be used volitionally by the patient. In order to achieve this end goal, indiscriminate use of the stereotyped response must first be brought under control. As depicted in Figure 9.1(C), the clinician stimulates the auditory and kinesthetic association through multiple input (1), but prohibits the patient from emitting any response. The patient's deviant motor pattern is subsequently altered (2), as contrasted with 9.1(B) (2), the unaltered pathological process. Once this is achieved, a closed set of verbal stimulus items based upon phonemic structures similar to the verbal stereotypy are used to stimulate the patient. As depicted in Figure 9.1(D), these stimuli form the corpus of multiple inputs (1). The stimulus activates the evocation of new motor patterns (2) similar to those of the perseverative utterance and eventually the patient is allowed to emit them (3) but only under carefully controlled situations.

Clinician as Controller Versus Facilitator

It is common knowledge that in aphasia the nonpropositional/nonvolitional use of language is preserved to a far greater degree than is propositional/volitional use of language. Likewise, the apractic patient performs relatively well with automatic speech tasks and may perfectly articulate the numbers one to five in rhythm, but when called upon to volitionally produce number 'four' out of sequence, may struggle and then fail to produce the word.

Because any volitional attempt at speech triggers the hypothesized automatic motor loop, i.e., the perseverative utterance shown in Figure 9.1(B), it is necessary to remove all volitional intent through a highly structured program, controlling and altering all of the patient's verbal output, seen in Figure 9.1(C). Because the patient is unable, the clinician must control what is allowed to emerge and when. Therefore, the clinician initially assumes the role of controller, not facilitator. In so doing, the patient ceases his struggle to volitionally verbalize or self-correct the stereotypies. Once these are controlled, thereby decreasing the motor loop's strength, the clinician can access and reimprint previously established motor patterns. Later on in the treatment hierarchy, the patient is allowed to assume more control. Thus, as more volitional tasks are introduced, more appropriate propositional communication skills emerge as in Figure 9.1(C). As stated by Basso,

Capitani and Vignolo, (1979), 'this passage from more automatic to volitional constitutes the core of rehabilitation. ...If an aphasic (*sic*) cannot bring forth an intended response by himself, it is sometimes possible to lead him to do so by eliciting a response first in a more automatic way and then more volitional ways by gradually withdrawing the facilitations incorporated in the stimuli' (p. 193). These tenets form the basic framework for MIPT.

Methodology

MIPT is divided into two levels, the first designed to reduce the patient's struggle and volitional attempts at initiating language and appropriate patterns of articulatory movement, and the second level which encourage the development of patient-initiated volitional control of verbal output. These levels, as well as their correlative steps of treatment, are summarized in Table 9.2. Table 9.3 more fully specifies the twenty-two steps that provide a hierachy of tasks which progressively increase in difficulty. In the section which follows, a detailed description of the therapy process is presented.

Level 1: Decreasing the volitional intent of speech

Step 1: Choice of target utterance and analysis of phonemes

Prior to selecting the initial stimulus word, it is necessary to analyze the patient's stereotypies. Typically verbal output is limited to one or more sounds, single syllable words, or two-word combinations. The automatisms are listed according to frequency of occurrence and their phonemic structure analyzed. The purpose of this is twofold:

1 To select the appropriate word for developing the STIMULUS RESPONSE SET (SRS)

Table 9.2: Organizational Framework of MIPT

Level I: Decreasing Volitional Intent of Speech	
Steps 1–3	Alterning motor loop via stimulus responses set (SRS)
Steps 4–5	Phoneme generalization
Steps 6–14	Word/phrase repetition 1:1
Level II: Increasing Volitional Intent of Speech	
Steps 15–18	Cue/responsive word and picture production
Steps 19–20	Spontaneous word and picture production
Steps 21–22	Cue/spontaneous phrase/sentence production

Table 9.3: Elaborated MIPT Therapy Steps

  1 Choice of target utterance and analysis of phonemes
  2 Developing the SRS and eliciting the target utterance
  3 Controlling all other perseverative utterances via SRS
  4 Phoneme generalization from perseverative utterances
  5 Expanded phoneme generalization
  6 Developing a 2:1 ratio within phoneme runs
  7 2:1 response ratio with rotating initial phonemes
  8 Consonant clusters
  9 Bisyllabic words
 10 Consonant clusters and multisyllabic words 2:1
 11 Rotating phoneme clusters and multisyllabic words
 12 Word repetition without phrase cue
 13 Developing phrases and short sentences 3–5:1
 14 Phrases and sentences 1:1
 15 Cue word reading
 16 Cue picture naming
 17 Responsive word reading
 18 Responsive naming of pictures
 19 Confrontation word reading
 20 Confrontation picture naming
 21 Assisted phrase production (without picture)
 22 Assisted phrase/sentence production (w/picture)

2 To identify target sounds for phoneme generalization.

The most frequently occurring word or sound, i.e., the strongest utterance in the patient's motor loop, is usually the initial stimulus and becomes the 'target' upon which the SRS control pattern is established. Should the patient's output be limited to recurring syllables such as /da/, this is used as the 'target'.

Step 2: Developing the SRS and eliciting the target utterance

The most critical phase in the program is the initial control and alteration of the perseverative utterance through the SRS. This is the point at which the patient relinquishes all volitional speech effort and the clinician assumes total control of the input–output set. The patient is *required* to watch the clinician's mouth as the target is repeated slowly eight to ten times, with slightly increased loudness and emphasis on the initial phoneme. Rhythmical tapping on the ipsilesional arm is also recommended during multiple input. Similar to MIT procedures (Sparks, Helm and Albert, 1974), a hand signal is used or the clinician's hand is held to the patient's mouth, indicating 'watch and listen but do not attempt verbalizations'. The patient is allowed to respond only when signaled. This pattern of watch, listen, wait, and respond when cued must be made clear to the patient.

Following the final input, but without breaking the rhythmic pacing of input, the patient is signaled to join in the next production. As the patient verbalizes, the clinician continues to repeat the word three to four times in choral fashion with the patient, yet louder than the patient. This procedure appears to encourage stabilization of the response. It is assumed that increased loudness on the part of the clinician prevents the patient from focusing on his/her own response, which in turn minimizes volitional attempts at altering the response. Using, for example, the word 'one' as the target, the procedure evolves temporarily as follows: the clinician begins the input by slowly repeating 'one, one, one, one, one, number one, one, one, one, one, number one ...'. Immediately, the patient is signaled to join the clinician and unison repetition continues until the patient's production has stabilized. At that point the clinician ceases production but continues to 'mouth' the word and tap as the patient produces the word three to four additional times. In most cases, a cue phrase should be inserted to facilitate comprehension and automatic response. For example, when eliciting the word 'door', the clinician may say 'door, door, open the door, shut the door, door, door...'. In so doing, one must be careful not to break the pace, causing a more volitional attempt on the part of the patient.

After the patient correctly produces the target, the clinician should repeat the process several times to strengthen the SRS. If the patient fails following the initial attempt, wait several minutes and try again. Should the patient utter a different recurring utterance present in his/her repertoire, the clinician immediately begins multiple input of this word as a new target.

Step 3: Controlling all other utterances via SRS

Next, all other recurring utterances are controlled through the SRS process.

Step 4: Phoneme generalization

Once verbalizations are produced within the confines of the SRS, the process of phoneme generalization begins. Assuming the SRS has been carefully programmed, this usually occurs fairly rapidly. Beginning with the initial target utterance, usually the strongest, ten new single syllable words with the same initial phoneme are introduced through multiple input as in Step 2. There is a tendency for patients to perseverate on the first new word elicited by the SRS. Thus, a thirty- to sixty-second delay should be observed prior to the introduction of another new target utterance. Subsequently, the initial phonemes of all other utterances are used to generate ten new words per phoneme. Finally, phonemes present in the final and medial positions are utilized to generate new words. All new words should be carefully chosen in order to present a variety of phonemes. It has been our experience that this reduces the patient's tendency to perseverate on a frequently utilized phoneme and also facilitates Step 5 which is directed towards expanded phoneme generalization.

If new words are presented with a cue phrase immediately preceding the required patient response, the use of cueing at a later level is easily facilitated. For instance, returning to the example of 'door', the clinician may say 'door, door, door, door, door, door, door, door, open the ...', with the clinician and patient responding, 'door'. Early on, a few patients experience greater difficulty when a cue phrase is utilized, possibly because this introduces too much noise into the system. In these cases only multiple input prior to the desired response is used.

Step 5: Expanded phoneme generalization

All phonemes present are next utilized to generate additional words. The process continues until all phonemes in the English language are produced consistently. Word lists should be balanced to assure that each consonant is produced in both the initial and final positions and words should be presented in phoneme-runs, i.e., ten words per initial phoneme. A time delay prior to the introduction of words with a new initial phoneme usually prevents perseveration of the previous phoneme. Should phoneme-runs of the initial phoneme /p/ be followed by runs of /m/, the patient may continue to produce the /p/ phoneme. Thus, word runs with an initial vowel are often a good break between consonant runs.

It has been our observation that the rules of distinctive features are nonpredictive for the application of MIPT. That is, they may work positively or negatively with patients. Proceeding from /f/ to /v/ would seem logical in terms of oral placement. However, if the voiced feature is not present elsewhere the perseverative production of /f/ will probably occur. The interjection of two or three words with an initial voiced consonant or preferably a vowel will usually precipitate successful production of /v/.

On occasion, patients may easily produce a particular phoneme in the initial position but not in the final position. Final production is usually developed by placing greater emphasis on that final phoneme, e.g., 'hatttt, hatttt'. Often, following a careful reanalysis of the word lists, a previously correct production will be found. That word is then presented via multiple input to again elicit the phoneme in the final position. Final position phoneme runs are then introduced, e.g., 'hot, hit, hat', to further stabilize production.

During this step the need for unison repetition will diminish until it can be eliminated. With many patients, input can likewise be reduced to five stimulus repetitions. However, the target response is a phonemically correct word without struggle and one must not be too eager to reduce input before the patient is ready. On the other hand, it is important that a particular word or phoneme not be overpractised or it will gain greater strength and tend to extinguish weaker phonemes. We have found that for most patients approximately ten words per phoneme (initial position) can be successfully repeated within a three month period, assuming therapy sessions are at least two to three times per week. Thus, following thirty-six therapy sessions, all vowels and consonants should be produced successfully in the initial position and the words should have good intelligibility.

Step 6: Developing a 2:1 response ratio within phoneme runs

At this point the patient should be able to repeat some 300 single syllable (CV, CVC, VC) words quite clearly. Multiple input is now progressively decreased until a 1:1 response ratio is developed during phoneme runs. Phrase cues should be carefully rotated to prevent the patient from becoming locked-in to any particular phrase.

Typically the patient with a primary severe apraxia of speech and mild aphasia is now easily distinguished from the patient with severe aphasia as his primary disorder. The former patient rapidly begins initiating spontaneous phrases and sentences, with fewer phoneme errors than one would anticipate. It is hypothesized that the early use of MIPT in the treatment process reimprints correct motor patterns and reduces dyspraxic errors later on in the recovery process. The patient with severe aphasia, however, may spontaneously elicit a few words and phrases, but for the most part will not show a significant increase in verbalizations until Steps 15 and 16 are reached. These are the steps in which output is facilitated through linguistic cueing.

Step 7: 2:1 response ratio with rotating phonemes

Next a 2:1 response ratio is developed while rotating phonemes. An example might be 'dog, hat, one, book'. As the number of inputs is decreased, ipsilesional hand/arm tapping is likewise eliminated.

Step 8: Consonant clusters

Consonant clusters are now introduced. A word such as 'black' is produced by presenting three to six words beginning with /b/ followed by the same number or more beginning with the /l/ phoneme. Words rhyming with the target, however, should be avoided, e.g., 'back', 'lack', since motor confusion appears to result. It is often advantageous to insert an intrusive vowel between members of the cluster and lengthen its duration, e.g., 'baaalack', in order to facilitate correct production. At least five inputs should be utilized during this step.

Step 9: Bisyllabic words

Bisyllabic words are developed in the same manner as monosyllables, commencing with five inputs and balancing phonemes for initial, medial, and final occurrence. The exact number of inputs necessary may vary depending on the patient's ability. Typically, compound words are more difficult than other bisyllabic words; thus, they are initially avoided. Later they are phased in along with three syllable words.

Step 10: Consonant clusters and multisyllabic words 2:1

The number of inputs is decreased to effect a 2:1 ratio for all consonant clusters and multisyllabic words in phoneme runs.

Step 11: Rotating phoneme clusters and multisyllabic words

This procedure is essentially the same as that described for monosyllabic words (see Step 7). Thus, a stimulus set may be as follows: 'table, window, yesterday'.

Step 12: Word repetition without phrase cues

During this step the phrase cue is eliminated from all inputs, resulting in repetition of single syllable, multisyllabic words, and clusters following a single input. The patient should be given practice in immediate responses and subsequently respond following latency periods of up to ten seconds.

Step 13: Developing phrases and short sentences

Once words are easily repeated at a 1:1 ratio, two-word combinations and later, longer phrases are introduced with multiple input of three to five times. Frequently, resumption of arm tapping for each word facilitates accurate production. Stimulus phrases should vary phonemically, semantically, and syntactically in order to prevent linguistic and motor speech perseverative behaviors.

Step 14: Phrases and sentences 1:1

During this step, phrases and sentences utilized in the preceding step are presented for immediate repetitions and subsequently with a latency period.

Level II: Increasing volitional intent of speech

Throughout steps 15–21 there is more allowance for variability, depending on the patient's capabilities and the clinician is encouraged to explore. Activities which result in excessive struggle, however, should be avoided.

Step 15: Cue word reading

Commonly used single syllable words from the previously developed word lists are initially presented in written form accompanied by a high probability concrete phrase cue such as 'open the...'. Cues should vary and progressively provide less information, e.g., 'here is a ...', 'he/she is ...', 'they wanted to ...'. In many cases 'pairing' a high probability with a low probability cue ('I fix my hair with a ...', 'This is a ...') stimulates self cueing by the patient. Typically, five words per initial phoneme are sufficient including clusters and multisyllabic words. If simple words are elicited initially, more complex words can be subsequently achieved with success.

Step 16: Cue picture naming

This step is essentially the same as the preceding one but now pictures are introduced. We have typically used colored photographs and line drawings including single pictures of objects and objects embedded within the context they are typically found.

Step 17: Responsive word reading

Cue phrases, previously used with word cards in Step 15, are now used to aid in generating responses to questions. Initially, ending a question with a preposition provides an easier transition for the patient as he moves up the hierarchy, e.g., 'What do you fix your hair with?'. At the onset a prompt may be needed, e.g., 'What do you stir with? A ...'.

Step 18: Responsive naming of pictures

This step is the same as Step 17 with the exception that pictures are used.

Step 19: Confrontation word reading

Words from stimulus items used in Step 15 are presented for the patient to read. If there is difficulty, a minimal cue such as 'Here is a ...' or 'This is a ...' should be provided and the response again elicited. Patients who continue to emit lexical confusions, semantic paraphasias or who fail to respond due to persistent reading impairment may be given a high probability cue followed by a delay and re-presentation of the written word.

Step 20: Confrontation picture naming

This step mimics Step 19 but taxes linguistic formulation to a greater extent in that the patient must name pictures rather than read names of objects.

Step 21: Assisted phrase production

As MIPT progressively encourages less cue-supported volitional attempts at speech, the clinician should make every effort to minimize struggle. Increasing ease of phonemic sequencing as well as establishing phrases which are not semantically or syntactically demanding are the goals of Step 21.

A simple phrase such as 'answer the phone' is initially introduced for repetition. The phrase is subsequently reintroduced followed by a probe such as 'when the phone rings I should...'. Varied sentence combinations can be developed from previous levels, or a packaged program such as the Helm Elicited Language Program for Syntax Stimulation can be utilized (Helm, 1981). In the latter case, action pictures would not be presented during this step. Progressively the initial presentation with repetition is eliminated.

Next, interrogatives are presented to the patient. Simple questions are posed such as 'Do you like candy?' or 'Do you watch television?'. The desired response incorporates phrasal elements of the question. Appropriate responses to the above questions would be 'Yes, I like candy' and 'No, I don't watch TV'. Thus, partial repetition is utilized but the patient also self-formulates part of the response.

Step 22: Assisted phrase sentence production

Action pictures are next presented to the patient along with a model phrase followed by a probe. An example would be 'Open the door'. 'When someone knocks I......'. Later questions can be phrased so as to more easily elicit an accurate response. For example, after presenting a picture of a girl eating an apple the clinician might say 'What does she like to eat?' vs 'What does she like?'.

At this point in the treatment program patients should be producing spontaneous output with varying degrees of phonemic, syntactic, and semantic efficiency. Those individuals demonstrating greater dyspraxic impairment should now be treated with traditional techniques appropriate to this disorder (see Chapter 6), whereas those with dysphasia should likewise benefit from an approach designed to modify dysphasic impairment.

Case Studies

In order to further assess the validity of this treatment technique, the USA Veterans' Administration Rehabilitation Research and Development Service funded a pilot project. Ten subjects, six or more months post onset and therefore past the spontaneous recovery period, were randomly assigned to two groups. Verbal output of these subjects consisted predominantly of stereotypies with some emitting an occasional appropriate word. One group was treated with traditional procedures for aphasia and apraxia of speech while the other group received MIPT. Comparison of pre- and post-treatment mean scores following fifty treatment sessions revealed a significant improvement in the verbal and nonverbal skills of the MIPT group while the traditional group failed to improve (Stevens, 1986). Two subjects who were part of the MIPT treatment group will be presented here.

Subject 1, was a sixty-three-year-old male six months post left carotid occlusion. CT scan revealed an area of decreased density in the left parietal area with some extension into the posterior frontal region. The stereotypies 'aya' and 'yup' were produced in response to all verbal stimulation. Pretreatment testing revealed an Aphasia Quotient (AQ) of 4.8 and Cortical Quotient (CQ) of 12.7 on the Western Aphasia Battery (WAB); (Kertesz, 1982), and a score of 34 on the Communicative Abilities in Daily Living (CADL) (Holland, 1980). A score of 175 out of a possible 1200 was obtained on a series of twelve simple baseline tasks (SBT). These tasks consisted of describing action pictures, confrontation naming, responsive naming, cue naming, responsive phrase production, word repetition, phrase repetition, word reading (objects and actions), word–picture matching, word discrimination of objects and actions, and word recognition. Following fifty treatment sessions with MIPT this subject was communicating in single words and short phrases. Retesting revealed an AQ of 74.4, CQ of 75.8, SBT score of 1128, and score of 113 on the CADL.

Subject 2, a fifty-three-year-old male six months post-onset, displayed global aphasia and dyspraxia following left middle cerebral artery infarct. Although a CT scan was not completed, neurological examination indicated probable subcortical as well as cortical damage. Traditional treatment for aphasia prior to enrollment in the research project had not resulted in improved verbal output, the latter of which was limited to the stereotypy 'right'. Pretreatment AQ was 0.3, CQ 0.6, CADL 6, and SBT 0.0. As with Subject 1, post-treatment scores revealed a significant improvement in verbal and nonverbal tasks following 50 sessions. AQ and CQ were 52.0 and 50.4, respectively, with a score of 99 on the CADL and 629 on the SBT. Spontaneous output consisted of single words and occasional phrases, with verbalizations occurring more frequently in response to specific questions.

Similar gains were achieved by the other three patients receiving MIPT. The improved language/communication scores as measured by the WAB AQ, CADL, and SBT could be explained based upon improved verbal expression abilities. The marked improvement in CQ scores in all five MIPT subjects following treatment, as well as the two reported above, was initially puzzling due to the fact that MIPT focuses solely on improving verbal skills. However, recovery of a variety of nonverbal abilities as reflected in the Performance Quotient (PQ) may be indirectly stimulated by MIPT. The combined PQ and AQ following treatment would therefore yield the higher CQ.

Conclusions

Stroke patients with spontaneous verbal output limited to one or more perseverative utterances and who are unable to repeat simple words or sounds are potential candidates for MIPT, despite poor performance on standardized aphasia tests. Although precise quantification of extent of verbal apraxia vs aphasia is not initially possible, the distinction usually becomes clear following three to four months of treatment. Those individuals with severe apraxia of speech accompanied by mild aphasia will demonstrate motor patterns of articulation enabling them to produce phrase level communication and they will, in turn, move more rapidly through the steps than their counterparts with severe aphasia accompanied by mild-moderate apraxia of speech.

The success of this technique would appear to substantiate an 'information processing hypothesis' as described by Santo Pietro and Rigrodsky (1986), i.e., one underlying process may be responsible for the phenomenon of oral–verbal perseverative responses. A stereotypy, once generated, may 'be retained in the working memory as stimulus traces which entered into "nonvolitional rehearsal process" interfering with the capacity of the short-term memory to add new items, or to search and retrieve from long-term memory' (p. 15). Additionally, results of the study by Santo Pietro and Rigrodsky (1986) revealed a phonemic pattern in certain perseverative responses although initially the errors appeared to be simple lexical errors. MIPT utilizes the nonvolitional perseverative utterance, alters the motor program, and stimulates 'phonemic carry-over' to generate new phonemic motor patterns via phoneme generalization.

MIPT is an exciting new technique, offering hope of more functional speech to those who previously did not respond to traditional treatment procedures. It must be stressed, however, that although the author developed and modified this approach over a thirteen-year period, resulting in the specific steps presented here, there are certain limitations inherent to any highly structured technique. As no two people are alike, one finds that, despite commonalities in test profiles, each individual with combined severe apraxia of speech and aphasia will respond in a slightly different manner to this approach.

The ultimate success of MIPT, as in any procedure, rests in the hands of the clinician. The perceptive clinician will observe subtleties in patient responses and modify this approach to meet the patient's individual needs. It is these nuances, if shared by clinicians, that will allow for continued modification and increased efficiency in the use of this technique.

References

ALAJOUANINE, T. (1956) 'Verbal realization in aphasia', *Brain,* **79**(1), pp. 1–28.

ALBERT, M., SPARKS, R. and HELM, N. (1973) 'Melodic intonation therapy for aphasia', *Archives of Neurology,* **29**, pp. 130–1.

BASSO, A., CAPITANI, E. and VIGNOLO, C.A. (1979) 'Influence of rehabilitation on language skills in aphasic patients: a controlled study', *Archives of Neurology,* **36**, pp. 190–6.

BENSON, F. (1979) *Aphasia, Alexia and Agraphia,* New York, Churchill, Livingston Inc.

BRUNER, R.J., SEEMULLER, E., SUGER, G. and WALLESCH, C.W. (1982) 'Basal ganglia participation in language pathology', *Brain and Language,* **16**, pp. 281–99.

HELM, N.A. (1981) *Helm Elicited Language Program for Syntax Stimulation,* Austin, Exceptional Resources.

HELM, N.A. and BARRESI, B. (1980) 'Voluntary control of involuntary utterances: a treatment approach for severe aphasia', in BROOKSHIRE, R. (Ed.) *Clinical Aphasiology: Conference Proceedings,* Minneapolis, BRK, pp. 308–15.

HELM-ESTABROOKS, N. (1983) 'Treatment of subcortical aphasias', in PERKINS, W. (Ed.) *Language Handicaps in Adults,* New York, Thieme Stratton Inc., pp. 97–103.

HILL, B. (1978) *Verbal Dyspraxia in Clinical Practice,* Australia, Pitman Publishing PTY, Ltd.

HOLLAND, A. (1980) *Communicative Abilities in Daily Living,* Baltimore, University Park Press.

KERTESZ, A. (1982) *Western Aphasia Battery,* New York, Grune and Stratton.

KORNHUBER, H. (1977) 'A reconsideration of the cortical and subcortical mechanisms involved in speech and aphasia', in DESMEDT, J. (Ed.) *Language and Hemispheric Specialization in Man: Cerebral Event-Related Potentials,* Basel, S. Karger, pp. 28–35.

KORNHUBER, H., BRUNNER, R.J. and WALLESCH, C.W. (1979) 'Basal ganglia participation in aphasia', in CREUTZFELD, O., SCHEICH, H. and SCHREINER, CHR. (Eds.) *Hearing Mechanisms and Speech,* Berlin, Springer-Verlag, pp. 183–8.

LEVY, J., NEBES, R.D. and SPERRY, R.W. (1971) 'Expressive language in the surgically separated minor hemisphere', *Cortex,* **7**, pp. 49–58.

MOSCOVITCH, M. (1973) 'Language and the cerebral hemispheres: reaction-time studies and their implications for models of cerebral dominance', in PLINER, P., KRAMES, L. and ALLOWAY, T. (Eds.) *Communication and Affect: Language and Thought,* New York, Academic Press, pp. 89–126.

SANTO PIETRO, M. and RIGRODSKY, S. (1986) 'Patterns of oral–verbal perseveration in adult aphasia', *Brain and Language,* **29**, pp. 1–17.

SELNES, O.A., KNOPMAN, D.S., NICCUM, N. and RUBINS, A.B. (1985) 'The critical role of Wernicke's area in sentence repetition', *Annals of Neurology,* **17**, pp. 549–57.

SHEWAN, C.M. (1980) 'Verbal dyspraxia and its treatment', *Human Communications,* **5**, pp. 3–12.

SHINDLER, A.O., CAPLAN, L.R. and HIER, D.B. (1984) 'Intrusions and Perseverations', *Brain and Language,* **23**, pp. 148–58.

SPARKS, R., HELM, N. and ALBERT, M. (1974) 'Aphasia rehabilitation resulting from melodic intonation therapy', *Cortex,* **10**, pp. 303–16.

STEVENS, E. (1986) 'Efficacy of multiple input phoneme therapy in the treatment of severe expressive aphasia', *Journal of Rehabilitation Research and Development-Rehabilitation R&D Progress Reports,* **24**, p. 338.

STEVENS, E. and GLASER, L. (1983) 'Multiple input phoneme therapy: an approach to severe apraxia and expressive aphasia', in BROOKSHIRE, R.H. (Ed.) *Clinical Aphasiology: Conference Proceedings,* Minneapolis, BRK.

WERTZ, R.T., LAPOINTE, L.L. and ROSENBEK, J.C. (1984) *Apraxia of Speech in Adults: The Disorder and its Management,* Orlando, Grune and Stratton.

PART FOUR
Treatment Programs and Techniques

Chapter 10

Clinical Management of Apractic Mutism

Marianne B. Simpson and Amy R. Clark

Many patients with apraxia of speech and coexisting aphasia present initially with mutism. Fewer verbally apractic–aphasic patients present with persisting mutism. The purpose of this chapter is to examine the mutism which occurs as a precursor to or persisting symptom of verbal apraxia. Specifically, the issues of differential diagnosis of apractic mutism from other neurogenic forms of mutism, and the assessment, treatment, and prognosis of patients with apractic mutism are discussed. Two case presentations of patients with initial apractic mutism are included to further illustrate the disorder.

Terms which over the years have been used to describe the condition we refer to as 'apractic mutism' include: cortical dysarthria (Bay, 1962), aphemia (Broca, 1865), pure motor aphasia (Brown, 1972), anarthric aphasia (Brown, 1977), anarthria (Lebrun, Buyssens and Henneaux, 1973; Vignolo, 1964), afferent motor aphasia (Luria, 1966) as well as other terms. We continue to encounter these terms in the current literature. Some terms such as 'pure motor aphasia', refer to a constellation of symptoms, among which mutism as an early symptom may be included.

The literature regarding mutism associated with apraxia of speech, aphemia, or aphasia is sparse (Mohr *et al.*, 1978; Mohr, 1980; Albert *et al.*, 1981; Schiff *et al.*, 1983; Crary, Hardy and Williams, 1985; and others). It is of interest that where this type of mutism is mentioned, it is usually discussed as a transient condition which ameliorates rapidly with no intervention. In our clinical practice, we have found this often to be the case. For some patients, however, the mute state persists and direct intervention is necessary.

In Chapter 1, Lebrun proposed that protracted mutism is the result of 'motor aphasia' which, in his view, is linguistically based. It is our opinion that, what Lebrun describes as 'motor aphasia', may, in fact, consist of at least two components: a linguistically-based aphasia plus a motor-based speech initiation/production deficit (a form of apraxia of speech). This speech initiation/production deficit, at times to the point of muteness, in fact, most often coexists with the syndrome of Broca's aphasia. Certainly the aphasic component complicates, or contributes, to the paucity of output in some patients. However, the inability for a mute patient to produce speech when accompanied by effortful, trial and error oral posturing behaviors and when lexical access does not seem to be the problem, appears to be attributable to a motor speech deficit.

Two of the factors which lend credence to this idea of a distinct motor speech component in Lebrun's 'motor aphasia' concept include the following clinical observations:

1 The mutism in these cases tends to respond best to speech initiation cueing (see Treatment section in this chapter)
2 The speech initiation/production difficulty improves at a different rate and to a different degree compared to the aphasic component.

It is this motor speech initiation/production deficit, not a linguistic one, in our opinion, that is responsible for long-term mutism such as that exemplified in our Case 2. In this case, the speech initiation difficulties remained fairly severe, while the aphasic deficits improved significantly.

Whether transient or long-lasting, the lost ability to speak is traumatic for the patient. Counselling and intervention with regard to the nature of the loss of speech and the prognosis provides the patient with a better understanding of the condition as well as with hope for improvement. Psychological trauma is thus reduced for both the patient and his/her family. Additionally, potential maladaptive, struggle behaviors may well be prevented when proper treatment for the mutism is provided.

The literature on treatment for apractic mutism is, to our knowledge, nonexistent. The information provided in this chapter on treatment of the mute state as a precursor to, or persistent symptom of apraxia of speech is based upon our combined twenty-one years of clinical experience with numerous mute patients. The influence of related scholarly literature and other skilled clinicians with whom we have had the privilege to work is obviously represented here as well. Our experience has taught us various approaches which have been most effective in the management of the person with apractic mutism. We present this information here in the hope that other clinicians may find it useful as well.

Neurogenic Mutism

The term 'mute' is commonly used to describe an individual who does not phonate under any circumstances, volitionally, reflexively, or emotively. Apractic mutism may be defined as the inability to program volitionally the initiation and/or maintenance of phonation and articulation for the purpose of verbal communication. Apractic mutism may be better understood after reviewing other forms of neurogenic mutism.

Akinetic mutism

Freemon (1971) described akinetic mutism as 'a disorder of consciousness characterized by unresponsiveness, but with the superficial appearance of alertness. The patient's eyes are open and he may seem to look at the examiner, but he neither speaks nor moves, nor is the examiner able to communicate with the patient' (p. 693). Freemon pointed out the importance of differentiating akinetic mutism from 'pseudoakinetic mutism'. The former is a disorder of consciousness associated with generalized slowing on electroencephalogram (EEG). The clinical picture varies from somnolence to an appearance of wakefulness. The patients may even follow some visual stimuli, however, no communication system can be established. Akinetic mutism is reportedly associated with damage to limbic structures (Brown, 1977), bilateral cingulate gyrus, basal ganglia, and/or certain nuclei in the thalamus (Freemon, 1971). According to Brown (1977), damage to these areas may result in disconnection or interruption of alerting influences from the thalamus to higher centers (p. 65).

The disorder called pseudoakinetic mutism, more commonly termed 'locked-in syndrome', resembles akinetic mutism in that the patient neither moves nor speaks. On closer evaluation, however, these patients show unimpaired consciousness, and they show normal activity on EEG. Their awareness often can be demonstrated through the use of a communication system of eye blinks or upward movements of the eyes. Cappa and Vignolo (1982) reported on psychometric evaluation of a patient who had been living in a locked-in condition for twelve years. Their findings suggested that locked-in syndrome is not associated with cognitive or language disturbances. Locked-in syndrome has been associated with a lesion in the base of the pons, usually sparing only occulomotor function. The mutism associated with this syndrome is actually the severest form of dysarthria.

The clinical importance of the differential diagnosis in these cases seems apparent. Akinetic mute patients are not able to utilize any form of communication. Therefore, they are not candidates for speech/language treatment. On the other hand, the mute patient with a diagnosis of locked-in syndrome (pseudoakinetic mutism) can benefit from professional assistance in the development of an appropriate nonoral communication system.

Dysarthria

Dysarthria is a speech disorder secondary to damage to the central nervous system (CNS). The CNS damage may cause weakness, slowness, dyscoordination, and/or aberration in tone of the speech musculature. The resulting movement disturbance may result in impairment of voice, nasal resonance, articulation and/or prosody. The site and size of the CNS lesion determines the nature and severity of speech motor subsystem involvement and, thus, the nature and severity of the dysarthria. Patients with severe dysarthria, for example, bilateral involvement of corticobulbar pathways, may present with initial or persistent mutism. Periodic follow-up by a speech/language clinician is strongly recommended for the patient with persistent mutism associated with severe dysarthria. Improvement in the patient's condition may warrant a trial of treatment for possible oral communication. We have personally treated two patients, initially mute with severe dysarthria (pseudoakinetic mutism), for whom oral communication treatment was appropriate and of moderate success as late as two and three years post-stroke (Simpson, Till and Goff, 1988). Mutism associated with severe dysarthria may also result from traumatic head injury. With recovery, whispered speech may emerge, followed by dysarthric speech (von Cramon, 1981).

True mutism

'True' mutism refers to a syndrome characterized by aspontaneity, not only of speech, but of other motor behaviors as well. Damasio, A. (1981) reported that these patients typically 'fail to indicate any desire to communicate by gesture, mimicry or writing... When probed about their abnormal behavior, they clearly give testimony to a strange experience of avolition but not to any problem with the actual composition of contents for verbal communication' (p. 53). This form of mutism may initially appear similar to apractic mutism or to transcortical motor aphasia. However, some degree of aphasic deficit is usually present in the latter two syndromes. The distinguishing feature in the 'true' mutism syndrome is the patient's disinclination to communicate in any form, even though his auditory comprehension, reading, and written language are intact. Recovery from this type of mutism proceeds directly into fluent speech with normal phonetic, syntactic, semantic, and prosodic features of language. The location of the lesion in 'true' mutism is found on the mesial aspect of the frontal lobe. These lesions involve the supplementary motor area and its surrounding tissue (Damasio, H., 1981, p. 38).

Aphasia

Aphasia is a disturbance of symbolic processing involving comprehension and formulation of language. It is usually present, at least to some degree, in patients with apractic mutism. One variety of aphasia, transcortical motor aphasia, warrants our attention here. Though not a true form of mutism, transcortical motor aphasia may initially appear similar to apractic mutism, and must be considered in the differential diagnosis. In both of these disorders, patients may not initiate speech. In contrast to the absence of speech in apractic mutism, in transcortical motor aphasia, speech repetition is preserved.

Mutism associated with right-hemisphere lesions

We have personally seen two patients with mutism resulting from right-hemisphere lesions. In both cases, language processing abilities were intact and the mutism responded to treatment techniques similar to those used for speech initiation difficulties in apractic mutism. The mutism lasted only two to three days. As the mutism resolved, a mild dysarthria was evidenced by one patient, much like the patient described by Damasio *et al.* (1982). The other's speech was dysprosodic, or 'aprosodic' as termed by Kent and Rosenbek (1982), marked by monotone and indistinct articulation. Long-term follow-up was not possible for either of our patients.

Apractic mutism

When apractic mutism, i.e., inability to program volitionally the respiratory, laryngeal, and articulatory behaviors for speech, is a part of the clinical picture, it is most commonly present during the earliest stages in the recovery period. Very often, by the time the speech/language clinician is consulted, the mute stage has passed. When mutism persists, it may be masking a variety of associated deficits. Apractic mutism most often coexists with at least some degree of aphasia. The coexisting aphasia may be minimal, such that, despite demonstrable language deficits, patients with apractic mutism may be able to comprehend high level verbal language and to write in sentences (see Case 1). Apractic mutism may, on the other hand, accompany a severe and persisting aphasia. Our clinical experience with patients who demonstrate persisting mutism with an accompanying aphasic component, provides the basis for our disagreement with Lebrun's point of view set forth in Chapter 1. He states that protracted mutism is a symptom of aphasia rather than of apraxia of speech. In order to treat these patients successfully, however, we have found that the aphasic and the apractic components must be approached differently and separately in treatment. The apraxia will not respond well to language remediation techniques that are appropriate for treatment of aphasia (see Chapter 5). Rather, the apraxia responds to specific treatment approaches directed towards the remediation of the initiation, sequencing, and/or spatial–temporal mechanisms underlying the disorder (see Chapter 2). Further, the recovery patterns differ. The motor planning/initiation difficulties improve at a different rate and to a different degree when compared to the aphasic symptomatology.

Two features which may emerge with verbalization and may accompany the classic pattern of apractic errors include:

1 Speech initiation difficulties
2 A distorted quality in articulation (Baxter *et al.*, 1980; Schiff *et al.*, 1983).

Often both of these features are present in the individual's speech, but usually there is a predominance of one feature over another.

The speech initiation difficulty usually responds best to automatic types of cueing such as sentence completion cues. As initiation abilities improve, self-initiated starter phrases, such as, 'I said...' or 'uh ...', may be helpful for the patient to utilize as a compensatory strategy (see Case 2). Once speech has been initiated, individuals with primarily speech initiation difficulties may be able to produce even multisyllable words clearly and, perhaps, fluently. However, the initial syllable, particularly one beginning with a vowel, is often omitted. During connected speech, the initiation deficit may result in disturbed prosody. The flow of the sentence is reduced to a word-by-word production as if each word requires a separate initiation effort. This characteristic is usually not apparent during production of more automatic utterances.

The distorted quality which may emerge in the speech of initially mute apractic patients can be mild or severe in nature. It may appear irregularly, or it may be a pervasive feature. Despite the pervasiveness of the distorted quality in the speech of some patients, the adequacy of nonverbal oral movements in vegetative or other automatic behaviors rules out weakness and/or gross coordination deficits as the underlying causes. Dysarthric speakers, on the other hand, show consistent weakness and/or gross coordination deficits for both nonverbal oral movements and in speech. Providing that a coexisting dysarthria is ruled out, when mutism emerges into speech with this distorted quality, treatment must, of course, be directed at the faulty programming of speech (see Chapter 6). In some cases, the initiation deficit and/or the distorted quality may resolve. In others, these features may persist despite appropriate treatment. Written communication, if at a functional level, may be a more practical means of expression (see Case 2).

Clinical Assessment

The clinician confronted with a mute patient who has known or suspected damage to the central nervous system often faces a diagnostic challenge. Modalities other than spoken communication must be thoroughly evaluated in order to arrive at a differential diagnosis regarding the nature of the mutism. In addition, the presence and influence of any coexisting disorders must be determined. When it appears that one is dealing with apractic mutism, the evaluation should:

1 Determine the existence and severity of aphasia, and, to the extent possible, that of apraxia of speech and dysarthria
2 Determine the presence and severity of any coexisting oral nonverbal (buccofacial) apraxia and limb apraxia
3 Provide sufficient information to guide the treatment approach
4 Provide information regarding the prognosis.

To that end, our assessment battery typically includes an aphasia evaluation, oral–peripheral evaluation, oral nonverbal apraxia battery, and limb apraxia battery.

During the initial assessment it is important to evaluate language competence first. We follow this with the oral–peripheral evaluation. The patient must have adequate auditory comprehension and sufficient motor strength to follow the instructions; otherwise, the inability to perform target behaviors to verbal command cannot reliably be interpreted as apraxia. If the patient demonstrates a significant deficit in comprehension, the balance of the evaluation must be modified. Alternate modes of instruction may then be utilized such as modeling of the desired response by the clinician.

The aphasia evaluation

The evaluation for aphasia has been thoroughly reviewed in other texts and need not be repeated here save several specific applications to the mute patient. All language modalities, i.e., comprehension, speaking, reading, writing, and gesture, should be assessed. This can be accomplished via administration of a standardized aphasia test or by nonstandardized assessment (see Helm-Estabrooks, 1984). The evaluation of auditory comprehension in the mute patient will depend exclusively upon reliable nonverbal response modes such as pointing, gesture, nodding the head, or writing. The assessment of reading comprehension is useful in helping to establish the presence or absence of aphasia. Further, it has treatment implications regarding the potential facilitating effect that graphic cues may have for speech. The patient with good or moderate reading abilities may find the pairing of the printed word with auditory and visual models facilitating to speech reorganization.

The mute patient may produce spoken language or vocalization when the utterance is automatic, emotive, overlearned, or appropriately cued. Dogged persistence in the complete administration of a formal verbal evaluation is inappropriate in such cases. The verbal portion of the evaluation should, more appropriately, include attempts to elicit overlearned social speech, rote sequences such as counting and days of the week, imitation, sentence completion, opposites, singing familiar tunes, reciting nursery rhymes, and so forth. Generally, natural and relaxed attempts to elicit verbal production are the most successful. In addition, the greater the support provided for the patient by way of cueing or simultaneous production, the greater the chance of eliciting verbalization (see Chapter 7).

We do not, then, expect to derive a good sense of the mute patient's underlying expressive language abilities from the evaluation of oral expression. Rather, we wish to determine whether phonation and/or speech can be elicited. If so, we note the effective stimulus conditions, the type, variety, and clarity of sounds or words produced, and the degree to which melody and prosody are preserved. This information will provide us with a starting point for treatment. A short speech sample, if obtained, also allows us to make limited perceptual judgements about the presence or absence of significant dysarthria.

The language formulation ability of the patient with apractic mutism is usually best determined through the evaluation of written expression. The typical patient with apractic mutism will be right handed with a right hemiparesis, and may need to be encouraged to write or print with his nonpreferred hand. Legibility is usually somewhat reduced, but is generally adequate to provide diagnostic information about the appropriateness and completeness of written language formulation, word retrieval, spelling and syntax.

Non-language batteries

Standardized and informal oral–peripheral, oral–nonverbal apraxia, and limb apraxia batteries have been discussed previously in this volume and elsewhere (DeRenzi, Pieczuro and Vignolo, 1966; Mateer and Kimura, 1977; Dabul, 1979; Wertz, LaPointe and Rosenbek, 1984, and others). Here, only specific applications to the evaluation of the mute patient will be addressed.

Oral–peripheral examination

Routine oral–peripheral evaluation will include assessment of facial sensation as well as strength, rate, and range of motion of the various structures and motor speech subsystems. These observations will usually provide sufficient information to rule out dysarthria of sufficient magnitude to be responsible for the complete absence of speech. The patient with a coexisting severe buccofacial apraxia may be unable to respond adequately to verbal instruction alone, even when auditory comprehension is adequate. These patients often require visual models and/or tactile stimulation to evoke desired responses.

In most severe cases of coexisting buccofacial apraxia, it is important to observe the patient's automatic and vegetative functions which involve speech structures. For example, behaviors such as licking lips, smiling, chewing, sucking, swallowing, coughing, and throat clearing should be observed. These observations may provide the only information initially available regarding aspects of motor execution including strength, rate and range of movement of the speech structures. When dysarthria, rather than apraxia, is the limiting disability, we typically see consistently reduced integrity of the speech musculature in automatic as well as in volitional responses. In oral apraxia, automatic, reflexive movements are superior to more planned, purposeful movements, implicating reduced volitional control and planning rather than weakness of the musculature.

Information about laryngeal functioning for speech, e.g., vocal quality, pitch, and intensity, will be minimal or nonexistent for the patient who cannot phonate at will. Laryngeal assessment should be attempted nonetheless. We have observed occasionally, mute patients who produce voice during the evaluation only when the clinician, armed with tongue depressor and penlight, probed the oral cavity and requested the traditional 'ahh'. This was apparently an automatic response since, minus the penlight and tongue blade, the same patients were unable to produce this vocalic segment.

The assessment of volitional control over respiration is of particular interest in the evaluation of mute apractic patients (see Mitchell and Berger, 1975, for further reading on volitional and automatic neural control of respiration). In treatment, one must occasionally resort to the restoration of the components of speech production such as control over respiration. The patient may be instructed to take a deep breath or sniff, and volitionally prolong exhalation or pant to demonstrate discrete control over inhalation and exhalation.

Oral nonverbal praxis battery

Apraxia of speech often coexists with oral nonverbal apraxia (see Chapter 2). In our clinical experience, treatment for the patient with severe apraxia can, at times, be approached through improving volitional control over nonspeech oral and lingual movements. This might include movements such as jaw opening, tongue elevation, and lip rounding. This approach has been reported by others (Luria, 1970; Rosenbek, 1978; Schuell, Jenkins and Jimenez-Pabon, 1964; and Wertz, LaPointe and Rosenbek, 1984). Establishing volitional control over oral, nonverbal movements which are components of articulate speech may provide a foundation upon which to base more direct speech treatment. This approach is most appropriate for patients with severe apraxia or those who are unable to respond to linguistic stimuli.

A thorough evaluation for oral praxis is therefore important in the assessment of the patient with apractic mutism. The examining clinician will want to note the nature and strength of the stimulus necessary to evoke the desired response. Can the patient respond to verbal command alone, or does he require a model of the desired behavior? Does he need a model with additional oral, tactile stimulation? The nature of the patient's responses should be noted as well. Are the behaviors observed only during 'automatic' acts, or can they be elicited from commands, that is, with more volitional intent? If elicited from commands, can the patient pretend, without the use of an object, or does he perform the act only when using an object? An example of this is the patient who is unable to demonstrate an ability to blow unless a lit match is present, and often only if he is holding the match with its impending threat. The assessment of wilful control over respiration is carried a step beyond that of the oral peripheral evaluation. Here we include nonverbal behaviors which require coordination of respiration with other components of the speech mechanism such as blowing, humming, and whistling.

Limb praxis battery

If a patient has demonstrated adequate understanding and sufficient strength, sensation, and coordination to enable him to follow instructions for limb gesture, failure to do so would then suggest disturbed volitional motor programming. This is termed limb apraxia. Limb praxis batteries are discussed in Chapters 2 and 4 as well as elsewhere (Duffy, 1974; Duffy and Duffy, 1981; Kertesz, 1982). When dealing with a mute patient, the limb praxis assessment gives the clinician an indication of the patient's potential to use that extremity for inter-systemic reorganization or gestural communication to augment, or, if necessary, to replace verbal communication (see also Chapter 12).

Prognosis

Wertz (1978) stated that 'since apraxia of speech typically results from a unilateral left hemisphere lesion, and since it typically coexists with aphasia, many of the prognostic variables that influence recovery from aphasia can be applied in predicting the future for patients demonstrating apraxia' (p. 69). The same holds true for patients with apractic mutism. Numerous discussions of the biographical, medical, behavioral, and treatment variables which influence recovery from aphasia and apraxia of speech can be found elsewhere in the literature

(Darley, 1972, 1975; Davis, 1983; Eisenson, 1949, 1981; Kertesz, 1979; Marquardt, 1982; Rosenbek, 1978; Sarno, 1980; Wertz, 1978; Wertz, LaPointe and Rosenbek, 1984) and in this text. When establishing a prognosis for the patient with apractic mutism, the interaction of these variables should be considered. Variables of specific prognostic interest for patients with apractic mutism include severity of coexisting aphasia, oral–nonverbal praxis ability, presence of other associated deficits, and duration of the impairments. The fewer and less severe the coexisting deficits, the better the prognosis.

The most critical factors in the clinical outcome of apractic mutism are the presence and the degree of coexisting aphasia. The aphasia accompanying apractic mutism may vary from severe to minimal. When apractic mutism coexists with severe aphasia, most individuals do not achieve a useful level of language. This is especially true in the presence of a significant auditory processing disturbance. There are, in essence, no words behind the silence once the mute state has passed. Individuals who, on the other hand, show relatively little concomitant aphasia usually progress to effective oral communication (see Case 1).

When apractic mutism is confounded by oral nonverbal apraxia, the rate at which each of these disorders resolves seems to have prognostic significance. Rapid improvement, within the first several days is a highly encouraging sign. Mohr (1980) reported that in patients with lesions confined to Broca's area, the mutism resolves in the first few days post onset. Rosenbek (1978) reported that mutism lasting even a few days portends a persisting problem. Vignolo (1964) considered oral–nonverbal apraxia and 'anarthria' (apractic mutism) which persist beyond two months to be an extremely poor prognostic sign. Our Case 2, who was twenty months post-stroke before phonating volitionally, is an example of a patient with a long mute period. Despite the establishment of some limited useful speech, severe word initiation deficits persisted, and written expression developed as the communicative avenue of choice.

Treating the Patient with Apractic Mutism

General principles

Treatment of the person with apractic mutism may be one of the most challenging of clinical experiences. It often provides clinicians with an opportunity to exercise some of their creative abilities.

The most important concept in the treatment of apractic mutism is the automatic versus volitional dichotomy. Given a disturbance in motor programming at a more volitional level, utilization of more automatic levels of language is the obvious avenue of choice. We find words to be the most successful stimuli in establishing verbal production in the mute patient. It appears as though isolated sounds and nonsense syllables require more, or different motor planning than do meaningful words. Nonmeaningful productions cannot capitalize on the familiarity of overlearned, more automatic levels of production such as the person's name or social greetings. Meaningful units, or words, on the other hand, seem to facilitate motor speech production. It seems that 'meaning is made to serve movement' (Rosenbek, Kent and LaPointe, 1984, p. 44). This is not to say that working directly on isolated sounds or movements is never appropriate. It is certainly appropriate as part of the treatment program for some patients.

In treating the patient with apractic mutism, it is extremely important for the clinician to create an atmosphere of acceptance. That is, an atmosphere in which an utterance which is less-than-perfect, perhaps far less-than-perfect, is acceptable. At times the patient may be able to produce only the vowel. Our objective at this point is for the patient simply to initiate speech. The quality or preciseness of the utterance will be addressed at a later time in the treatment program.

The initial clinical assessment provides essential information as to what types of cues and tasks are most facilitating. The patient's background and interests may also serve to guide the selection of specific, familiar words or subject matter for treatment (Wallace and Canter, 1985).

Establishing word production

With most patients, we aim initially for word production from some type of 'running start' cue. This includes sentence completion or 'cloze' cues such as 'Wind the ____' (watch) or 'Let's go ____' (home), or paired associates, e.g., 'down and ____' (up) or 'high and ____' (low). Visual augmentation of these auditory cues by objects, pictures or, when appropriate, the printed form of the target word is important. Other very helpful accompanying cues include relevant gestures and the patient's utilization of cues from the clinician's oral postures.

Phrase and sentence completion cues are usually most successful when the target word is produced by the clinician one, two or, better yet, three times, then followed by the phrase to be completed by that target word. The clinician's intonation may be a critical factor in the facilitating effect of these cues. The phrase or 'running start' must be delivered in such a manner that it is 'left hanging', in need of finalization with the target word. Another running start cue is provided by what we term a 'starter phrase', such as, 'I said...' followed by the desired word. This type of starter phrase is usually less facilitating initially, but is a strategy which some patients are able to learn to utilize themselves at a later time for word initiation. Thereby, the need to rely on the clinician for these starter cues is eventually eliminated. This technique seems to be useful specifically for the speech initiation difficulty, overcoming what Luria and Hutton (1977) have referred to as 'inertia'.

Rote productions such as counting, singing, reciting nursery rhymes, or prayers may facilitate verbalization. If such 'automatic' speech is stimulable, this can be relied upon extensively at first to provide the patient with a successful experience of speaking again. These utterances may then be eased from rote sequences into sentence completion responses, e.g., 'Row, row, row your ____', or 'Give us this day our daily ____'. From here, clinician cues are systematically faded and increasingly volitional productions are encouraged as progress allows.

The key to this treatment approach is that automaticity must give way to more propositional levels of word production. Rote series production and sentence completion are modified to more direct production of selected words such as simultaneous production, imitation, or delayed imitation. Sentence completion cues give way to 'weaker' carrier or starter phrases, e.g., 'a piece of apple ____' (pie) moves to 'a piece of ____' then to 'I'd like some ____' or even 'That's a ____'. It has been our experience, however, that it is usually necessary to retain visual (object or picture), graphic (printed word), and some auditory cues, for a significant portion of the apraxia treatment with any patient.

If this direction is not successful, it may be that a trial with Melodic Intonation Therapy (MIT) (Albert, Sparks and Helm, 1973) would provide the vehicle needed to re-establish verbal production (see Chapter 6 in this text). Another approach to elicit words in the patient with apratic mutism who produces words at reflexive or emotive levels involves 'Voluntary Production of Involuntary Utterances' (Helm and Barresi, 1980). For example, if the person reflexively utters 'no' or even curses (we accept *anything* at this point), he/she is immediately encouraged to repeat the same utterance more volitionally while the speech mechanism is, so-to-speak, engaged (see also Chapter 9).

Re-establishing elements of speech

For patients with persistent (resistent) mutism, for whom elicitation of the more automatic levels of language has not been successful, re-establishment of some of the components of speech production may be the next choice. These speech components include phonation, non-verbal–oral and lingual movements, and volitional control of respiration.

The re-establishment of volitional phonation can be approached utilizing vegetative or relatively automatic responses which involve laryngeal sound. These include grunting on command or imitatively or as an accompaniment to physical resistance. Resistive techniques such as arm wrestling, or pushing against a stationary object facilitate glottal closure, which may be instrumental in achieving phonation. Vocalization accompanying a sigh ('ah', 'oh' or 'mmm'), laugh, or cough may be attempted under volitional control. Attempts may even be made to prolong labile behaviors, such as vocalization accompanying laughing or crying. Humming while chewing may also be attempted. We have tried, but not found success with, using an electrolarynx applied to the laryngeal area to provide focal sensory stimulation for voice production. Creative clinicians have probably tried other novel methods to elicit phonation. Many techniques may fail, but just one that works is all that is needed as a key to open the way to the re-establishment of the ability to program phonation. Success may be quite sporadic initially, but with persistent efforts, phonation, almost without exception, becomes more consistent.

If possible, working initially with mouthed speech without phonation or whispered speech, may be a helpful predecessor to re-establishing verbalization in the mute patient. Direct work with control of nonverbal oral and lingual movements may be the only avenue of treatment open for some patients with persistent apractic mutism who are unable to respond to speech stimuli. Improved ability to assume volitional, speech-related jaw, lip, and tongue positions may benefit later attempts at speech.

Establishing voluntary control of respiration may be a difficult process in the person with apractic mutism. Tasks such as blowing a tissue away from the face, blowing out a match, blowing bubbles through a straw, or biofeedback with air flow may be used to attempt to bring respiration under more volitional control. This behavior might then be utilized in attempts to phonate. Later, this may be incorporated along with appropriate articulatory postures to achieve production of speech segments, especially vowels and consonants marked by the feature of continuancy.

When components of speech, e.g., respiration, phonation, or articulation at the level of production of oral postures, become replicable and more consistent, the focus of treatment moves to combining these stimulable elements toward speech sound or word production. Phonation may be added to a phonetic posture, e.g., humming in /m/ posture. An oral posture and phonation may be combined with vowel production, e.g., bilabial plus /i/ for 'me'. A core vocabulary can thereby be created from a limited phonetic repertoire. Procedures as outlined in Chapter 9 may also be appropriate.

The emerging utterance

As more consistent phonation emerges, some patients' utterances may be limited to vowels. Treatment may at first necessarily be limited to improving consistency, accuracy, and expanding the patient's repertoire of vocalic segments. One can even use words as stimuli in these cases, accepting the target vowel in the word as meeting the initial criteria for success. With continuing treatment, certain consonants often become stimulable. The nature of the cueing support provided for the patient is particularly important in re-establishing consonant production (see Chapter 7). Usually diphthongs are not stimulable until later in the course of treatment. Diphthongs often do not emerge until after some consonant production is established. Initially, diphthongs seem to require discrete, sequential production of the two vowels of which the diphthong is comprised.

As phoneme production becomes more consistent, the stimulable phonemes can be incorporated into stimulus words. The cueing system which provided the vehicle for success must then be gradually and systematically withdrawn as discussed in Chapter 7. In general, when treating a person with apractic mutism, inconsistent, limited abilities are brought to consistency, and phonetic repertoires are gradually and systematically expanded.

Selection of stimuli for verbal production

The nature of the words chosen as stimuli is a critical factor in the success or failure of treatment efforts with the mute patient. First and foremost, the words must be useful and relevant for the patient. Adjunctively, however, only words which are phonetically programmable should be chosen. There appears to be a relatively consistent hierarchy of difficulty among phonemes for the majority of patients with apraxia. For a summary of the research concerning relative difficulty of selected phonetic segments, see Wertz, LaPointe and Rosenbek (1984, p. 59). When speech emerges from a mute state, the concept of a hierarchy of difficulty must be considered in order to provide the optimum conditions for success.

In general, we, as others, have found the simpler and more visible the movement, the greater the likelihood of success. A CV word, e.g., 'bow', is easier than a CVC combination, e.g., 'boat'. Although it appears to be a relatively simple movement, the /h/ phoneme tends to be difficult for many of these patients. It appears as though the timing and coordination required of the breath stream with the oral posture in this sound may be the problem.

We find some individual variation in the hierarchy of difficulty or emerging order of phoneme production following the mute period in apraxia. However, initially, we see vowels, with the exception of /æ/ and diphthongs, appearing with greater ease than consonants. Next to appear are voiced bilabials, some lingual–alveolars, anterior plosives, labiodentals, glides, some continuants, then velars (/k/ and /g/), fricatives, affricates, and, finally, blends. This hierarchy of difficulty or pattern of re-emerging sounds is variable from patient to patient and may change in each patient over time. Clinicians must systematically explore each patient's individual hierarchy initially and at frequent intervals throughout the course of treatment. At any given time, the patient's phonemic repertoire is incorporated into an ever-expanding vocabulary. One exception to the relatively consistent hierarchy of difficulty of sounds is found in persons with predominant speech initiation problems. In these cases, the phonemic repertoire may be relatively preserved.

In the selection of response stimuli, the clinician must take into consideration the emerging repertoire of sounds and the complexity and the component features of the target sounds. Successes and failures and careful analysis of stimulus and response variables are utilized to guide the course of treatment.

Counselling

A final consideration in the treatment of patients with apractic mutism is appropriate patient, family, and staff counselling. The inability to speak is usually frightening to the patient, and is often the primary concern of the patient's family once he is medically stable. Because of the absence of spoken language, families of these patients are particularly unaware of the patients' underlying language abilities or disabilities. They frequently assume that the patient is understanding everything they say; that his reading is intact; and that he would express himself graphically were his dominant upper extremity useful. Family members or hospital staff often request spelling boards and other devices requiring an intact language system, being unaware as to whether or not these devices are appropriate.

As soon after the evaluation as possible, the clinician should discuss the findings with the patient, with his significant others and with the attending hospital staff. This discussion should include an explanation of the nature of the mutism, the extent of aphasia and other coexisting disorders, the prognosis, and the best methods of immediately enhancing communication with the patient. For patients with minimal coexisting aphasia, writing is generally the most functional mode of communication at the outset, and should be depended upon as long as necessary.

The family of the patient who has a significant coexisting aphasia will need instruction to simplify their spoken input to the patient, and supplement it with visual and gestural cues whenever possible. They will also need to know the extent to which the patient is able to communicate graphically. If writing is nonfunctional, alternatives should be explored to enhance communication while speech is being restored. One viable alternative, as language comprehension permits, is to ask simple, direct yes/no questions to which the patient can respond nonverbally. The patient who is not limited by a significant limb apraxia may be encouraged to use gestural communication. Drawing is another alternative which is often overlooked as a means of expressive communication (Lyon and Helm-Estabrooks, 1987).

Family members are frequently eager to learn how they can help the patient in his/her speech recovery. While we seldom wish to place them in the role of the clinician, there are advantages to having family members understand and practise appropriate stimulation. We must prevent the development of maladaptive struggle behaviors. Placing the patient's speech attempts in the spotlight may be counterproductive. Since the earliest speech forthcoming from a patient with apractic mutism is usually overlearned, i.e., social speech and automatic utterances, it is often appropriate for family members to provide opportunities for this type of speech in a natural and relaxed way as a part of daily conversation. Family sing-a-longs may also be instrumental in eliciting vocalization from the patient. When patients with apractic mutism begin to speak or phonate spontaneously they often do so infrequently and at reflexive, emotive, or automatic levels. Family and staff can capitalize on such times by gently encouraging the patient to attempt the utterances again more purposefully.

Finally, it is most appropriate to include family members in the therapy session from time to time. The patient's speech usually emerges under cued conditions long before it is evident spontaneously. Opportunities to observe the patient speaking under cued conditions can be both encouraging and instructive to family members.

Concluding Remarks

Treatment of the mute apractic patient may be one of the more challenging and worthwhile clinical experiences. Treatment of these patients requires a disciplined approach, yet, at the same time, it can call upon the clinician's creativity.

Each patient is different in his or her symptomatology and accompanying deficits. Each, therefore, requires a somewhat different treatment approach. A thorough assessment of the patient's speech, language, oral motor, and gestural abilities along with careful data collection provide the necessary information to guide the treatment approach. Careful selection of stimuli and cueing as well as analysis of the data collected throughout the course of management help to keep the treatment appropriate along the way.

Case Presentations

The following case examples represent problems and outcomes a clinician may encounter when treating persons with apractic mutism. Both patients were mute initially. Included in each case example is information regarding extent of coexisting aphasia, the treatment approach, course in treatment, and communication outcome.

Case 1

This male patient was 48 years old at the time of his left-hemisphere stroke. He had a high school education and had worked as a cryptographer, a printer, and a bartender. He showed a mild paresis of the right upper extremity which lasted less than one week. He was initially described as unable to speak, but appeared to understand what he heard.

On examination five days post onset, the patient showed slight weakness of his right face on grimace, but tongue movements showed normal range of movement and strength. A moderately severe nonverbal apraxia was present for oral, lingual, and laryngeal movements. Voluntary control over respiration was demonstrated for inhalation and exhalation. Even after extensive stimulation, the patient was rarely able to produce vocal sound.

Mild–moderate aphasia was apparent. He was 70 per cent accurate in comprehending two elements of auditory information at a time, but complexly worded sentences were not consistently comprehended. Initially, the patient wrote in single words or occasionally in phrases in order to communicate. This writing contained spelling errors. Reading comprehension was accurate for simple sentences but, with increased syntactic complexity, was incomplete.

The aphasia improved relatively rapidly. The Porch Index of Communicative Abilities (PICA) (Porch, 1981) was administered at one month post-stroke. The Overall score was at the 65th percentile. The 39th percentile was attained for Verbal subtests, while Graphic and Gestural subtests were at the 84th and 73rd percentiles, respectively. At one-and-a-half months post-stroke, the patient was accurate on ten of twelve items on the Complex Ideational Material on the Boston Diagnostic Aphasia Examination (BDAE) (Goodglass and Kaplan, 1983) and five out of ten were accurate on paragraph level reading on the same test. At four months post-onset he was 100 per cent accurate on auditory comprehension on the Complex Ideational Material subtest.

Verbal recovery was considerably slower. Speech initiation was severely disturbed. The patient attempted to speak, but no phonation or utterance was forthcoming. Automatic, overlearned speech and sentence completion were utilized in order to facilitate more consistent verbalization. Articulatory accuracy was initially disregarded in order to encourage any utterance, as most responses were obviously attempts at the target word. It was felt that highly cued word production with low emphasis on articulatory accuracy was needed to reduce the effortful behaviors associated with speech initiation.

This gentleman learned techniques quickly, successfully reducing effort associated with speaking. As consistency of overlearned word production was achieved and longer utterances were produced spontaneously, it was apparent that syntax was not disturbed. There was, however, a distorted quality to this man's speech which improved somewhat at the single word level. This distorted quality was still present six years post-stroke and reduced speech intelligibility to approximately 80 per cent.

Case 2

This left-handed male was a high school graduate with some college education. He was an insurance agent for ten years and an independent truck driver for twenty years. He suffered a left CVA when he was 54 years old. CT scan showed massive infarct in the distribution of the left middle and anterior cerebral arteries. The patient was left with a dense right hemiplegia, severe aphasia, and was essentially mute. He initially showed left-sided gaze and stereotypic movement of the left arm, often accompanying episodes of apparent agitation or frustration.

One week post-stroke the patient had an NG tube in place and followed very few simple commands. He was inaccurate on identifying objects when named. A severe oral nonverbal apraxia was demonstrated. He was aphonic except for labile episodes which were accompanied by phonation. When he was encouraged to continue phonating volitionally during or after a labile episode, phonation ceased. The patient showed no comprehension of printed single words or simple printed commands. He did not write, nor did he copy simple geometric figures or words. The patient was not treated at the time of the initial evaluation due to severe emotional lability and distractability.

He was re-evaluated at two months post-stroke and again at four months. Speech and language evaluation was essentially unchanged. In addition, there were more frequent episodes of emotional lability which were accompanied by phonation (a loud whine).

At nineteen months post-onset, interfering behaviors had reduced to the point where trial speech and language treatment could be initiated. Attempts at phonation were initially unsuccessful. These attempts included singing, counting, sentence completion cues, attempts at humming while chewing, manual pressure on the diaphragm, electrolarynx stimulation to the larynx, and volitional attempts to prolong phonation which accompanied labile reactions. In addition, resistive techniques such as arm wrestling and having the patient push against the wheelchair with his left arm were employed to facilitate phonation. Attempts to control respiration volitionally were equally unsuccessful. These included blowing out a burning match and blowing bubbles through a straw. Arm wrestling finally elicited a very inconsistent grunt beginning one month after initiation of treatment which was twenty months post-stroke.

In treatment, imitation of mouth movements continued separately from attempts at phonation. At first, nonverbal–oral movements such as mouth opening, grimace, and pucker of the lips were practised. As these improved in consistency, oral postures for certain sounds were incorporated, e.g., positions for /o/, /i/, /a/, and /m/. This was followed by combining two movements in sequence still without phonation. Approximately seven weeks after initiation of treatment this patient finally whispered his first word, 'home', after a sentence completion cue. Inconsistent whisper was soon accompanied by voicing, initially only with resistive techniques. The repertoire of words slowly increased, but severe word initiation deficits were apparent. A sentence completion cue was, therefore, the most reliable cue for initiation of speech. In order to eliminate reliance on the clinician for the initiation cue, a self-cue was eventually established. The patient would utter (aloud or silently) 'I said...' followed by the target word or phrase.

Aphasia (language) treatment was provided in addition to treatment for the apractic mutism. The patient showed significant improvement in his language abilities. He improved from forty out of a possible seventy-two on the BDAE auditory comprehension Subtest A to seventy correct after two months in treatment. Written naming improved from zero out of ten at one month, to seven out of ten at two months post-initiation of treatment. On Reading Sentences and Paragraphs on the BDAE, he scored four out of ten at one month and nine out of ten at five months into treatment.

The PICA was administered at twenty-two months post CVA. This was one month after the patient had produced his first word. The Verbal response mean was at the 43rd percentile. Graphics were at the 76th percentile and the Gestural modality mean was at the 75th percentile. The Overall score was at the 60th percentile.

The patient was discharged from individual treatment after eight months of therapy. Frequency of self-initiated speech began to decline after that time, but could be encouraged with reminders. Written expression continued to improve. Occasional contacts with this patient up to five years post-stroke showed writing to be the expressive avenue of choice. Single written words evolved into phrases followed by some complete sentences. Minor spelling and grammatical errors persisted in writing, however. The patient spoke intermittently, but seemed to be more inclined to reach for a pen and paper to express himself.

The course of recovery for this patient showed a differential improvement between the apraxia of speech (speech initiation difficulties) and the aphasic symptomatology. The former showed minimal improvement, while the latter, as seen in auditory comprehension, reading comprehension and written language, showed significant improvement. Unlike Lebrun (Chapter 1), we feel the different rate and degree of recovery of the two components, coupled with the responsiveness of the mutism to motor speech initiation/programming techniques, tends to support the theory that a motor-speech component (as opposed to aphasia) is the primary cause of prolonged mutism in patients such as this one.

This is not to imply that the aphasic and apractic components do not interact and influence one another. It would be artificial and neurologically unsound to reduce spoken language to dichotomous processes which are completely independent. Indeed, language improvements must allow these patients to derive more benefit from treatment instructions directed at the motor-speech component and to better formulate the linguistic aspects of spoken language.

Acknowledgment

Marianne Simpson and Amy Clark express their gratitude to the Veterans' Administration, Long Beach, California, for support and resources provided in the preparation of this chapter.

References

ALBERT, M.L., GOODGLASS, H., HELM, N.A., RUBENS, A.B. and ALEXANDER, M.P. (1981) 'Clinical aspects of dysphasia', in ARNOLD, B.E., WINCKEL, F. and WYKE, B.D. (Eds.) *Disorders of Human Communication, 2*, New York, Springer-Verlag.

ALBERT, M., SPARKS, R. and HELM, N. (1973) 'Melodic intonation therapy for aphasia', *Archives of Neurology*, **29**, pp. 130–1.

BAXTER, S.D., SIMPSON, M., GREENBAUM, H. and PRIBRAM, H. (1980) 'Phonological realization disorders in aphasia with three-dimensional computed tomography'. Paper presented to the Academy of Aphasia, South Yarmouth, Massachusetts (unpublished).

BAY, E. (1962) 'Aphasia and non-verbal disorders of language', *Brain*, **85**, 411–26.

BROCA, P. (1865) Quoted by BROWN, J.W. (1979) 'Language representation in the brain', in STEKLIS, H. and RALEIGH, M. (Eds.) *Neurobiology of Social Communication in Primates*, New York, Academic Press, pp. 133–95.

BROWN, J.W. (1972) *Aphasia, Apraxia and Agnosia*, Illinois, Charles C. Thomas.

BROWN, J. (1977) *Mind, Brain and Consciousness*, New York, Academic Press.

CAPPA, S.F. and VIGNOLO, L.A. (1982) 'Locked-in syndrome for 12 years with preserved intelligence', *Annals of Neurology*, **11**, p. 545.

CRARY, M.A., HARDY, T. and WILLIAMS, W.N. (1985) 'Aphemia with dysarthria or apraxia of speech?', *Clinical Aphasiology: Conference Proceedings*, Minneapolis, BRK Publishers.

DABUL, B. (1979) *Apraxia Battery for Adults*, Tigard, CC Publications.

DAMASIO, A. (1981) 'The nature of aphasia: Signs and syndromes', in SARNO, M.T. (Ed.) *Acquired Aphasia*, New York, Academic Press.

DAMASIO, A., DAMASIO, H., RIZZO, M., VARNEY, N. and GERSH, F. (1982) 'Aphasia with nonhemorrhagic lesions of the basal ganglia and internal capsule', *Archives of Neurology*, **39**, pp. 15–20.

DAMASIO, H. (1981) 'Cerebral localization of the aphasias', in SARNO, M.T. (Ed.) *Acquired Aphasia*, New York, Academic Press.

DARLEY, F.L. (1972) 'The efficacy of language rehabilitation in aphasia', *Journal of Speech and Hearing Disorders*, **37**, p. 3.

DARLEY, F.L. (1975) 'Treatment of acquired aphasia', in FRIEDLANDER, W.J. (Ed.) *Advances in Neurology*, **7**: *Current Reviews of Higher Nervous System Dysfunction*, New York, Raven Press.

DAVIS, G.A. (1983) *A Survey of Adult Aphasia*, Englewood Cliffs, Prentice-Hall.

DE RENZI, E., PIECZURO, A. and VIGNOLO, L.A. (1966) 'Oral apraxia and aphasia', *Cortex*, **2**, pp. 50–73.

DUFFY, J.R. (1974) 'Comparison of brain injured and non-brain injured subjects on an objective test of manual apraxia'. Doctoral dissertation, University of Connecticut (unpublished).

DUFFY, J.D. and DUFFY, J.R. (1981) 'Three studies of deficits in pantomimic expression and pantomimic recognition in aphasia', *Journal of Speech and Hearing Research*, **24**(1), pp. 70–84.

EISENSON, J. (1949) 'Prognostic factors related to language rehabilitation in aphasic patients', *Journal of Speech and Hearing Disorders*, **14**, p. 262.

EISENSON, J. (1981) 'Issues, prognosis and problems in the rehabilitation of language disorders in adults', in CHAPEY, R. (Ed.) *Language Intervention Strategies in Adult Aphasia*, Baltimore, Williams and Wilkins.

FREEMON, F.R. (1971) 'Akinetic mutism and bilateral anterior cerebral artery occlusion', *Journal of Neurology, Neurosurgery and Psychiatry*, **34**, pp. 693–8.

GOODGLASS, H. and KAPLAN, E. (1983) *The Assessment of Aphasia and Related Disorders*, 2nd ed., Philadelphia, Lea and Febiger.

HELM, N. and BARRESI, B. (1980) 'Voluntary control of involuntary utterances: A treatment approach for severe aphasia', in BROOKSHIRE, R. (Ed.) *Clinical Aphasiology: Conference Proceedings*, Minneapolis, BRK Publishers.

HELM-ESTABROOKS, N. (1984) 'Treatment of the aphasias', *In-Services in Neurology*, **4**(2), p. 196.

KENT, R.D. and ROSENBEK, J.C. (1982) 'Prosodic disturbance and neurological lesion', *Brain and Language*, **15**, pp. 259–91.

KERTESZ, A. (1979) *Aphasia and Associated Disorders: Taxonomy, Localization and Recovery*, New York, Grune and Stratton.

KERTESZ, A. (1982) *The Western Aphasia Battery*, New York, Grune and Stratton.

LEBRUN, Y., BUYSSENS, S.E. and HENNEAUX, J. (1973) 'Phonetic aspects of anarthria', *Cortex*, **9**, pp. 126–35.

LURIA, A.R. (1966) *Higher Cortical Functions in Man*, New York, Basic Books, Inc.

LURIA, A.R. (1970) *Traumatic Aphasia: Its Syndromes, Psychology and Treatment*, The Hague, Mouton.

LURIA, A.R. and HUTTON, J.T. (1977) 'A modern assessment of the basic forms of aphasia', *Brain and Language*, **4**, pp. 129–52.

LYON, J.G. and HELM-ESTABROOKS, N. (1987) 'Drawing: its communicative significance for expressively restricted aphasic adults', *Topics in Language Disorders*, **8**(4), pp. 61–71.

MARQUARDT, T.P. (1982) *Acquired Neurogenic Disorders*, Englewood Cliffs, Prentice-Hall.

MATEER, C. and KIMURA, D. (1977) 'Impairment of nonverbal oral movements in aphasia', *Brain and Language*, **4**, pp. 262–76.

MITCHELL, R.A. and BERGER, A.J. (1975) 'Neural regulation of respiration', *American Review of Respiratory Disease*, **III**, pp. 206–24.

MOHR, J.P. (1980) 'Revision of Broca's aphasia and the syndrome of Broca's area infarction and its implications in aphasia theory', *Clinical Aphasiology: Conference Proceedings*, Minneapolis, BRK Publishers, pp. 1–16.

MOHR, J.P., PESSIN, M.S., FINKELSTEIN, S., FUNKENSTEIN, J., DUNCAN, G.W. and DAVIS, K.R. (1978) 'Broca's aphasia: pathologic and clinical aspects', *Neurology*, **28**, pp. 311–24.

PORCH, B.E. (1981) *The Porch Index of Communicative Ability*, 3rd ed., Palo Alto, Consulting Psychologists Press.

ROSENBEK, J.C. (1978) 'Treating apraxia of speech', in JOHNS, D.F. (Ed.) *Clinical Management of Neurogenic Communication Disorders*, Boston, Little, Brown and Company.

ROSENBEK, J.C., KENT, R.D. and LAPOINTE, L.L. (1984) 'An overview and some perspectives', in ROSENBEK, J.C., MCNEIL, M.R. and ARONSON, A.E. (Eds.) *Apraxia of Speech: Physiology, Acoustics, Linguistics, Management*, San Diego, College Hill Press.

SARNO, M.T. (1980) 'Review of research in aphasia: Recovery and rehabilitation', in SARNO, M.T. and HOOK, O. (Eds.) *Aphasia: Assessment and Treatment*, New York, Masson Publishing USA, Inc.

SCHIFF, H.B., ALEXANDER, M.P., NAESER, M.A. and GALABURDA, A.M. (1983) 'Aphemia: clinical-anatomic correlations', *Archives of Neurology*, **40**, 720–7.

SCHUELL, H., JENKINS, J.J. and JIMENEZ-PABON, E. (1964) *Aphasia in Adults: Diagnosis, Prognosis, and Treatment*, New York, Harper and Row.

SIMPSON, M.B., TILL, J.A. and GOFF, A.M. (1988) 'Long-term treatment of severe dysarthria: A case study', *Journal of Speech and Hearing Disorders*, **53**, pp. 433–40.

VIGNOLO, L.A. (1964) 'Evolution of aphasia and language rehabilitation: A retrospective exploratory study', *Cortex*, **1**, p. 344.

VON CRAMON, D. (1981) 'Traumatic mutism and the subsequent reorganization of speech functions', *Neuropsychologia*, **19**(6), pp. 801–5.

WALLACE, G.L. and CANTER, G.J. (1985) 'Effects of personally relevant language materials on the performance of severely aphasic individuals', *Journal of Speech and Hearing Disorders,* **50**, pp. 385–90.

WERTZ, R.T. (1978) 'Neuropathologies of speech and language: An introduction to patient management', in JOHNS, D.F. (Ed.) *Clinical Management of Neurogenic Communicative Disorders*, Boston, Little, Brown and Company.

WERTZ, R.T., LaPOINTE, L.L. and ROSENBEK, J.C. (1984) *Apraxia of Speech in Adults: The Disorder and Its Management*, Orlando, Grune and Stratton, Inc.

Chapter 11

Use of Augmentative Communication Devices with Apractic Individuals

Kathryn M. Yorkston and Patricia F. Waugh

The communication disability resulting from severe apraxia of speech may be so extensive that apractic individuals may not be able to meet their communication needs. Augmentative communication is the general term referring to all communication that supplements or augments speech (Vanderheiden and Yoder, 1986). Augmentative approaches are typically divided into two major categories — 'unaided' or gestural approaches and 'aided' or approaches requiring a board, a book, or a mechanical or electronic device. It is the aided approaches and their application with apractic speakers that will be the focus of this chapter.

Historical Perspective

Historically, the field of augmentative communication has developed as three diverse areas have converged (Vanderheiden and Yoder, 1986). The first of these areas is the use of language boards in the cerebral palsied population (Dixon, 1965; Feallock, 1958; McDonald and Schultz, 1973; and Vicker, 1974). The second area involves the use of sign and gesture approaches with hearing impaired individuals. The final area, originally based chiefly in Europe, involved the development of typing and environmental control systems for individuals who used natural speech but who were severely physically handicapped (Copeland, 1974). During the past decade, there has not only been a tremendous growth in the technology of augmentative communication devices (Brandenburg and Vanderheiden, 1987), but also a growing trend towards application of technology in populations not previously served by the field of augmentative communication (Blackstone, 1986; Musselwhite and St Louis, 1982; Schiefelbusch, 1980; Silverman, 1980). Not only are physical limitations less of a barrier to control of communication devices, but also cognitive and linguistic limitations no longer preclude the use of augmentative communication devices (Beukelman, Yorkston and Dowden, 1985; Hooper and Hasselbring, 1985; Meyer, 1983; Mirenda and Dattilo, 1987; Romski, Sevcik and Joyner, 1984; Warren and Datta, 1981; Yorkston and Dowden, 1984).

Current Trends

Changing technology

One of the important trends that has allowed us to serve the communication needs of apractic individuals is the changing device characteristic brought about by increasingly sophisticated and flexible technology. Some devices do not require spontaneous spelling skills to prepare messages, relying instead on more transparent symbol systems. Devices are becoming increasingly flexible with vocabulary and symbol set selection individualized for the user. Many devices now have speech output, a feature that facilitates learning in cognitively or linguistically limited users. Devices are now becoming truly portable, a mandatory feature for ambulatory users. In short, the technology is changing and providing us with an increasing number of options.

Expanding view of communication competence

Light (1988) has suggested three broad areas of communication needs which augmentative approaches must address if communication competence is to be achieved. The first of these areas is the communication of needs and wants. Here the content of the messages are relatively predictable. Thus, meeting these types of communication needs is straight forward. The second general area is information transfer. Here the content of the message is somewhat less predictable especially with individuals with adult onset disorders who have retained extensive background knowledge and interests. Because of the relative unpredictability of these messages, many of the traditional augmentative devices used for nonreaders are inadequate for achieving this communication need. The final area of communication need that must be served by an augmentative communication approach is the area of social contact. Light (1988) suggests that although most of our research and clinical attention has focused on developing approaches to meet communication needs and to transfer information, a communication approach that facilitates the maintenance of social contact may be extremely important especially when the disability has been acquired in adulthood. In summary, when assessing the effectiveness of any augmentative communication approach its ability to meet the broadest range of communication needs must be verified.

Multicomponent augmentative communication systems

A trend that is closely associated with our broadening view of communication competence is an increasing appreciation of the necessity for multicomponent augmentative communication systems (Beukelman, 1987; Kraat, 1986). We all use multiple communication approaches. For the able-bodied, the list of these approaches would include gestures, pencils, typewriters, computers, telephones, etc. Individuals communicating through augmentative techniques use multiple modes of communication to a greater extent than do able-bodied individuals. It is unrealistic to seek a single augmentative communication approach that will meet all the communication needs of the user.

Approaches to Intervention

Dictated to a large extent by the specific needs and capabilities of the client, a number of approaches to augmentative intervention have been suggested. Beukelman and Garrett (1988) list four approaches to intervention with aphasic individuals including:

1 Comprehensive communication systems
2 Controlled communication systems
3 Writing systems
4 Augmented communication input.

Because apractic speakers who require communication augmentation are typically severely involved and often exhibit a coexisting aphasia, many of the general approaches suggested for aphasic speakers are also appropriate for apractic speakers. In the following discussion, we will adopt some of the approaches used with aphasic individuals, modify others, and add still other approaches specifically for apractic individuals.

Augmented responses

System characteristics

At times a combination of apraxia of speech, limb apraxia, and aphasia make it impossible for an individual to respond using natural speech or gestures. For such severely involved individuals, a voice output communication aid (VOCA) with a small number of preselected responses may serve as a useful treatment tool in helping them to develop an accurate means of indicating choice. A number of VOCAs are commercially available (Brandenburg and Vanderheiden, 1987) and reports of their use with apractic speakers is beginning to appear in the literature (Rabidoux, Florance and McCauslin, 1980). For severely involved individuals who are early post-onset and receiving regular speech treatment, we have found the Talking Word Board system particularly useful. The Talking Word Board consists of several components which are commercially available and which can easily be assembled. The list of components, which appear assembled in Figure 11.1, include the following:

Apple IIe computer: This standard Apple package consists of the computer, a disk controller card, and one disk drive.

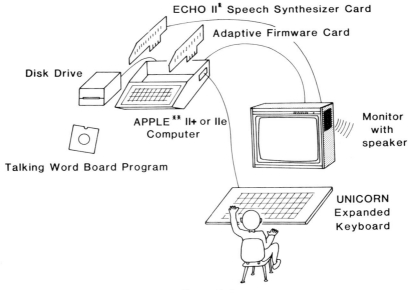

Figure 11.1

Adaptive Firmware Card (manufactured and distributed by Adaptive Peripherals, 4529 Bagley Ave. N., Seattle, WA, 98102): This card allows physically disabled users to run standard, unmodified software for the Apple computer, using any of sixteen input methods including linear scanning and Morse code. The card also permits use of expanded keyboards to access the computer. The redefinition function permits the user to individualize the output in the expanded keyboard mode, thus creating a customized keyboard arrangement. For more details about the Adaptive Firmware Card see Schwejde and Vanderheiden (1982).

Talking Word Board Program (available through Adaptive Peripherals, 4529 Bagley Ave. N., Seattle, WA, 98102): This software is compatible with the Echo II card described below and allows the Unicorn keyboard to serve as an individualized picture, word, and phrase board.

Unicorn Keyboard (available through Unicorn Engineering Co., 6201 Harwood Avenue, Oakland, CA 94618): This is a flat keyboard with touch sensitive keys arranged in eight rows by sixteen columns.

Echo II Speech Synthesizer (Street Electronics, 1140 Mark Avenue, Carpenteria, CA 93013): This is a text-to-speech system that converts normal English text directly to speech.

The core of the Talking Word Board is the software which allows the user to create any number of custom keyboards. Plastic overlays can be customized with up to 128 characters, words, phrases, symbols, pictures and so forth to suit the particular needs of the user. For example, during initial phases of response establishment, we might create an overlay with only two items: a large 'yes' on the left and 'no' on the right. The keyboard would be programmed so that if the client selected any of the locations on the right side of the board, the word, 'no', would be produced and on the left side of the board, 'yes'. For others, we might create an overlay with a combination of pictures and printed messages to facilitate drill work on auditory and reading comprehension. The keyboards can be changed as easily as calling up a new file from the software and changing the plastic overlay.

The Talking Word Board system is both symbol- and content-free so that symbol sets are completely flexible and can be selected commensurate with the user's cognitive, linguistic and visual skills. For example, with some individuals, written words and phrases are most appropriate. With other individuals, a less arbitrary symbol set, such as line drawings or Picsyms (Carlson, 1983), may be used. For those individuals with severe cognitive limitations, actual photographs depicting the message may be appropriate. For some individuals a combination of symbol sets may best meet their communication needs. The size of the target locations may be changed depending on the motor control and vision of the user. For example, for individuals with severe motor control problems each target location can be made up of four squares rather than a single square. The message types may be completely individualized. Specific vocabulary or messages can be created for each user. Finally, different files with individualized vocabularies and display arrangements can be created and stored on the computer disk. Thus, if a clinician is working with three different patients using the Talking Word Board, a different file or level within each file can be created for each of them.

Candidacy

Candidates for the use of such a system in treatment typically exhibit severe apraxia of speech complicated by limb apraxia and/or aphasia. They often will be unreliable in responding to simple yes/no questions with natural speech or gestures. This failure to respond is often attributed to poor auditory comprehension skills, but may also be due, at least in part, to inability to formulate an adequate response. They appear to benefit from the additional cueing provided by the visual presence of the symbol and auditory signal of the speech synthesized word. We have found augmented response devices particularly useful early in recovery when alternative response modes are just being established. Frequently such feedback can be faded, and more portable communication books are developed.

Case presentation

At the age of 70 years, Lillian suffered a left CVA with resultant right hemiparesis, severe aphasia, apraxia of speech, and limb apraxia. At one month post-onset, she was unable to imitate oral movements, sounds, or syllables. Some automatic words were noted in conversation ('yes', 'no', 'well', and 'okay'). Lillian's gestures were noncommunicative because of perseveration and an obvious limb apraxia. Treatment was begun with the goal of increasing reading and auditory comprehension skills, so that a picture and word communication book could be developed for her. One of our initial goals was to improve her ability to respond to yes or no questions. A number of problems appeared to interfere with her ability to do so. First, she exhibited obvious auditory comprehension deficits on both materials that related to personal topics and on standard testing materials. Second, Lillian appeared to have no reliable output mode. Her verbal output was limited to only a few stereotyped words. She had a tendency to answer 'no' to all questions. The gestural mode was also severely limited in that she had difficulty imitating positive or negative head nods. When using head nods, she frequently nodded 'yes' while saying 'no' or used head nods to indicate 'yes' and 'no' to the same question. To make matters more confusing for her partners, she would occasionally appear to change her mind about her responses and first give a signal 'yes', then followed by a 'no'. At times, she would give her response and appear to follow it with a comment about the adequacy of her response. For example, she would indicate 'yes', then signal 'no' as if to say, 'That was a difficult question', or 'I didn't do well on that one'. Thus, responses were both undifferentiated and unreliable, and communication partners were often misled.

One way of providing Lillian with a reliable output mode would be to have her point to the written words, 'yes' and 'no'. Lillian had demonstrated the ability to accurately point to the words, 'yes' and 'no', after the clinician had said the words. We felt that use of printed words would provide a differentiated response. Unfortunately, the accuracy of her responses to yes or no questions when she pointed to the written words was less than 50 per cent.

After some training to use a VOCA to signal 'yes' and 'no', Lillian responded to personal yes or no questions with 90 per cent accuracy as compared to 60 per cent accuracy when she pointed to the printed words. Treatment was continued using the device as an output mode for Lillian until her accuracy in responding to personal questions was nearly 100 per cent. Eventually, the synthesized speech cues were eliminated and we returned to the use of the printed cards, which were arranged in the same order as they had been on the device.

At the time of discharge from the rehabilitation unit at three months post-onset, Lillian continued to exhibit severe nonfluent aphasia complicated by oral, verbal, and limb apraxia. Both verbal and gestural (head nods) responses to yes or no questions remained difficult to differentiate. However, she could reliably answer personal questions by pointing to the printed words, 'yes' and 'no'.

Comprehensive communication system

System characteristics

Comprehensive communication systems are multicomponent augmentative communication systems designed for individuals who wish to 'go anywhere and say anything' (Beukelman and Garrett, 1988). Such systems, when they are designed for severely apractic/aphasic individuals, typically include the following components:

1 Natural speech: a limited repertoire of spoken words, often highly practiced or stereotypic expressions communicating different messages depending on their delivery
2 Communication book: containing basic communicate needs that cannot be communicated in other ways, content words suggesting personal interests, names of people and locations, maps and household floor plans, a chronology of life events, a new information section for 'current events', and instructions for new partners
3 Spelling system: either an alphabet board or scratch paper for identification of the first letters of unique words
4 Drawing system: paper and pen for sketching new ideas (Lyon, 1986)
5 Gestural system: usually idiosyncratic gestures that initially occurred spontaneously, when these gestures are identifiable they are practiced and their use is encouraged
6 Well-instructed partners: frequent partners are instructed to accept whatever communication mode is effective in getting the messsage across. They are also trained in communication breakdown resolution strategies

Candidacy

Candidates for this communication approach are individuals who 'communicate much better than they talk' (Holland, 1977.) Thus, they are individuals whose high communication drive places them in a variety of communication situations, but whose comprehension skills and world knowledge far outstrip their expressive ability. They have some natural speech, some identifiable gestures, some spelling and drawing skills, but none of these areas are strong enough to carry the full burden for communication of all messages. They are usually mobile enough to be independent in self-care activities. They are patient with their communication partners' inability to interrupt garbled messages and appear to even enjoy the give and take that is involved in the resolution of communication breakdown. In summary, although they are severely impaired, they exhibit residual areas of strength. They are a challenge to serve adequately because of their dynamically changing vocabulary needs and their mobility.

Case presentation

Ruth is the type of individual just described. When she was referred to our Augmentative Communication Center, she was a 45–year-old ambulatory woman, twelve years post-onset of severe left cerebrovascular accident (CVA). Members of her healthcare team noted in their referral that she had little speech but was highly communicative and appeared to understand all that was said to her. Their question was, 'Could she benefit from one of the new talking computers that are now available?'.

Our evaluation led us to describe her deficits as moderately severe, nonfluent aphasia accompanied by a severe apraxia of speech. Ruth arrived at our facility with three communication word books, which had been provided to her during the past twelve years. The most recent word book consisted of lists of words under a variety of main categories. It contained over 300 entries in approximately twenty different categories, most of which were content words designed primarily to communicate predictable needs. In addition to her communication books, Ruth printed words in order to transfer information and to maintain social contact. Although her printing contained numerous misspellings, Ruth found this mode of communication to be relatively efficient, flexible, and portable. Further, it allowed her access to a broader range of vocabulary. Ruth's strategy was to attempt an approximation of the word and have the communication partner guess the content of her message. For example, Ruth wished to express the fact that she had been a volunteer at a neighboring hospital. She printed the letters, 'V-A-L' and waited for her communication partner to interpret her meaning. After several incorrect guesses, Ruth corrected her printed message to read 'V-O-L', which eventually led to a successfully communicated message. This admittedly limited approach to communication served Ruth well in most social situations. In these situations, the goal was not to exchange large amounts of information precisely and rapidly but to simply have a few minutes of social contact.

Another communicative approach that Ruth used in some situations was a gestural one. With a moderate aphasia, it is not surprising that Ruth was unable to learn a highly symbolic gestural system in which a gesture is an arbitrary symbol for the concept it conveys. Ruth evidenced some limited concrete gestures, such as head on hand to indicate 'tired' or pointing to her wrist to indicate 'it's time for ... '. Further, she was very expressive in the coverbal behaviors, such as head nods, smiles, and eye contact that serve to regulate conversation (Katz, LaPointe and Markel, 1978).

Though communication was slow and required extensive partner participation, Ruth appeared to be a functional communicator utilizing a combination of word books, gestures, some simple printed messages, and yes or no responses to questions from her partners. The question we faced in our evaluation was whether or not the use of an augmentative communication device would improve Ruth's daily communication. We decided not to recommend the portable speech output system that was available at the time we served Ruth despite the fact that she had demonstrated the ability to operate it in structured communication situations. Our reasons included the following. First, Ruth's message needs were so highly variable and unpredictable that programming appropriate messages into the device would have been difficult. Ruth's limited spelling skills would have made programming a prohibitively difficult task for her to do independently. Second, portability was a problem. She found that even her small notebooks were cumbersome to carry with her and felt that a portable speech output system would have been even more inconvenient. Finally, a discussion with her family indicated that they preferred well-established communication strategies (yes or no responses, gestures, limited printing) to the augmentative communication device. We attributed this preference to the fact that Ruth's multicomponent communication system required a great deal of partner participation. This participation was not viewed by the family as an inconvenience. Rather, extended conversational exchange needed for Ruth to transfer information also served as an important means of establishing and maintaining social contact.

Approaches for specific situations

Characteristics of the approach

Specific communication situations are often an important enough aspect of an individual's life that the development of an approach to meet communication needs of that situation is warranted. Beukelman and Garrett (1988) list the following features of such a communication approach: a means of topic selection, a list of control phrases, and a topic-specific dictionary of words or other symbols. Often such topic-specific communication approaches can take advantage of current technology because message content is sufficiently predictable for dictionaries of appropriate messages to be 'programmed' into electronic devices.

Candidacy

Candidates for such specific communication approaches are typically characterized by the same features characteristic of the candidate for the multicomponent communication approaches just described. In addition, however, candidates for specific approaches are able to identify one or two communication situations that are extremely important to them. The following case will illustrate such a specific situation.

Case presentation

Dallas had suffered a left CVA at the age of 47 years which left him with severe verbal apraxia and moderately severe aphasia. He had received an extensive period of traditional speech therapy which included the development of a multicomponent augmentative communication system described in more detail elsewhere (Beukelman, Yorkston and Dowden, 1985). Included among the components of this approach was a communication book, which initially involved only pictures but later had developed into an elaborate combination of word lists and photographs. He used several gestures meaningfully and could verbally produce a small number of well-drilled words and phrases.

Prior to his stroke, Dallas had owned and managed a successful interior design firm. He continued to participate in this business following his stroke. At the time of his discharge from active speech treatment at nine months post-onset, there was no electronic augmentative communication system that would incorporate all of the features he would require which included portability, speech output, and whole-message retrieval of unique entries. Approximately three years later, the Handivoice 130, a portable speech synthesizer with a single programmable level, became commercially available and its appropriateness to meet some specific communication needs for Dallas was evaluated. We interviewed Dallas, his wife, his business assistant, and his Division Vocational Rehabilitation counselor in order to identify his communication needs and found that we could identify a number of important needs related primarily to his interior design business that were not being met. For example, Dallas reported the need to speak a greater number of phrases intelligibly and quickly when interviewing his clients. He required conversational management phrases, which would allow him to control the conversation during decision-making. We became convinced that the Handivoice 130 could meet some limited, but specific needs.

Dallas's training to use the system included two different tasks. First, Dallas, his wife, and his business assistant needed to learn how to operate the system, including programming the fifth level with messages appropriate for business interaction. Dallas learned to accurately select the desired message, to shift from level to level, and to perform other operations such as clearing the memory of the system. The second training task was a more challenging one; to select the messages which would be programmed into the memory of the system. We began to create our list by interviewing Dallas, his wife, and his business assistant. Dallas selected a small number of these messages and began to practice their rapid and accurate retrieval. The initial 'control' messages included the following:

> This is going to be fun.
> Let's decide this later.
> Let's move on.
> When will that be done?
> When will we meet again?

Among the content words that Dallas selected for practice were: 'contract', 'drawings', 'model', and 'proposal'. Other messages already programmed in the Handivoice 130 were highlighted for Dallas's use: 'How are you?', 'Thank-you', 'Table', 'Elevator', and 'Lunch'. In a follow-up session several months later, Dallas used his 'favorite' messages promptly and effectively in natural communication situations. When new messages are added, Dallas first practiced retrieving them as part of his daily 'exercises'. Once he became comfortable with his ability to retrieve them quickly and accurately, he and his assistant made note of the number of times they were useful to him in natural settings. Those that did not prove to be useful were deleted as others were added.

It was interesting to note the types of messages that Dallas found useful. Many of them were conversational control phrases, which allowed him to initiate, direct, and terminate portions of conversations. The Handivoice 130, with its rapid retrieval of whole messages and speech output, is more suited to the delivery of these types of messages than any of the other communicative approaches that Dallas is currently using. Other of Dallas's most frequently used messages are content words. He does not formulate grammatically complete sentences by combining words and phrases. Rather, he selects a content word and embelishes its meaning with gestures. An example will illustrate his sophisticated use of multiple communicative modes. It was apparent that Dallas frequently used the message, 'lunch'. When we offered to program a number of more complete messages related to lunch ('Shall we go to lunch?', or 'I don't want lunch now'), he indicated that he did not need those messages. He showed us that he would retrieve that spoken word, 'lunch', and then point to his watch for the message, 'It's time for lunch'. He would retrieve the word, 'lunch', and raise his eyebrows in order to ask if his listener might be interested in going to lunch. In short, he used the Handivoice 130 to express a concept that was not easily gestured and then expressed a series of related concepts by combining them with gestures.

Supplemented speech

Characteristics of the approach

Alphabet supplementation is an approach initially suggested for use by language-intact, severely dysarthric individuals (Beukelman and Yorkston, 1977; and Yorkston, Beukelman and Bell, 1988). Individuals use an alphabet board to point to the initial letter of each word as they say the word. Thus, not only are listeners provided extra cues in the form of the initial letter, but dysarthric speakers reduce their overall speaking rate. Alphabet supplementation may serve a different purpose for selected apractic speakers. Use of gestures to 'deblock' the speech of apractic individuals has often been suggested (Rosenbek, 1985). The alphabet supplementation approach may serve the same deblocking function. In addition, identification of initial letters may serve as phonetic placement cues for certain apractic individuals.

Candidacy

Candidates for the alphabet supplementation approach typically do not exhibit major word finding or grammatical formulation problems. Rather, their speech is marked by frequent articulatory errors which interfere significantly with both the flow and intelligibility of their speech. Speakers are acutely aware of their breakdowns and will frequently attempt to repair them even when the listener has understood the message. Candidates for this technique need sufficient spelling skills to accurately indicate the initial letter of words.

Case presentation

Tom was a 38-year-old biologist when a left-hemisphere tumor was diagnosed and surgically removed leaving him with severely apractic speech and mild aphasia. Regular speech treatment was initiated two weeks post-surgery. At that time, Tom was alert, cooperative, and quite frustrated by his inability to produce understandable speech. His speech attempts were characterized by multiple articulatory errors, frequent revisions of misarticulated sounds, and groping or searching for the initial articulatory position of a word. Inability or difficulty in initiating the first sound of a word was a major problem; struggling behavior lasting for ten to fifteen seconds to produce the initial sound of a word was characteristic. Often his struggle did not lead to an accurate production. Thus, his conversational speech was extremely slow and nearly unintelligible. Initial evaluation of language skills revealed only mild deficits. For example, he could write the names of common objects, read, understand paragraph length materials, and spell at a level beyond tenth grade on standardized tests.

Tom benefited from a number of cueing strategies (see Chapter 7) including seeing the printed word and watching the clinician's production of the word. He also benefited from more subtle cues including the first letter of the words and seeing the appropriate articulatory posture for the initial phoneme. Because of his good spelling skills and the benefits he appeared to derive from phonetic placement, the alphabet supplementation approach was demonstrated to Tom and his wife. Within one session, Tom was using it to construct whole sentences which were understandable to his partners. Tom's instructions when using the approach were to point to the initial letter of each word as he said the word. If the initial letter of the word was difficult, he was to 'ignore' that part of the word and try to get as much of the rest of the word as possible. For example, if he was attempting the word, 'gate', he would point to the 'g' and say, 'ate'. Rather than attempting 'perfect' productions, focus was placed on getting the message across to his partner as quickly and efficiently as possible. The initial effect of the alphabet supplementation was a reduction in struggle behavior. Many words were produced without the first phoneme, but listeners' understanding was maintained because Tom was identifying the missing letter for them. As Tom continued to use the approach and continued to improve, he appeared to take more and more advantage of the letters as phonetic placement cues. For example, as he pointed to an initial 't', he would adopt the correct posture for that phoneme. Tom used the approach successfully for approximately three weeks, until he no longer needed it.

Concluding Remarks

In the introduction to this chapter, three trends were identified as contributing to our increasing ability to serve severely apractic speakers using augmentation communication approaches. These trends included advances in technology, an expanding definition of communication needs, and use of multicomponent augmentative communication systems. If we are to continue to improve service to apractic individuals, each of these trends must continue. In the area of technology, content-free and symbol-free voice output devices need to become truly portable if they are to serve the needs of ambulatory apractic individuals. We also must seek to better understand the communicative needs of adults with acquired apraxia. Questions such as the following must be addressed. Which augmentative communication approaches best serve the user when communicating predictable messages, when providing unique information, when engaging in friendly conversation with family or acquaintances? Apractic–aphasic individuals exhibit a unique pattern of newly acquired deficits and residual skills and knowledge. As we continue to serve this population, it will no doubt become obvious that no single approach to augmentative communication will compensate for all the deficits and take advantage of the residual skills. We, therefore, must seek multicomponent approaches in an effort to meet the broadest range of communication needs in this population.

Acknowledgments

Dr Yorkston and Ms Waugh acknowledge support in part for preparation of their chapter from Research Grant No. G008200076 from the National Institute of Handicapped Research, Department of Education, Washington, DC 20202. Dr David Beukelman and Ms Pat Dowden are thanked for their helpful suggestions.

References

BEUKELMAN, D. (1987) 'When you have a hammer, everything looks like a nail', *Augmentative and Alternative Communication*, **3**(2), pp. 94–96.

BEUKELMAN, D. and GARRETT, K. (1988) 'Augmentative communication for adults with acquired severe communication disorders', *Augmentative and Alternative Communication*, **4**, pp. 104–21.

BEUKELMAN, D. and YORKSTON, K. (1977) 'A communication system for the severely dysarthric speaker with an intact language system', *Journal of Speech and Hearing Disorders*, **42**, 265–70.

BEUKELMAN, D., YORKSTON, K. and DOWDEN, P. (1985) *Communication Augmentation: A Casebook of Clinical Management*, San Diego, College-Hill Press.

BLACKSTONE, S. (Ed.) (1986) *Augmentative Communication: An Introduction*, Rockville, MD, American Speech-Language-Hearing Association.

BRANDENBURG, S. and VANDERHEIDEN, G. (1987) *Communication, Control, and Computer Access for Disabled and Elderly Individuals: Communication Aids*, Boston, College-Hill Publications/Little, Brown and Co.

CARLSON, F. (1983) *Picsyms Workshop Manual*, Omaha, NE, Meyer Children's Rehabilitation Institute.

COPELAND, K. (1974) *Aids for the Severely Handicapped*, London, Spector Publishing.

DIXON, C. (1965) 'Some thought on communication boards', *Cerebral Palsy Journal*, **26**, pp. 12–13.

FEALLOCK, B. (1958) 'Communication for the non-verbal individual', *American Journal of Occupational Therapy*, **12**, 60–63.

HOLLAND, A. (1977) 'Some practical considerations in aphasia rehabilitation', in SULLIVAN, M. and KANSMERS, M.S. (Eds.) *Rationale for Adult Aphasia Therapy*, Lincoln, University of Nebraska Medical Center.

HOOPER, E. and HASSELBRING, T. (1985) 'Electronic augmentative communication aids for the nonreading student: Selection criteria', *Journal of Special Education Technology*, **7**, pp. 39–49.

KATZ, R., LAPOINTE, L. and MARKEL, N. (1978) 'Coverbal behavior and aphasic speakers', in BROOKSHIRE, R. (Ed.) *Clinical Aphasiology Conference Proceedings*, Minneapolis, MN, BRK Publishers, pp. 164–73.

KRAAT, A. (1986) 'Developing intervention goals', in BLACKSTONE, S. (Ed.) *Augmentative Communication: An Introduction*, Rockville, MD, American Speech-Language-Hearing Association, pp. 197–266.

LIGHT, J. (1988) 'Interaction involving individuals using augmentative communication systems: State of the art and future directions for research', *Augmentative and Alternative Communication*, **4**, pp. 66–82.

LYON, J. (1986) 'Drawing: It's communicative significance for expressively restricted aphasic adults', A presentation at the annual convention of the American Speech-Language-Hearing Association Convention, Detroit.

MCDONALD, E. and SCHULTZ, A. (1973) 'Communication boards for cerebral palsied children', *Journal of Speech and Hearing Disorders*, **38**, pp. 73–88.

MEYER, L. (1983) 'Unique contributions of microcomputers to language intervention with handicapped children', *Seminars in Speech and Language*, **5**, pp. 23–35.

MIRENDA, P. and DATTILO, J. (1987) 'Instructional techniques in alternative communication for students with severe intellectual handicaps', *Augmentative and Alternative Communication,* **3**(3), pp. 143–52.

MUSSELWHITE, C. and ST LOUIS, K. (1982) *Communication Programming for the Severely Handicapped: Vocal and Non-vocal Strategies,* San Diego, College-Hill Press.

RABIDOUX, P., FLORANCE, C. and MCCAUSLIN, L. (1980) 'Use of a Handivoice in the treatment of a severely apractic, non-verbal patient', in BROOKSHIRE, R. (Ed.) *Clinical Aphasiology Conference Proceedings,* Minneapolis, MN, BRK Publishers.

ROMSKI, M., SEVCIK, R. and JOYNER, S. (1984) 'Nonspeech communication systems: Implications for language intervention with mentally retarded children', *Topics in Language Disorders,* **5**, pp. 66–81.

ROSENBEK, J. (1985) 'Treating apraxia of speech', in JOHNS, D. (Ed.) *Clinical management of neurogenic communication disorders,* Boston, Little, Brown and Co., pp. 267–312.

SCHIEFELBUSCH, R. (Ed.) (1980) *Nonspeech Language Intervention,* Baltimore, University Park Press.

SCHWEJDE, P. and VANDERHEIDEN, G. (1982) 'Adaptive Firmware Card for the Apple II', *Byte,* **7**, pp. 276–317.

SILVERMAN, F. (1980) *Communication for the Speechless,* Englewood Cliffs, NJ, Prentice Hall, Inc.

VANDERHEIDEN, G. and YODER, D. (1986) 'Overview', in BLACKSTONE, S. (Ed.) *Augmentative Communication: an Introduction,* Rockville, MD, American Speech-Language-Hearing Association, pp. 1–28.

VICKER, B. (1974) *Nonoral Communication System Project 1964/73,* Iowa City, Campus Stores Publishers, University of Iowa.

WARREN, R. and DATTA, K. (1981) 'The return of speech 4 1/2 years post head injury: A case report', in BROOKSHIRE, R. (Ed.) *Proceedings of the Clinical Aphasiology Conference,* Minneapolis, BRK Publishers, pp. 301–8.

YORKSTON, K. and DOWDEN, P. (1984) 'Nonspeech language and communication systems', in HOLLAND, A. (Ed.) *Language Disorders in Adults,* San Diego, College-Hill Press, pp. 283–312.

YORKSTON, K., BEUKELMAN, D. and BELL, K. (1988) *Clinical Management of Dysarthric Speakers,* Boston, College-Hill Publications, Little, Brown and Co.

Index